The ADA Practical Guide Substance Use Disorders Safe Prescribing

T0176786

Andrew Taylor O'Neil (September 2, 1991–September 9, 2014)

This book is dedicated to Andrew – high-school valedictorian, Eagle Scout with highest honors, naturalist, intellectual, humorist, friend and teacher to all, brother, and most importantly an amazing, caring, giving, and loving son. No parent could ever be more proud of a son than I am of you. You are forever in the hearts of all that ever met you.

Dad

The ADA Practical Guide to Substance Use Disorders and Safe Prescribing

Edited by

Michael O'Neil, PharmD

Professor and Vice-Chair, Department of Pharmacy Practice
Drug Diversion, Substance Abuse, Pain Management Consultant
South College School of Pharmacy
Knoxville, TN, USA

WILEY Blackwell **ADA** American Dental Association®
America's leading advocate for oral health

Published by John Wiley & Sons, Inc., Hoboken, New Jersey
Published simultaneously in Canada

The contents of this work are intended to further general scientific research, understanding, and discussion only and are not intended and should not be relied upon as recommending or promoting a specific method, diagnosis, or treatment by health science practitioners for any particular patient. The publisher and the author make no representations or warranties with respect to the accuracy or completeness of the contents of this work and specifically disclaim all warranties, including without limitation any implied warranties of fitness for a particular purpose. In view of ongoing research, equipment modifications, changes in governmental regulations, and the constant flow of information relating to the use of medicines, equipment, and devices, the reader is urged to review and evaluate the information provided in the package insert or instructions for each medicine, equipment, or device for, among other things, any changes in the instructions or indication of usage and for added warnings and precautions. Readers should consult with a specialist where appropriate. The fact that an organization or Website is referred to in this work as a citation and/or a potential source of further information does not mean that the author or the publisher endorses the information the organization or Website may provide or recommendations it may make. Further, readers should be aware that Internet Websites listed in this work may have changed or disappeared between when this work was written and when it is read. No warranty may be created or extended by any promotional statements for this work. Neither the publisher nor the author shall be liable for any damages arising herefrom.

For general information on our other products and services or for technical support, please contact our Customer Care Department within the United States at (800) 762-2974, outside the United States at (317) 572-3993 or fax (317) 572-4002.

Wiley also publishes its books in a variety of electronic formats. Some content that appears in print may not be available in electronic formats. For more information about Wiley products, visit our web site at www.wiley.com.

Library of Congress Cataloging-in-Publication Data

The ADA practical guide to substance use disorders and safe prescribing / edited by Michael O'Neil.
    p. ; cm.
  Practical guide to substance use disorders and safe prescribing
  American Dental Association practical guide to substance use disorders and safe prescribing
  Includes bibliographical references and index.
  Summary: "This is in addition to a variety of legal regulations dentists must follow regarding the storage and record keeping of controlled substances"—Provided by publisher.
  ISBN 978-1-118-88601-4 (paperback)
  I. O'Neil, Michael (Pharmacist), editor. II. American Dental Association, issuing body. III. Title: Practical guide to substance use disorders and safe prescribing. IV. Title: American Dental Association practical guide to substance use disorders and safe prescribing.
  [DNLM: 1. Dental Care–United States. 2. Substance-Related Disorders–United States. 3. Dental Offices–organization & administration–United States. 4. Dentist-Patient Relations–United States.
5. Drug Prescriptions–standards–United States. 6. Drug and Narcotic Control–United States. WM 270]
  RK701
  617.6061–dc23   2015006921

Cover images (clockwise from top middle): © iStockphoto/JurgaR; © iStockphoto/mphillips007; © iStockphoto/KarenMower; © iStockphoto/Bunyos; © Stephen Wagner, used with permission

Set in 9.5/12pt Palatino LT Std by Aptara Inc., New Delhi, India

Printed in Singapore

10 9 8 7 6 5 4 3 2 1

Contents

Contributors

Carlos M. Aquino
DEA Compliance Consultant
Milford, MA, USA
Retired Police Department Officer
Retired Drug Enforcement Agent, DEA

James H. Berry, DO
Addiction Psychiatrist
Medical Director – Chestnut Ridge Center
Inpatient Services
Assistant Professor – Department of
Behavioral Medicine and Psychiatry
West Virginia University
Morgantown, WV, USA

Matthew Cooke, DDS, MD, MPH
Assistant Professor
Departments of Dental Anesthesiology &
Pediatric Dentistry
University of Pittsburgh School of Dental
Medicine
Pittsburgh, PA, USA
and
Departments of Oral & Maxillofacial Surgery &
Pediatric Dentistry
Virginia Commonwealth University School of
Dentistry
Richmond, VA, USA

Amanda Eades, PharmD
Assistant Professor/Clinical Pharmacist
University of Illinois at Chicago
Chicago, IL, USA

Elliot V. Hersh, DMD, MS, PhD
Professor Pharmacology
Director – Division of Pharmacology and
Therapeutics
University of Pennsylvania School of Dental
Medicine
Philadelphia, PA, USA

William T. Kane, DDS, MBA, FAGD, FACD
General Dentistry
Dexter, MI, USA

William J. Maloney, DDS
Clinical Associate Professor
Department of Cariology and Comprehensive
Care
New York University College of Dentistry
New York, NY, USA

**Sarah T. Melton, PharmD, BCPP, BCACP,
CGP, FASCP**
Associate Professor of Pharmacy Practice
Gatton College of Pharmacy at ETSU
Johnson City, TN, USA

Paul A. Moore, DMD, PhD, MPH
Professor – Pharmacology and Dental Public
Health
University of Pittsburgh School of Dental
Medicine
Pittsburgh, PA, USA

Michael O'Neil, PharmD
Professor and Vice-Chair
Department of Pharmacy Practice
Drug Diversion, Substance Abuse and Pain
Management Consultant
South College School of Pharmacy
Knoxville, TN, USA

Ralph A. Orr
Director
Virginia's Prescription Monitoring Program
Henrico, VA, USA

George F. Raymond, DDS
Clinical Instructor
Department of Cariology and Comprehensive
Care
New York University College of Dentistry
New York, NY, USA

Carl Rollynn Sullivan, MD
Professor and Vice-Chairman
Director, Addictions Programs
WVU School of Medicine
Department of Behavioral Medicine &
Psychiatry
Morgantown, WV, USA

Frank Vitale, MA
National Director
Pharmacy Partnership for Tobacco Cessation
Pittsburgh, PA, USA

Preface

Health-care practitioners have become inundated by an array of patients with multiple medical conditions that are further complicated by pain/sedation management issues, substance use disorders (SUDs), and worries of drug diversion. Pain management, whether for acute or chronic pain, has become a primary concern for dental practitioners. Practitioners often feel pressured by patient survey results *and patients* to "overprescribe" controlled substances. With the rise in opioid addiction there has been a significant increase in medication-assisted treatment, including use of methadone and buprenorphine products. These agents have proven efficacy *in both* the treatment of opioid addiction and pain. However, evidence-based studies evaluating treatment of patients *with concurrent opioid addiction and acute or chronic pain* are lacking. Opioid or alcohol addiction treatment medications, such as naltrexone, have complicated opioid analgesia in many patients.

The plethora of substances being abused in society today includes household products such as paints and "cleaners" to combinations of heroin, cocaine, and other medicinal agents. Public health risks of medication misuse and substance abuse have reached epidemic proportions. When patients present to the dental practitioner with a history of SUD or recent substance abuse, routine procedures are no longer routine. Dental practitioners treating patients under the influence of substances may put both the patients and themselves at unnecessary risk of complications. Use of routine local anesthetics, such as lidocaine with epinephrine, now has the potential to put the methamphetamine addict in a life-compromising situation. Data supporting definitive management of patients with acute pain and SUD are limited. Recognizing patients with SUD, intervening, and directing them to appropriate treatment require time and expertise.

All dental office staff must now look for drug diversion behaviors on a daily basis. Unknowingly, dental practitioners may become victims of various scams and schemes. Recognition, prevention, deterrence, detection, and reporting of potential criminal behaviors interrupt the daily work flow for many dental practices. Prescription drug fraud and "Dr Shopping" are only two of the many diversion activities dental practitioners must address. A significant rise in prescription fraud has created an environment of fear and frustrations for pre-scribers, patients, law enforcement agencies, and local communities.

Dental practitioners must be fully prepared to manage a variety of patients with complex analgesic/sedation needs and SUD and, at the same time, protect themselves and their staff from drug diversion activities.

The purpose of this book is multifactorial:

1. Review basic elements of SUD, acute pain/sedation management, and drug diversion.
2. Provide clinical tools proven to aid in the identification, interviewing, interven-tion, referral, and treatment of SUD.

3. Summarize evidence-based literature that supports what, when, and how to prescribe controlled substances to patients with SUD (e.g., analgesia, sedation).
4. Discuss key federal controlled-substance regulations that frequently impact dental practitioners.
5. Provide checklists that will help prevent drug diversion in dental practices.

In completing this challenge, dental prac-titioners will be better prepared to care for patients, protect the community, and safeguard their own practices.

Michael O'Neil

Acknowledgments

I am forever indebted to the chapter authors of this book. Their work, patience, and commitment to excellence are nothing less than exceptional. Managing patients in an environment of increasing frequency of substance use disorders, drug diversion, and pain is often an overwhelming endeavor. The expertise offered by the chapters is practical and evidence based and will guide dental practitioners in their day-to-day practices. I wish to acknowledge the American Dental Association (ADA) staff editors of this book for their excellent and timely work. These include Amy Lund, Senior Editor, Kathryn Pulkrabek, Manager/Editor Professional Products, Alison Siwek, Manager, Dentist Health and Wellness, and Carolyn Tatar, Senior Manager of Product Development and Management. I wish to thank Carolyn Tatar for her direction in this project.

I would also like to thank the Wiley publishing team of Rick Blanchette, Nancy Turner, and Jennifer Seward for their due diligence and commitments to making this book a success.

I am indebted to Alison Siwek for her insights and perspectives regarding the many concerns of dental practitioners working with the ADA. The authors and I would like to thank the ADA leadership for their recognition of the need to create this book to educate their members.

Michael O'Neil

Substance Use Disorders, Drug Diversion, and Pain Management: The Scope of the Problem

Michael O'Neil, PharmD

Introduction

The practice of dentistry has become increasingly complicated by multiple factors, including increasing numbers of patients with substance use disorder (SUD), patients receiving chronic pain medications, and prescription drug-related crime (see Box 1.1). In January 2012, the Centers for Disease Control (CDC) announced that the USA is experiencing an epidemic of prescription drug-related overdoses with the majority of these involving prescription opioids.[1] Findings from the 2011 National Health and Aging Trends Study reported bothersome pain afflicts half of the community-dwelling US older adult population and is associated with significant reduction in physical function, particularly in those with multisite pain.[2] National Survey on Drug Use and Health (NSDUH) 2012 data indicate that 6.8 million people aged 12 or older are current nonmedical users of psychotherapeutic drugs and that 4.9 million of these were users of pain relievers.[3] The NSDUH 2012 data also indicate

> ### Box 1.1 Factors Complicating the Practice of General Dentistry
>
> - Chronic pain management.
> - Misuse of prescription medication.
> - SUD associated with prescription medications.
> - SUD associated with illicit substances.
> - SUD associated with alcohol.
> - Psychiatric disorders (diagnosed and undiagnosed).
> - Opioid maintenance treatment programs (methadone, buprenorphine).
> - Aging population.
> - Polypharmacy (use of multiple medications to treat the same condition).
> - Patient criminal activity.

that the rate of current illicit drug (e.g., cocaine, marijuana, inhalants) use among persons aged 12 or older was 9.2%. In 2012, the NSDUH survey revealed an estimated 22.2 million persons aged 12 or older were classified as having an SUD in the past year (8.5% of the population aged 12 or older). Other results from this

The ADA Practical Guide to Substance Use Disorders and Safe Prescribing, First Edition. Edited by Michael O'Neil.
© 2015 American Dental Association. Published 2015 by John Wiley & Sons, Inc.

survey are include 2.8 million people were classified as having an SUD of both alcohol and illicit drugs, 4.5 million had an SUD associated with illicit drugs but not alcohol, and 14.9 million an SUD associated with alcohol but not illicit drugs. Overall, 17.7 million had an SUD associated with alcohol and 7.3 million had an SUD associated with illicit drugs.[3]

The extent of the overlap of pain management, SUD, prescription drug misuse, and drug diversion in the same patient has not been well defined. However, patients commonly present with more than one of these clinical and ethical challenges at any given office visit or hospital admission. Individual motivations and behaviors leading to the abuse, misuse, and diversion of prescription drugs, illicit drugs, and alcohol vary significantly. This chapter will provide an overview of SUD, prescription drug misuse, drug diversion, pain management, and cultural considerations in patients involved in these activities. Key terminology used throughout this book is also defined.

Definitions

Acute Pain

Acute pain comes on quickly, can be moderate to severe in intensity, and generally lasts a short period of time (e.g., from days up to 3 months). Acute pain is considered a beneficial process, warning of potential harm to the body from injury or medical conditions. Acute pain is most commonly nociceptive, modulated by mediators such as prostaglandins, substance P, and histamines, or neuropathic, characterized by alterations in the transmission pathways of nerves.

Addiction

Addiction is a primary chronic disease of brain reward, motivation, memory, judgment,

and related circuitry. Dysfunction in these circuits leads to characteristic biological, psychological, social, and spiritual manifestations that frequently result in destructive and life-threatening behaviors.[4] Addiction is influenced by multiple factors, including, but not limited to, genetics, environment, sociology, physiology, and individual behaviors.

Addiction is characterized by the inability to consistently abstain, impairment in behavioral control, craving, diminished recognition of significant problems in behavior and interpersonal relationships, and a dysfunctional emotional response. Like other chronic diseases, addiction often involves cycles of relapse and remission. Without treatment or engagement in recovery activities, addiction is progressive and can result in disability or premature death.[4]

Chronic Pain

Chronic pain generally refers to intractable pain that exists for 3 months or more and does not resolve in response to treatment. Some conditions may become chronic in as little as 1 month. Chronic pain may be continuous or reoccurring, persisting for months or even a lifetime. While the exact duration and characteristics of acute and chronic pain may overlap considerably depending on a patient's medical condition, dental practitioners should recognize that specific timelines for the diagnosis of acute versus chronic pain may be integrated into federal and state legislation and into state board regulations to promote safe pain management practices and safe medication prescribing guidelines.

Drug Diversion

Drug diversion may be defined as the intentional transfer of a substance, or possession of a substance, or alteration of legitimate medication orders outside the boundaries designated by the Food and Drug Administration, federal Drug Enforcement Administration (DEA), or state regulatory board. Drug diversion may involve prescription or over-the counter (OTC) medications or illicit substances. These illegal activities are usually motivated by financial incentives, SUD behaviors, or other activities, such as sharing medications with the intent to help. Examples include a patient selling or giving their prescription medication to someone else, altering the original information on a prescription without the prescriber's consent, or theft of medications.

Drug Misuse

Drug misuse may be defined as taking a prescribed or OTC medication for nonprescribed purposes, in excessive doses, shorter intervals than prescribed or recommended, or for reasons other than the original intent of the prescription. Examples include doubling the dosage, shortening dosing intervals, or treating disorders for which the medication was not prescribed.

Opiates and Opioids

Opiates refer to natural substances derived from the poppy plant. Opioids function in a similar manner to opiates but are either synthetic or partially synthetic derivatives of opiates. For the purpose of this text, the term opioid will be used interchangeably for opiate.

Prescriber–Patient Mismatch

Prescriber–patient mismatch is defined as the inconsistency in treatment goals or expectations of treatment between the prescriber and the patient. Examples include analgesia, sedation, or anxiolysis.

Substance Abuse

Substance Abuse is a maladaptive pattern of chemical use (e.g. alcohol, medications, marijuana, cocaine, solvents, etc.) leading to clinically significant impairment or distress, as manifested by one (or more) of the following, occurring within a 12-month period:

- Recurrent chemical use resulting in a failure to fulfill major role obligations at work, school, or home
- Recurrent chemical use in situations in which it is physically hazardous
- Recurrent chemically-related legal problems
- Continued chemical use despite having persistent or recurrent social or interpersonal problems caused by or exacerbated by the effects of the chemical

The substance abuse culture consists of individuals whose sole intent is to alter in any number of ways their mood, psychological sense of well-being, physical sense of well-being, or their personal connection with the world around them.[5]

Substance Dependence

Substance dependence may be defined as persistent use of alcohol, other drugs, or chemicals despite having problems related to use of the substance. It is a maladaptive pattern of chemical use, leading to clinically significant impairment or distress, as manifested by three (or more) of the following, occurring within a 12-month period:

- Tolerance, as defined by either of the following:
  - a need for significantly increased amounts of the substance to achieve intoxication or desired effect;
  - significantly diminished effect with continued use of the same amount of the substance.
- Withdrawal, as manifested by either of the following:
  - the characteristic withdrawal symptom for the substance (see Chapter 2);

- the same (or a closely related) substance is taken to relieve or avoid withdrawal symptoms.
- The substance is often taken in larger amounts or over a longer period than was intended.
- There is a persistent desire or unsuccessful efforts to cut down or control substance use.
- A great deal of time is spent in activities necessary to obtain the substance, use the substance, or recover from its effects.
- Important social, occupational, or recreational activities are given up or reduced because of substance use.
- The substance use is continued despite knowledge of having a persistent or recurrent physical or psychological problem that is likely to have been caused or exacerbated by the substance.[5]

Box 1.2 SUD Symptoms List

- Taking the substance in larger amounts or for longer than you meant to take it.
- Wanting to cut down or stop using the substance but not managing to be successful.
- Spending a lot of time getting, using, or recovering from use of the substance.
- Cravings and urges to use the substance.
- Not managing to do what you should at work, home, or school because of substance use.
- Continuing to use the substance, even when it causes problems in relationships.
- Giving up important social, occupational, or recreational activities because of substance use.
- Using substances again and again, even when it puts you in danger.
- Substance dependence.
- Developing tolerance.
- Developing withdrawal symptoms.

Substance Use Disorders

In May 2013, The American Psychiatric Association redefined terminology previously used in the Diagnostic and Statistical Manual of Mental Disorders Text Revision (DSM-IV TR) guidelines regarding diagnostic classifications of Substance Dependence and Substance Abuse Disorders. SUD in DSM-5 combines the DSM-IV-TR categories of substance abuse, substance dependence and addiction disorders into a single disorder measured on a continuum from mild to severe. Nearly all SUDs are diagnosed based on the same overarching criteria which have not only been combined, but strengthened. (For example, in DSM-IV TR, a diagnosis of substance abuse previously required only one symptom, in DSM-5 a diagnosis of mild SUD requires two to three symptoms from a list of 11 [see Box 1.2]. SUD may be best described as a continuum of substance abuse and the disease of addiction.[6]

Substance Use Disorder, Drug Misuse, Drug Diversion, and Pain Management in the Dental Community

The terms psychological or psychiatric dependency and addiction are often used interchangeably with SUD, the term used in this book. Although the terms *chemical, medication, drug, substance, chemical substance,* or *illicit substances* are often used interchangeably, in this book the term *substance* is used when generally referring to products that are being abused or misused. Differences are only likely to occur based on federal and state classifications or medically accepted use.

Substance Use Disorder

Dental practitioners likely observe many patients at various stages of the *substance abuse–disease of addiction* continuum known as SUD. Specific patient behaviors may range from subtle exaggerations of pain severity with the intent to acquire more medications, to patients presenting in an exaggerated euphoric or dissociative state. Although the impact of opioid abuse and misuse on health care has been evaluated,[7] the financial and workload burden of these behaviors has not been well characterized in the practice of dentistry. However, in a comprehensive statewide survey of dentists by O'Neil, 75% of dentists surveyed suspected 1–20% of their patients had a drug addiction or drug abuse disorder and 94% of dental practitioners altered their prescribing practices of opioid analgesics if the patient acknowledged an SUD.[8] These survey results suggest SUD likely impacts patient management and the prescribing practices of dentists.

Medication Misuse

Prescription drug misuse has been identified as a significant health-care problem. Individuals self-medicating with prescription drugs outside of the boundaries of the original intent of the prescription appears to be a significant contributing factor in the development of SUD. Recent survey data from the SAMSHA in 2012 indicated 6.8 million Americans aged 12 or older (or 2.6%) had used psychotherapeutic prescription drugs without a prescription or in a manner or for a purpose it was not prescribed in the past month.[3] Individuals may misuse drugs by self-prescribing unused or expired drugs. The impact of self-medicating with prescription drugs by patients for dental procedures or dental pain has not been well described in the USA. Excessive opioid prescribing by dental practitioners has been suggested in the dental literature, and these surveys have reported a wide dosing range of opioid analgesics for identical or similar dental procedures.[9,10] Multiple factors may influence excessive prescribing (see Box 1.3). Dental practitioners should be aware of prescription medication misuse and abuse behaviors (see Box 1.4). These behaviors are

---

Box 1.3   Potential Influential Factors of Excessive Prescribing

- Limited guidelines for appropriate drug and dosage selection for specific disease states or dental procedures.
- Subjectivity of individual patient *or dentist's* perception of pain severity.
- Patient assertiveness or aggressiveness toward prescriber.
- Complicated patient pathology.
- Lack of knowledge of pharmacologic principles and treatment options.
- Prescriber–patient mismatch.
- Provider availability.
- Patient or prescriber convenience.

Box 1.4   Common Prescription Drug Misuse and Abuse Behaviors in Dental Patients

- Requesting refills or running out of medications early.
- Repeated frequent or unnecessary office visits.
- Obvious powder or tablet fragments in nostrils.
- Impaired patients at initiation of office visit.
- Request from members of the family (spouse, parent) or patient's friends (boyfriend, girlfriend) for more medications.
- Family members or patient friends demanding to be present when asking for medications (excluding young children).
- Patients reporting multiple allergies to **only** less potent opioids and nonsteroidal anti-inflammatory drugs (NSAIDs).

---

discussed in more detail in Chapter 8. Ultimately, the most effective pharmacological agent, with minimal side effects or adverse effects, should be prescribed with the lowest dose possible for the minimal amount of time to achieve a reasonable effect such as analgesia, anxiolysis, or sedation. The impact of SUD on dental health and the dental community will be discussed in Chapter 6.

Clinical Consideration

Prescribing of any medication requires comprehensive patient histories, examinations, screening prior to prescribing or dispensing medications, and patient education regarding medication misuse.

Alcoholism

Alcohol-related SUD is the most common of all SUDs in society today. In 2012, the NSDUH found that slightly more than half (52.1%) of Americans aged 12 or older reported being current drinkers of alcohol.[3] This information translates to an estimated 135.5 million current drinkers in 2012.[3] Other results in this same survey indicated nearly one-quarter (23.0%) of persons aged 12 or older were binge alcohol users in the 30 days prior to the survey. This translates to about 59.7 million people. Heavy drinking was reported by 6.5% of the population aged 12 or older, or 17.0 million people.[3] The cost of excessive alcohol consumption in the USA in 2006 reached $223.5 billion according to the CDC in a 2006 study.[11] The CDC defines excessive alcohol consumption, or heavy drinking, as consuming an average of more than one alcoholic beverage per day for women, and an average of more than two alcoholic beverages per day for men, and any drinking by pregnant women or underage youth.[11] The exact costs of alcohol abuse and addiction to the dental health-care system have not been well elucidated. Because many dental patients are seen routinely for preventive as well as treatment services, dental practitioners may have the greatest opportunity to recognize potential alcohol SUD behaviors. This recognition at a minimum should result in a recommendation or referral to a local substance treatment center, substance abuse counselor, or primary-care physician for evaluation. See Box 1.5 for common signs and symptoms of potential alcohol-associated SUD. Chapter 2 will discuss the diseases of alcoholism and other SUDs.

Box 1.5   Common Signs and Symptoms of Potential Alcohol-Associated SUD

- Alcohol odor on breath or clothes during normal day hours.
- Slurred speech.
- Oversedation *before* office procedures start.
- Clumsiness, imbalance while walking.
- Unexplainable loud and argumentative behavior.
- Reduced effects of anesthetics during procedures.

Drug Diversion

Drug diversion presents in various forms, from simple self-prescribing and using someone's leftover prescription medications, to criminal activity to acquire more medications to sell or abuse. The penalties and punishments for these behaviors vary significantly.

Box 1.6 lists the most common types of drug diversion. For the purpose of this textbook,

Box 1.6   Common Types of Drug Diversion

- Counterfeit medications/misbranding.
- Robbery/burglary.
- Trafficking/transport of illegal medications.
- Prescription forgeries (written or verbal)
- Sharing prescription medications.
- Internet scams avoiding state, federal, and national drug control regulations.
- Fraudulent or "fake" patient schemes, injuries, or complaints.
- Selling prescriptions or prescription medications.
- Personnel/office staff theft of medications from offices, hospitals, stock supplies.
- Doctor/dentist/pharmacy shopping with intent to deceive.
- Knowingly overprescribing medications by prescribers.
- Health-care fraud.
- Extortion/coercion.
- Self-prescribing leftover medications/misuse.

information provided will focus on common prescription drug diversion methods related to dental practices. An important concept for all health-care practitioners to understand is that an individual demonstrating specific drug diversion behavior frequently may not have an SUD. Various drug diversion behaviors are commonly motivated by other factors, such as financial incentives or sex.

Dental practitioners are likely to be victims of fraudulent patient schemes, written or phoned-in prescription forgeries or "dentist/pharmacy shoppers with the intent to deceive the dental practitioner or pharmacy." The actual impact of drug diversion behavior on the dental community is not well defined. However, a statewide survey by O'Neil revealed that nearly 60% of dentists surveyed suspected they were victims of prescription drug diversion or fraud by their patients by methods such as theft of prescription pads, fake phoned-in prescriptions, altered refill or pill quantity on prescriptions, or false "stolen prescription" reports.[8] When taking this information into consideration, time spent addressing these aberrant patient behaviors by dental practitioners and their office staff likely would have a significant impact on dental practitioner and office staff time. Chapter 8 will discuss in greater detail the various patient drug diversion schemes and scams as well as intervention and prevention strategies. Chapter 11 will discuss *dental practitioner* behaviors frequently involved in SUD.

Pain Management in Dentistry

Effective prevention and minimization of pain is a primary focus of all dental practitioners. Prescriptions for analgesics lead the list of prescribed medications by dental practitioners. Most prescribing is for acute pain, although occasionally analgesics or muscle relaxants may be prescribed for more chronic pain conditions, such as trigeminal neuralgia or temporomandibular joint disorders. Acute pain management in dentistry may be influenced by underlying chronic, nondental-related pain,

diseases, or injuries. Although the reported incidence of chronic pain in the USA varies, most pain specialists would agree that at least 100 million Americans suffer annually with chronic pain.[12] As life expectancies continue to increase in the USA, dental practitioners should expect an increase in patients on *chronic* analgesics for chronic pain now requiring medications for acute pain management. Similarly, the opioid-addicted population continues to rise, and many of these patients are maintaining a successful addiction recovery through opioid-based treatment programs with methadone or buprenorphine. Chapter 4 will discuss dental treatment considerations for acute pain in patients receiving opioid therapy for chronic pain and opioid-based addiction treatment.

Although the actual medications used to manage dental-associated pain are generally limited to two major classes of medications, (NSAIDs and opioid analgesics, actual prescribing patterns may vary considerably between practitioners prescribing for the same indication. Multiple factors certainly influence the quantity of medications and duration of pain medication therapy. See Box 1.7 for a list of some common considerations that may influence analgesic prescribing. Unless otherwise contraindicated, NSAIDs remain the first-line

---

Box 1.7   Common Considerations That May Influence Analgesic Prescribing

- Complexity of dental pathology.
- Perceived physical forces required for extractions and procedures.
- Duration of procedures.
- Combined pathologies, such as injury and infection.
- Patient pain sensitivity.
- Patient allergies and medication tolerance.
- Drug–drug interactions.
- Drug–disease interactions.
- Underlying diseases.
- Patient analgesic preferences.
- Prescriber analgesic preferences.

drug therapy of choice for most dental pain, including prophylaxis, dental-procedure-induced pain, infection, or structural damage.[13] However, many dental practitioners remain reluctant to prescribe them as first-line agents. Variability in analgesic prescribing in dentistry will likely be reduced as national and state regulatory boards continue to promote "best practices" for pain management and as evidence-based studies are published in the dental literature. Chapter 3 will further discuss acute pain management considerations in dental practice.

Understanding the Cultures of Substance Use Disorder, Drug Misuse, and Drug Diversion

Individuals' motivations leading to the abuse, misuse, and diversion of drugs vary significantly. Although most health-care practitioners, licensing boards, and law enforcement agencies focus their efforts on controlled substances under DEA regulation, it is important to recognize that a significant amount of prescription and OTC drug misuse, abuse, and diversion occurs with drugs such as muscle relaxants, anticonvulsants, antipsychotics, and antibiotics not regulated by the DEA. Understanding the cultures associated with these behaviors is a key step to help facilitate education, treatment, and prosecution of these individuals. The cultures of SUD, drug misuse, and drug diversion can be divided into four categories. Each culture has its own characteristics. These categories include the sharing culture, the income-driven culture, the substance abuse culture, and the addiction culture. Categories may be identified based on the *intent* of the individual. Each category can be further divided to identify subpopulations.[14]

The Sharing Culture

The sharing culture may be defined as the giving, lending, or borrowing of prescription medication to anyone *other than* whom

the prescription was intended. The intent of the sharing culture is to help treat illness, symptoms of an illness, or a perceived psychiatric or physical problem that may or may not have been appropriately diagnosed by a health-care practitioner. The sharing culture is characterized by the patient's perception that prescription medications are safe simply because the medical or dental practitioner prescribed them and a pharmacist or prescriber dispensed them. There is little recognition that the sharing of prescriptions is illegal and a type of drug diversion. Sources of these medications include leftover prescriptions, expired medications, or discontinued medications. Subcategories include adult-to-adult sharing or adult-to-child/adolescent sharing.[14]

The Income-driven Culture

The income-driven culture consists of patients, prescribers, and pharmacists. Medication theft, prescription forgeries, dentist/doctor/pharmacy shopping, and illegal Internet acquisition of medications are all methods individuals use to obtain prescription medications. The income-driven culture is motivated by financial gain and items or services that may be traded, such as other drugs or sex. However, at the community level, prescription drug sales may be a major source of income that an individual uses to pay utility bills or to buy food. Other characteristics include individuals who may never abuse any of the drugs they sell nor have they been diagnosed with legitimate medical or dental problems.[14]

The Substance Abuse Culture

The substance abuse culture consists of individuals whose sole intent is to alter in any number of ways their mood, psychological sense of well-being, physical sense of well-being, or their personal connection with the world around them. This culture can be further categorized into two subgroups: experimenters and mood modifiers. Experimenters try substances to evaluate whether or not they "like" or "dislike" the way a substance makes them feel. If the experience is perceived as positive and then leads to a more routine use of the substance, the individual may be categorized as a mood modifier. Mood modifiers may use these substances to enhance social, academic, or work performances. Prolonged abuse or misuse of substances by mood modifiers frequently leads to the disease of addiction.[14]

The Addiction Culture

The addiction culture consists of individuals who meet the diagnostic criteria for this disorder. Addiction behaviors may include substance seeking, compulsion to use, loss of control, craving, and continued use in spite of known negative consequences. This culture may be further divided into active addicts, who are abusing medication and not in recovery, and addicts who are in recovery. These categories may be further divided based on selective substance use behaviors.[14]

Combinations of Cultures

In reality, it is not unusual for dental practitioners to have patients in more than one culture. For example, active addicts may share their medications with friends or family to minimize withdrawal symptoms between "highs." An individual may also sell part of their own prescription in order to obtain food for their family while maintaining their own drug habit with the remaining drug. The complexity of these cultures makes identification, prevention, treatment, and prosecution difficult. Dental practitioners and their office staff are likely to interface with all types of professionals involved in dealing with these various behaviors.[14] Box 1.8 contains a list of resources that dental practitioners and office staff can interface with when necessary to optimize patient outcomes or simply report aberrant behaviors.

Box 1.8 Office Ready-Access List for Dental Practitioners

Law enforcement/regulatory agencies
- Local police department.
- State drug task force.
- DEA.
- State Board of Pharmacy.
- State dental board.

Specialists
- Addiction specialist for methadone/buprenorphine.
- Pain specialist.
- Community pharmacist.
- Substance abuse counselor.
- Local addiction treatment centers.
- Drug information center/poison center.
- Local hospital or emergency room.

Summary

In summary, dental practitioners are at the center of a very complex, demanding profession that requires, at a minimum, significant skills in dental and surgical procedures, knowledge of medical diagnoses, recognition of concurrent medical and psychiatric disorders, advanced communication and interview skills, and advanced knowledge in pharmacology, pharmacotherapy, pain management, drug diversion, and SUD. Dental practice is further complicated by the multitude of social issues and personalities of patients who visit the dental practitioner's office daily and cause difficulties in the dental practice. Safe prescribing of medications and recognition of SUD must be accomplished by dental practitioners staying up to date and knowledgeable about federal and state regulations. The following chapters will serve as a clinician's guide to help dental practitioners understand and successfully practice fundamental concepts involving SUD, pain and sedation management, and drug diversion prevention. These chapters will emphasize out-patient management of dental patients.

References

1. CDC Grand Rounds: prescription drug overdoses—a U.S. epidemic. Morb Mort Wkly Rep 2012;61(01):10–13. http://www.cdc.gov/mmwr/preview/mmwrhtml/mm6101a3.htm. Accessed January 5, 2015.

2. Patel KV, Guralnik JM, Dansie EJ, Turk DC. Prevalence and impact of pain among older adults in the United States: findings from the 2011 National Health and Aging Trends Study. Pain 2013;154(12):2649–57.

3. Substance Abuse and Mental Health Services Administration. Results from the 2012 National Survey on Drug Use and Health: Summary of National Findings. NSDUH Series H-46, HHS Publication No. (SMA) 13-4795. 2013. Substance Abuse and Mental Health Services Administration, Rockville, MD. http://media.samhsa.gov/data/NSDUH/2012SummNatFindDetTables/NationalFindings/NSDUHresults2012.pdf. Accessed January 5, 2015.

4. American Society of Addiction Medicine. The definition of addiction. 2011. http://www.asam.org/advocacy/find-a-policy-statement/view-policy-statement/public-policy-statements/2011/12/15/the-definition-of-addiction. Accessed January 5, 2015.

5. Diagnostic and Statistical Manual of Mental Disorders, 4th ed., text revision, DSM-IV-TR. 2000. American Psychiatric Association,

6. The Diagnostic and Statistical Manual of Mental Disorders, 5th ed., DSM-5. 2013. American Psychiatric Association.

7. Manchikanti L, Boswell MV, Hirsch JA. Lessons learned in the abuse of pain-relief medication: a focus on health care costs: impact on healthcare costs. Expert Rev Neurother 2013;13(5):527–43. http://www.medscape.org/viewarticle/803051_6. Accessed January 5, 2015.

8. O'Neil M. Dentists' experiences with drug diversion and substance use disorders. Accepted for poster presentation, ADEA Annual Conference, March 2015.

9. Mutlu I, Abubaker AO, Laskin DM. Narcotic prescribing habits and other methods of pain control by oral and maxillofacial surgeons after impacted third molar removal. J Oral Maxillofac Surg 2013;71(9):1500–3. doi: 10.1016/j.joms.2013.04.031.

10. O'Neil M. A statewide survey of opioid prescribing practices in dentistry: clinical implications. JADA 2015; under review.

11. CDC. Excessive drinking costs U.S. $223.5 billion. 2014. http://www.cdc.gov/features/alcoholconsumption./ Accessed January 5, 2015.

12. American Academy of Pain Medicine. AAPM facts and figures on pain. http://www.painmed.org/patientcenter/facts_on_pain.aspx. Accessed January 5, 2015.

13. Hersh EV, Kane WT, O'Neil MG, Kenna GA, Katz NP, Golubic S, Moore PA. Prescribing recommendations for the treatment of acute pain in dentistry. Compend Contin Educ Dent 2011;32(3):22, 24–30.

14. O'Neil M, Hannah KL. Understanding the cultures of prescription drug abuse, misuse, addiction, and diversion. W V Med J 2010;106(4 Spec No):64–70.

Understanding the Disease of Substance Use Disorders 2

James H. Berry, DO and Carl Rollynn Sullivan, MD

Introduction

Substance use disorder (SUD) includes some of humanity's most common and destructive disease states. The range of physical, emotional, social, familial, legal, financial, and spiritual problems associated with SUD is vast and frequently uncompromising to patients and families. Unfortunately, identification and treatment of these patients is often complicated by their own denial, rationalization, or minimization of their condition. This has traditionally been compounded by a society where alcoholic or addicted patients were often morally stigmatized as "bad" or "weak" people rather than having a disease and in need of medical help. But this attitude is changing as scientific discovery has significantly enhanced our understanding of the neurophysiology of addiction. In the last 40 years, we have been able to identify the meso-limbic reward pathway as the primary site of dysfunction and have begun to understand the primary role of

"craving" as the mediator to ongoing drug or substance usage. Researchers have mapped the receptors for all the major classes of addicting drugs and have developed medication treatments to specifically target those areas of dysfunction. Equally important has been the development of evidence-based psychotherapies to assist in the goal of psychosocial recovery of the individual and family suffering with an SUD. In this chapter we will present a concise overview of our current understanding of SUD.

Definitions

Addiction

Addiction is a primary chronic disease of brain reward, motivation, memory, judgment, and related circuitry. Dysfunction in these circuits leads to characteristic biological, psychological, social, and spiritual manifestations

The ADA Practical Guide to Substance Use Disorders and Safe Prescribing, First Edition. Edited by Michael O'Neil.
© 2015 American Dental Association. Published 2015 by John Wiley & Sons, Inc.

that frequently result in destructive and life-threatening behaviors. Addiction is influenced by multiple factors, including, but not limited to, genetics, environment, sociology, physiology, and individual behaviors.

Addiction is characterized by inability to consistently abstain, impairment in behavior control, craving, diminished recognition of significant problems in behavior and interpersonal relationships, and a dysfunctional emotional response. Like other chronic diseases, addiction often involves cycles of relapse and remission. Without treatment or engagement in recovery activities, addiction is progressive and can result in disability or premature death.[1]

Ambivalence

One of the most important concepts to understand regarding a person suffering from SUD is ambivalence. Ambivalence is the coexistence of both positive and negative feelings and thoughts towards an action. This often results in no action being taken. Working through this ambivalence is a normal part of life as individuals negotiate many of the choices made as human beings. In SUD, however, this process results in significant internal conflict that keeps people engaged in many behaviors that they often know are not healthy.

Cross-addiction

Cross-addiction occurs when a person gives up one substance and becomes addicted to another. This can occur immediately after the initial substance is discontinued or in the future. Because all reinforcing substances activate the reward pathway in the brain as discussed later, a person predisposed to addiction is at risk regardless of the substance. This is an important concept for the dental practitioner to understand as one must be very cautious in prescribing a

controlled substance to a recovering alcoholic, for example.

Medication-assisted Therapy

Taking into account that SUD is a disease, several evidence-based medications have been developed to treat this disease. This chapter will highlight many of these pharmacotherapies. Medication-assisted therapy is a term most commonly used in reference to medications used in the treatment of opioid-use disorders.

Medical Model

Much stigma has been attached to addiction throughout history. People suffering from addiction have been considered morally or spiritually weak and that the problem is primarily a social problem. The medical model of addiction recognizes that SUD is a health problem with features that parallel other chronic disease states. There are genetic predispositions, environmental factors, and organ (brain) susceptibilities that factor into the development and course of this disease. Furthermore, treatment outcomes are similar to other chronic diseases, such as type 2 diabetes mellitus, hypertension, and asthma.[2]

Psychological Therapy or Psychotherapy

Psychotherapy is the informed and intentional application of clinical methods and interpersonal stances derived from established psychological principles for the purpose of assisting people to modify their behaviors, cognitions, emotions, and/or other personal characteristics in directions that the participants deem desirable.[3]

Tolerance

Tolerance may be defined by either a need for markedly increased amounts of the substance to achieve intoxication or desired effect or a markedly diminished effect with continued use of the same amount of the chemical.[1]

Transtheoretical Model of Change

Understanding behavior change is a process that occurs in specific stages with specific implications for each stage and is helpful in approaching the addicted patient. DiClemente and Prochaska developed the transtheoretical model of change (Figure 2.1), which identifies five stages of change.[4] As illustrated in the figure, a person moves from the initial stages of not recognizing a problem exists or being unwilling to make a change, to understanding there is a problem and identifying that change needs to occur, to preparing to make a change and taking action, and finally sustaining the change. The treatment implications are clear. It will not be beneficial to approach an individual who is in the precontemplation stage as if they were in

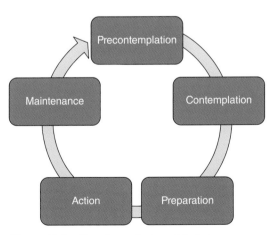

Figure 2.1   Transtheoretical model of change.

the action stage. To do so would invite considerable resistance from the patient, further frustration for the clinician, and potentially damage the therapeutic alliance.

Withdrawal

Withdrawal is an unpleasant physiologic phenomenon characterized by a wide range of signs and symptoms. Physiologic systems, such as the cardiovascular system or central nervous system (CNS) have adapted to function normally in the presence of substances not endogenous to the physiologic system. This usually occurs over a prolonged period of time. Abrupt discontinuation of the substance produces a hyperactive response by the same physiologic system. For example, long-term CNS depression by a substance will likely produce CNS stimulation upon withdrawal. Diazepam, a CNS depressant, will likely produce increased anxiety or agitation upon withdrawal in a patient who has physiologically adapted to being on the medication for a prolonged period of time.

Epidemiology: Drug/Alcohol

According to the 2012 National Survey on Drug Use and Health (NSDUH), an estimated 22.2 million persons aged 12 or older met criteria for an SUD in the past year (8.5% of the population aged 12 or older). Of these, 2.8 million met criteria for alcohol and illicit drugs, 4.5 million for illicit drugs but not alcohol, and 14.9 million alcohol but not illicit drugs. (Note: NSDUH used Diagnostic and Statistical Manual of Mental Disorders (DSM-)IV abuse/dependence criteria, not DSM-5 SUD criteria.[5])

Age and Gender

Many studies have demonstrated that exposure to drugs and alcohol during adolescence increases the risk of developing problems with substances as an adult.[6] According to the NSDUH, among adults, age at first use of marijuana was associated with illicit SUDs. Among those who first tried marijuana at age 14 or younger, 13.2% met criteria for an illicit drug use disorder, higher than the 2.2% of adults who had first used at age 18 or older. The first use of alcohol was also associated with an alcohol use disorder. Among those who first tried alcohol at age 14 or younger, 16.1% met criteria, which was higher than the 3.6% of adults who had first used alcohol at age 18 or older. Adults who had their first drink before age 21 were seven times more likely to have an alcohol use disorder than those who had their first drink at age 21 or older. This highlights the importance of screening youth for substance use and making treatment accessible, as well as providing education regarding the risks.

Rates of SUD were also associated with age. In 2012, the rate of SUD among adults aged 18–25 (18.9%) was higher than that among youths aged 12–17 (6.1%) and among adults aged 26 or older (7.0%). The rate of alcohol use disorders among youths aged 12–17 was 3.4%, 14.3% for adults aged 18–25, and 5.9% for those aged 26 or older.[5] Furthermore, there is a growing body of evidence and concern for alcohol and substance use among the elderly population.[7,8]

Interestingly, the results from the NSDUH demonstrate a gender difference among adults compared with youth. Males have almost double the rate of an SUD for adults aged 18 or older, whereas the rate is equal for youth aged 12–17.[5]

Clinical Consideration

Early age abuse of substances such as alcohol or marijuana have a high association with SUD later in life when compared with individuals that began abusing these same substances as adults.

Treatment

The NSDUH also surveyed the rates of people obtaining substance use treatment. In 2012, 4 million received treatment for a problem related to the use of alcohol or illicit drugs. Of these, 1.2 million received treatment for the use of both alcohol and illicit drugs, 1 million received treatment for the use of illicit drugs but not alcohol, and 1.4 million received treatment for the use of alcohol but not illicit drugs. There were differences in where the individuals obtained treatment. The majority of people received treatment at a self-help group (2.1 million) or at a rehabilitation facility as an outpatient (1.5 million). An equal number (1 million) received inpatient treatment at a rehabilitation facility as those that got care as an outpatient at a mental health clinic. The numbers of persons who received treatment at other locations were 1 million at a rehabilitation facility as an inpatient, 1 million at a mental health center as an outpatient, 861 000 at a hospital as an inpatient, 735 000 at a private doctor's office, 597 000 at an emergency room, and 388 000 at a prison or jail.[5]

Pathophysiology/Brain Pathways

The mesolimbic reward pathway is known as the reward center of the brain for food, water, sex, social interactions, and other positive responses. This pathway connects the midbrain to the limbic system or emotion center of the brain to the prefrontal cortex (PFC), an area associated with higher cognitive and emotional control (Figure 2.2). The mesolimbic reward pathway has significant connectivity to the memory storage areas of the brain in the amygdala and hippocampus. Dopamine is the predominant neurotransmitter associated with this complex pathway. The nucleus accumbens (NAcc) is a small portion of the brain that regulates pleasure, motivation, and other survival behaviors. The NAcc is situated in the

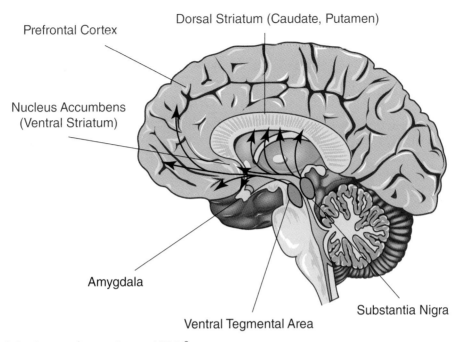

Prefrontal Cortex

Dorsal Striatum (Caudate, Putamen)

Nucleus Accumbens
(Ventral Striatum)

Amygdala

Ventral Tegmental Area

Substantia Nigra

Figure 2.2   Brain pathways. *Source:* NIDA.[9]

limbic system and plays a central role in this reward circuit. Virtually all substances of addiction act through specific receptor modulations along this pathway to either directly or indirectly exert their reinforcing effects by inducing dopamine bursts primarily in the NAcc. In the nonaddicted state there exists a balance between the cognitive decision-making and restraint of the PFC and the instinctual, libidinal, survival function of the limbic system's reward center. *Repetitive substance usage induces alterations in this homeostasis that leads to changes in craving, motivation, reward perception, behavior control, salience attribution, and memory.*[10, 11] These substance-induced brain alterations are the neurophysiologic hallmarks of SUD.

Signs, Symptoms, Behavior

The various substances of abuse have predictable signs and symptoms of withdrawal and intoxication. These often depend upon the category of medications in which the substance is placed. For example, cocaine and amphetamines are both stimulants and have similar effects on the human body. Frequently, the intoxicating effects of a substance will be the opposite of the withdrawal. Opioids are a case in point. During use, the pupils will constrict, and during withdrawal they will dilate. It is important to note that withdrawal, regardless of whether or not it is life threatening, can be very uncomfortable and often results in the dependent individual returning to use despite the horrible consequences.

Alcohol

Most Americans have used alcohol at some point in their lifetime and are familiar with the intoxication effects. For those who have not experienced these effects first hand, many have witnessed in others or seen examples of drunkenness portrayed in media. Signs/symptoms of intoxication are listed in Box 2.1.

> **Box 2.1   Signs and Symptoms of Alcohol Intoxication**
>
> - Slurred speech
> - Incoordination/unsteady gate
> - Stupor/coma
> - Memory loss
> - Attention impairment
> - Nystagmus
> - Somnolence
> - Impaired judgment

The degree of impairment is related to the blood alcohol concentration (BAC), with a low concentration generally resulting in mild euphoria and relaxation and a high concentration potentially resulting in a coma or death. In general, after the consumption of one standard drink, the BAC peaks within 30–45 min. (A standard drink is defined as 12 oz of beer, 5 oz of wine, or 1.5 oz of 80-proof distilled spirits, all of which contain the same amount of alcohol.) BAC is routinely measured as milligrams per deciliter or milligram-percent. A 70 kg person metabolizes about 2/3 to 1 oz of 90-proof spirits or 8–12 oz of beer per hour. Table 2.1 highlights common effects based on BAC. It is important to note that frequent users of high amounts of alcohol may develop a tolerance to the intoxicating effects and may appear strikingly unaffected with an elevated BAC.

Alcohol withdrawal can be life threating and, therefore, require medical attention. Signs and symptoms may occur following a few hours to a few days after one stops drinking (see Box 2.2).

> **Box 2.2   Signs and Symptoms of Alcohol Withdrawal**
>
> **Mild to Moderate**
> - Sweats
> - Tachycardia
> - Tremors
> - Insomnia
> - Anxiety
> - Psychomotor agitation
>
> **Severe**
> - Generalized tonic clonic seizures
> - Delirium tremens ("DTs")
> - Hallucinations

Benzodiazepines

Benzodiazepines are a class of medications that are frequently used to treat anxiety and aid in relaxation and sleep. They are similar to alcohol in their mechanism of action and, therefore, have similar intoxicating and withdrawal effects. They can be habit forming, result in

Table 2.1   Clinical Correlation of BAC

BAC (mg%)	No. of drinks/h	Effects
30	1	Little or nothing
50	~2	Relaxation or lowering of inhibitions
80[a]	~3	Legally intoxicated and subjected to driving under the influence
100	4–5	Slurred speech, awkwardness, drowsiness
150–300	6–10	Staggering gait, blackout, passing out, irrational behavior
400	Fifth to a quart of whiskey	Coma
500		Death

[a]A BAC of 80 mg% is considered legally drunk and may subject to regulatory action in the USA.

dependence, and, like alcohol, precipitate life-threatening withdrawal.

Death is unlikely during intoxication in a patient who has overdosed on benzodiazepines alone. However, it is important to note that combining benzodiazepines with other substances that cause respiratory depression significantly increases the risk of death. Unfortunately, it is common for benzodiazepine misusers to use with other substances of abuse, such as alcohol and opioids.

When considering the severity of impending withdrawal it is helpful to know how long the patient has been on benzodiazepines and at what dosage. There is little chance of withdrawal in patients who have been on benzodiazepines for ≤2 weeks. However, >90% of long-term users (8 months–1 year) have withdrawal symptoms. Short-acting/high-dose agents typically have more severe withdrawal.

Post-acute withdrawal from benzodiazepines is a further phenomenon that is described in the literature and clinical experience that is marked by long-lasting symptoms. These symptoms can be very distressing for the patient and difficult for the provider to manage (see Table 2.2).

> **Clinical Consideration**
>
> Patients with a known history of daily alcohol abuse or benzodiazepine use/abuse for several weeks may be at risk of life-threatening withdrawal events such as seizures, especially if known doses of benzodiazepines or number of daily drinks of alcohol is large. Often times, these individuals may require hospital admission for treatment.

> **Clinical Consideration**
>
> Dental practitioners should avoid prescribing benzodiazepines to patients with known alcohol use disorders owing to the potential for stimulating similar brain pathways that potentially may exacerbate cravings for alcohol.

Opioids

For many people who have taken prescription opioid pain medication as prescribed, it is difficult to understand why an individual would misuse these drugs, since they may cause mental dulling and have other undesirable side

Table 2.2 Symptoms of Post-acute Withdrawal from Benzodiazepines[12]

Symptoms	Usual course
Anxiety	Gradually diminishing over a year
Insomnia	Gradually diminishing over a year
Depression	Few months
Perceptual symptoms – tinnitus – paresthesia – pain in limbs	Gradually diminishing over a year, but occasionally permanent
Motor symptoms – muscle pain, weakness, cramps, tremor, jerks, blepharospasm	Gradually diminishing over a year, but occasionally permanent
GI symptoms – gaseous distention, pain, alternating diarrhea and constipation	Gradually diminishing over a year, but occasionally permanent

effects (see Box 2.3). However, for many individuals they may be energizing, cause euphoria, and with prolonged use over time may result in dependence. Appendix 2.A lists common opioid analgesics and their brand names.

Box 2.3   Signs and Symptoms of Opioid Intoxication

- Drowsiness or coma
- Slurred speech
- Memory or attention impairment
- Euphoria
- Energy or increased alertness
- Pupillary constriction
- Impaired judgment
- Head nodding
- Bradycardia
- Low blood pressure

Like alcohol, high doses of opioids can result in significant respiratory depression in an opioid-naive patient, especially *in combination* with other substances such as benzodiazepines. Withdrawal results in flu-like and other symptoms that can be very distressing, but, unlike alcohol and benzodiazepines, they do not result in a life-threating withdrawal. Withdrawal signs/symptoms can occur within minutes to several days and are listed in Box 2.4.

Box 2.4   Signs and Symptoms of Opioid Withdrawal

- Dysphoria/dissociation
- Agitation
- Nausea/vomiting/diarrhea
- Deep muscle, bone, joint aches
- Lacrimation
- Rhinorrhea
- Pupillary dilation
- Piloerection
- Sweats
- Frequent yawning
- Low-grade fevers
- Insomnia
- Tachycardia

Stimulants

Stimulants such as cocaine, amphetamine, and methamphetamine are commonly used in a binge manner where the user will use several times in a day and/or for several days in a row to achieve a steady "high"; the subsequent "crash" results in a significant "low." Stimulants also include prescription drugs such as methylphenidate (Ritalin®, Concerta®) or dextroamphetamine (Adderall®) or over-the-counter medications like pseudoephedrine. Stimulant use can cause life-threating conditions such as a myocardial infarction or stroke. Box 2.5 lists signs/symptoms of stimulant intoxication.

Box 2.5   Signs and Symptoms of Stimulant Intoxication

- Hypervigilance or pressured speech
- Euphoria
- Anxiety
- Tension, anger, or aggression
- Impaired judgment
- Tachycardia, chest pain, or arrhythmias
- Pupillary dilation
- Elevated blood pressure
- Sweats or chills
- Nausea or vomiting
- Respiratory depression
- Confusion
- Seizures or dystonia
- Dyskinesia
- Stereotyped movements such as skin picking
- Transient paranoia, delusions, hallucinations

Withdrawal from stimulants is typically not life threating and rarely requires medical intervention, although, like the substances just mentioned, it can be quite distressing. Signs and symptoms of stimulant withdrawal develop within a few hours to days after cessation (see Box 2.6).

Box 2.6   Signs and Symptoms of Stimulant Withdrawal

- Dysphoria
- Fatigue
- Vivid, unpleasant dream
- Insomnia, or hypersomnia
- Increased appetite
- Psychomotor retardation
- Anxiety or irritability

Cannabis

For many years cannabis has been the leading illicit substance of abuse in the USA. With the changing legal landscape regarding this intoxicating weed, this could become the leading licit substance of abuse. Regardless, dental practitioners are likely to treat a number of patients who are frequent users both now and in the future. Signs/symptoms of cannabis intoxication are listed in Box 2.7.

Box 2.7   Signs and Symptoms of Cannabis Intoxication

- Impaired motor coordination
- Euphoria
- Anxiety
- Paranoia
- Impaired judgment
- Sensation of "slowing" and slowed reaction time
- Irritated conjunctiva
- Increased appetite
- Xerostomia
- Tachycardia

Dependence and withdrawal from cannabis was a subject of debate for many years. Enough evidence now exits to definitively describe a predictable withdrawal pattern that is now included in the DSM-5. The signs/symptoms develop within a week of cessation and are listed in Box 2.8.

Box 2.8   Signs and Symptoms of Cannabis Withdrawal

- Irritability, anger, or aggression
- Nervousness or anxiety
- Sleep difficulty
- Decreased appetite or weight loss
- Restlessness
- Depressed mood
- Abdominal pain
- Tremors
- Sweats or chills
- Fever
- Headache

Nicotine

In the USA there is an almost universal understanding that tobacco smoking is harmful and deadly, and yet some patients will continue to smoke despite the associated risks. The withdrawal symptoms that occur within a few hours of the last cigarette are just too unpleasant to ignore and are relieved quickly when tobacco is inhaled (see Box 2.9).

Box 2.9   Signs and Symptoms of Nicotine Withdrawal

- Irritability, frustration, or anger
- Anxiety
- Difficulty concentrating
- Increased appetite
- Restlessness
- Depressed mood
- Insomnia

Chapter 7 will discuss nicotine and tobacco cessation in greater detail.

Hallucinogens, Designer Drugs, Inhalants

This is a very large and diverse group of "abusable" substances. The hallucinogens typically produce intense sensory experiences which are mostly auditory or visual disturbances. LSD, mescaline, mushrooms and certain "designer drugs" all share this ability. Some of these drugs have more of a stimulatory effect on the CNS, but many will have both "psychedelic" and stimulant effects. Many of the "designer drugs" (e.g., MDMA "Ecstasy", MDPV/mephedrone "bath salts") are known compounds that have been chemically altered to enhance their desired effects. There is a constantly changing array of mind-altering chemicals being evaluated, with new ones becoming popular all the time.

The inhalants are likely the most diverse group of all "abusable" substances. These substances are often easily obtained and can be found under the cabinets in virtually every home. They are solvents, cleaners, repellents, fuels, anesthetics, room odorizers, and adhesives. Inhalants are used by mostly younger people because of the ease of access. The substances are usually placed into a cloth or bag and then inhaled deeply by the user. There is no universal effect, but it has been noted that inhalant intoxication looks most like alcohol intoxication.

> **Clinical Consideration**
>
> Dental practitioners may observe residue of paints or solvents, or redness/irritation around the nose or mouth in patients that are abusing inhaled commercial products.

Treatment Methods

Behavioral Modifications and Counseling

Motivational Interviewing

Miller and Rollnick developed motivational interviewing (MI) as an effective and evidence-based approach to address ambivalence.[13] This approach is widely used in the field of addiction treatment. This chapter does not allow an adequate discussion of MI, but motivation is not simply an intrinsic phenomenon but an "interpersonal process" that can be affected by the clinician's interaction with the patient.[13] This understanding helps avoid the trap of assuming that someone is either inherently motivated or not motivated to get better and that there is not much that can be done if they are not motivated. It is this trap that often results in frustration on the part of the clinician and poor treatment for the patient. The therapeutic alliance that exists between the clinician and patient can be a vehicle of change toward healthy behavior and a predictor of successful outcomes.[14] The mnemonics "OARS" and "FRAMES" highlight some MI principles and techniques that clinicians use to encourage change:

OARS

Open-ended questions
Affirming statements
Reflective listening
Summarizing

FRAMES

Give personal **F**eedback
Patient has **R**esponsibility for change
Give **A**dvice in a nonjudgmental manner with permission
Present a **M**enu of options to the patient to choose from
Express **E**mpathy
Support **S**elf-efficacy

> **Clinical Consideration**
>
> Incorporating the OARS or FRAMES principles into routine discussions with patients abusing or suspected of abusing substances may be a helpful intervention strategy for dental practitioners and staff.

Cognitive Behavioral Therapy

Cognitive behavioral therapy (CBT) is a psychosocial intervention that seeks to address an individual's faulty thinking, labeled "cognitive distortions," as well as their maladaptive behaviors. The practice of CBT was initially used to manage depression and anxiety. As these techniques proved helpful, they began to be applied to more disorders, such as SUD.[15] CBT helps individuals recognize that thoughts and behaviors, for a large part, have been learned over time and these can be modified to foster a greater state of health. The main goals of CBT are helping patients identify how cognitive distortions can affect emotional experiences and subsequently change behavioral responses. Relapse prevention is a significant area of focus that helps one to identify specific "triggers" which increase the risk of relapse and to develop effective coping techniques to minimize this risk.[16]

Contingency Management

Contingency management is a behavioral intervention grounded on the theory that positive behaviors will be reinforced with positive rewards. Practitioners of this technique will offer incentives (such as vouchers or gifts) to reward healthy behaviors (such as abstinence and compliance with treatment). Studies of substance users have demonstrated that using contingency management can be successful in keeping people in treatment and reducing their substance use.[17]

Alcoholics Anonymous

Perhaps the most widely known program to address alcoholism is Alcoholics Anonymous (AA). AA has been in existence since 1935 and has had faithful participation throughout much of the world. The primary purpose of AA is "to stay sober and help other alcoholics to achieve sobriety.[18] Sobriety is sought by working through 12 steps on a path towards spiritual awakening (12-step table, Table 2.3). The testimonies of success in AA have engendered similar programs such as Narcotics Anonymous for drug addiction. Twelve-step facilitation is the intervention used by clinicians to help patients become engaged in 12-step programs. The

Table 2.3   The 12 Steps of AA[18]

1. We admitted we were powerless over alcohol—that our lives had become unmanageable.
2. Came to believe that a Power greater than ourselves could restore us to sanity.
3. Made a decision to turn our will and our lives over to the care of God as we understood Him.
4. Made a searching and fearless moral inventory of ourselves.
5. Admitted to God, to ourselves and to another human being the exact nature of our wrongs.
6. Are entirely ready to have God remove all these defects of character.
7. Humbly asked Him to remove our shortcomings.
8. Made a list of all persons we had harmed, and became willing to make amends to them all.
9. Made direct amends to such people wherever possible, except when to do so would injure them or others.
10. Continued to take personal inventory and when we were wrong promptly admitted it.
11. Sought through prayer and meditation to improve our conscious contact with God as we understood Him, praying only for knowledge of His will for us and the power to carry that out.
12. Having had a spiritual awakening as the result of these steps, we tried to carry this message to alcoholics and to practice these principles in all our affairs.

Table 2.4   **Clinical Considerations Prior to Administering or Prescribing to Patients with a History of SUD**

Is the medication in the class of medications or substances that was/is the patient's preferred substance of abuse? If yes, do you absolutely need to administer or prescribe this medication? (Addiction IS NOT a contraindication to prescribe the medication if the benefits outweigh the risks.)

Is the patient in a treatment program for drug or alcohol addiction or under a treatment center/prescriber contract for pain or anxiety management? If yes, dental practitioners optimally should consult with the treatment center or practitioner enforcing the contract to discuss preferred treatment options.

Will the medication being administered result in a positive drug screen that potentially could compromise treatment contracts? If yes, dental practitioners *and patients* should discuss this issue with personnel responsible for the treatment contract *before* the procedure when possible.

NSAIDS remain the first-line oral agents of choice for the management of acute pain in dental procedures unless otherwise contraindicated.

For patients with a history of alcohol, benzodiazepine, or barbiturate addiction, controlled substances such as benzodiazepines or barbiturates are not recommended for light sedation or anxiolysis due to the *potential* for stimulating similar pathways in the brain that promote craving. Alternative agents, such as antihistamines (diphenhydramine or hydroxyzine), may be considered if light sedation is required. Anecdotally, patients in recovery from alcohol or benzodiazepine addiction have reported a significant increase in cravings after receiving nitrous oxide inhalation for light sedation or anxiolysis.

clinician encourages attendance in 12-step meetings, and the focus of therapy sessions is helping the patient process each step. Thoughts, feelings, cravings, relapses, and other important issues are dealt with, and recovery assignments are given to work on between sessions.

Medications for Substance Use Disorder

Currently, there are no definitive medical cures for the disease of addiction. Various pharmacologic treatments are available for many, but not all, types of SUD. Evidence-based medicine supports psychotherapy alone or the combination of psychotherapy and pharmacotherapy to produce the best patient outcomes in the treatment of medication- or substance-based addictions. Pharmacological intervention of addiction alone without appropriate psychotherapy offers minimal benefits for most individuals.

Since pharmacologic therapy is not curative, the primary goals of pharmacological treatment of addiction are to decrease cravings of the

particular substance or substances, to eliminate the compulsions to abuse, to deter euphoria or desired effects that drive addiction, and to prevent activation of the reward pathways.

Table 2.4 provides a list of important clinical considerations prior to the dental practitioner administering or prescribing medications to a patient with a history of alcohol or drug addiction.

Medications used to pharmacologically manipulate the reward or behavior pathways are now briefly listed and discussed. Key points for dental practitioners are highlighted as they apply to dental practices.

Alcohol

The following medications are approved by the US Food and Drug Administration (FDA) for treatment of alcohol dependence:

- Disulfiram—Antabuse®
  - Acetaldehyde dehydrogenase—blocks conversion of acetaldehyde to acetic acid.

- Dopamine beta-hydroxylase—blocks conversion of dopamine to norepinephrine (psychosis has been rarely reported).
- Usual daily dose is 250–500 mg orally.
- Side effects include drowsiness, headache, metallic taste, hepatitis, diarrhea.
- Avoid in patients who are actively drinking.
- Alcohol–disulfiram reaction—due to rapid buildup of acetaldehyde. Symptoms include nausea, vomiting, warmth and flushing, sweating, throbbing headache, tachycardia, hypotension, shortness of breath, vertigo, syncope.

- Acamprosate—Campral®
  - N-Methyl-D-aspartate blocker and may decrease alcohol-induced receptor hyperactivity.
  - Usual daily dose is 333 mg, two tabs orally three times a day.
  - Side effects—diarrhea.
  - Acamprosate may decrease patient cravings associated with alcohol addiction.
- Naltrexone—ReVia®
  - Opioid antagonist—blocks reinforcing properties of alcohol.
  - Usual daily dose is 50 mg orally.
  - Side effects—nausea, vomiting, headache, anxiety, fatigue, insomnia, elevated liver function tests (LFTs).
- Depo-naltrexone—Vivitrol®
  - Opioid antagonist—blocks reinforcing properties of alcohol.
  - One injection of 380 mg intramuscularly every month.
  - Side effects—nausea, vomiting, headache, anxiety, fatigue, insomnia, elevated LFTs, pain or redness at injection site.

Naltrexone is a pharmacological treatment used to suppress cravings and compulsions of alcohol and opioid-based addictions. This therapy has significant clinical ramifications for the dental practitioner. Patients receiving naltrexone therapy should be prescribed nonsteroidal anti-inflammatory drugs (NSAIDS) or alternative non-opioid-based pharmacotherapy as first-line agents whenever possible since naltrexone specifically blocks the receptors responsible for opioid analgesia. If opioid therapy is deemed clinically necessary due to potential contraindications to NSAIDs, such as allergies or if patients have moderate to severe pain, opioid doses may need to be increased due to receptor blockade by naltrexone. Patients with alcoholism *may* also have opioid addiction, and use of opioids in these patients without prior approval from their addiction treatment center could be a violation of their treatment contract leading to dismissal from the treatment center. Patients presenting with a naltrexone agent in their medication lists should be evaluated for the purpose of the naltrexone and potential contract violations.

> **Clinical Consideration**
>
> When possible, patients receiving daily naltrexone should discontinue their naltrexone at least 72 h before any procedure requiring post-procedure opioid analgesia.

Benzodiazepines

There are no FDA-approved medications used to treat benzodiazepine addiction. Pharmacological treatment has focused on symptomatic management of long-term withdrawal states. Frequently used medicines include gabapentin, pregabalin, carbamazepine, valproate, propranolol, and trazodone.[19–23]

Opioids

The following medications are FDA approved for the treatment of opioid dependence. Figure 2.3 shows the range of opioid receptor activation/inactivation for various opioid agonists/antagonists.

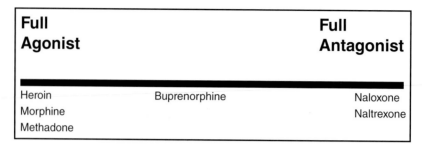

Full Agonist		Full Antagonist
Heroin	Buprenorphine	Naloxone
Morphine		Naltrexone
Methadone		

Figure 2.3 Opioid receptor activation/inactivation.

Methadone—CII (Methadose®, Dolophine®)

Since the early 1970s, medication-assisted treatment (MAT), primarily in the form of methadone, has been used to treat opioid addicts. Methadone treatment is regulated by the Substance Abuse and Mental Health Services Administration and the medication is distributed in certified clinics. The critical part of methadone treatment occurs during the induction.

- Typically the patient is started on about 30 mg/day with day 1 maximum of 40 mg orally.
- Common side effects—dry mouth, constipation, nausea or loss of appetite, feeling anxious or restless; insomnia, weakness or drowsiness; decreased sex drive.
- Methadone has a half-life of 24 h. Therefore, it takes four to five half-lives before steady state is reached.
- The goal is to establish the dosage that will keep the patient free from withdrawal symptoms for a 24 h period.
- The average oral dose of methadone is 70–120 mg/day.
- Avoid use of concurrent benzodiazepines due to risk of overdose and death.
- It is unknown how long a patient should remain on methadone, though some patients have been treated successfully for decades.

Methadone maintenance therapy creates various clinical challenges for the dental practitioners. The most common problem is the reluctance for patients to share with their dental practitioners the fact that they are being prescribed methadone for opioid addiction. This reluctance is multifactorial in origin. The most common factors include embarrassment or shame and fear of not receiving adequate analgesia. Caution should be used in prescribing any opioid to methadone treatment patients for potential contract violations with methadone treatment centers, as well the risk of stimulating opioid cravings. Discussion between treatment center and the dental practitioner is recommended if opioid therapy is warranted. *The dental practitioner should not assume that chronic methadone treatment for opioid addiction will adequately treat acute dental-related pain.* This is discussed in more detail in Chapter 4.

> **Clinical Consideration**
>
> Other than anecdotal reports, there are no evidence-based studies that show opioid addicts *in recovery and in acute pain* have an increased risk of relapse when treated with opioids when compared with patients not receiving opioid analgesics. *The stress of acute pain may be more likely to contribute to relapse.*

Buprenorphine—CIII

Buprenorphine mono product—generic mono-buprenorphine tablets (often referred to as "Subutex®," though brand name discontinued by manufacturer in 2011). Buprenorphine/naloxone tablets (4/1 ratio)—generic tablets, buprenorphine/naloxone film (4/1 ratio)—Suboxone®.

- All forms of buprenorphine approved for opioid treatment are to be used sublingually.
- Only approved office-based MAT for opioid dependence. Physician must have US Drug Enforcement Administration waiver in order to prescribe buprenorphine products.
- A recent consensus panel of the American Society of Addiction Medicine noted that the combination buprenorphine/naloxone should be used for induction, stabilization, and maintenance.
- The mono-product buprenorphine should be reserved only for use in pregnant women who need maintenance treatment and the rare individual who is allergic to buprenorphine/naloxone.
- Average daily dose is 12–16 mg. At 16 mg, 90% of the μ receptors are occupied. A patient on more than 16 mg/day should generate a serious reevaluation of the patient's treatment status.
- Side effects—headache, nausea, sweating, constipation, stomach pain, problems sleeping; sublingual irritation.
- Avoid use of concurrent benzodiazepines due to risk of overdose and death.
- It is imperative that all patients on buprenorphine be engaged in a psycho-educational addiction treatment program.
- Length of treatment—the optimal length of time that a patient should remain on buprenorphine is unknown. At this point it is recommended that patients should continue until the patient is engaged in healthy recovery.[24]

The same clinical considerations for methadone should be applied to patients receiving buprenorphine treatment.

Clinical Consideration

Dental practitioners should not assume that *daily* doses of methadone or buprenorphine for the treatment of opioid addiction provide adequate analgesia for acute dental pain.

Naltrexone (ReVia®, Vivitrol®)

- Naltrexone 50 mg tablets—ReVia®, naltrexone 380 mg monthly injection—Vivitrol®.
- Naltrexone is a long-acting oral opioid antagonist. When taken correctly it completely blocks the reinforcing properties of ingested opioids.
- In order to avoid precipitating opioid withdrawal a patient must be opioid free for several days before starting naltrexone.
- Oral dose is 50 mg daily.
- Naltrexone should be an ideal medication for the treatment of opioid addiction. However, 30 years of clinical experience has shown that compliance with the medication is a persistent problem for most patients.[25]
- The injectable form of naltrexone, Vivitrol®, was developed as a way of trying to increase medication compliance.
- Side effects—nausea, vomiting, headache, anxiety, fatigue, insomnia, elevated LFTs, injection-site reactions.

Stimulants, Hallucinogens, Cannabis, Inhalants

There are no FDA-approved medications to treat stimulant, hallucinogen, cannabis, or inhalant SUDs. Treatment generally consists of engaging the patient in a psycho-educational addiction treatment program.

Tobacco

Chapter 7 will provide a review of psychological and pharmacologic management of nicotine addiction.

Summary

The dental practitioner should understand that SUD is a complicated and chronic disease that has many underlying causes and complications. Advances in the neurosciences have demonstrated this is a brain disease that requires a comprehensive approach to treatment. Fortunately, there are many pharmacologic as well as psychosocial therapeutics available to help manage this disease. Guilt, shame, denial, fear of legal or clinical repercussions, and so on may preclude a patient from being open and honest regarding their substance use and seeking treatment. By being aware of the signs, symptoms, and behaviors of substance use, the dental practitioner may recognize a potential problem and assist in a patient obtaining necessary treatment. Furthermore, the dental practitioner should remain vigilant to assess for a history of SUD and potential pharmacologic treatments when considering prescribing controlled substances as access to these substances can result in negative outcomes for some patients.

Appendix 2.A: Common Opioid Analgesics and their Brand Names

Generic name	Dosage form	Brand name
Buprenorphine	Transdermal patch	Butrans
Buprenorphine	Sublingual tablet	Subutex
Buprenorphine/naloxone	Sublingual tablet, sublingual film	Suboxone
Buprenorphine/naloxone	Sublingual tablet	Zubsolv
Butorphanol	Nasal spray	Stadol NS
Codeine/APAP	Tablet	Tylenol w/Codeine #3
Codeine/APAP	Tablet	Tylenol w/Codeine #4
Codeine/APAP	Suspension	Capital w/Codeine
Codeine/caffeine/butalbital/APAP	Capsule	Fioricet w/Codeine
Codeine/caffeine/butalbital/aspirin	Capsule	Fiorinal w/Codeine
Codeine/caffeine/butalbital/aspirin	Capsule	Ascomp w/Codeine
Codeine/guaifensin	Syrup	Mytussin AC
Codeine/guaifensin	Syrup	Guaifenesin AC
Codeine/guaifensin	Solution	Dex-Tuss
Codeine/guaifensin	Syrup	Cheratussin AC
Codeine/guaifensin	Solution	Codar GF
Codeine/Promethazine	Syrup	Phenergan w/Codeine
Codeine/promethazine/phenylephrine	Syrup	Phenergan VC w/Codeine
Fentanyl	Transdermal patch	Duragesic
Fentanyl	Spray	Subsys
Fentanyl	Buccal film	Onsolis
Fentanyl	Nasal spray	Lazanda
Fentanyl	Buccal tablet	Fentora
Fentanyl	Lozenge	Actiq
Fentanyl	Sublingual tablet	Abstral
Hydrocodone	ER capsule	Zonhydro ER
Hydrocodone/APAP	Tablet	Zydone
Hydrocodone/APAP	Elixir	Zolvit
Hydrocodone/APAP	Solution	Zamicet
Hydrocodone/APAP	Tablet	Xodol
Hydrocodone/APAP	Tablet	Vicodin
Hydrocodone/APAP	Tablet	Vicodin HP
Hydrocodone/APAP	Tablet	Vicodin ES
Hydrocodone/APAP	Tablet	Norco
Hydrocodone/APAP	Elixir	Lortab Elixir
Hydrocodone/APAP	Tablet	Lortab
Hydrocodone/APAP	Tablet	Lorcet
Hydrocodone/APAP	Tablet	Lorcet Plus
Hydrocodone/APAP	Capsule	Lorcet HD
Hydrocodone/APAP	Elixir	Hycet

(continued)

Generic name	Dosage form	Brand name
Hydrocodone/chlorpheniramine	Solution	Vituz
Hydrocodone/chlorpheniramine	Suspension	Tussionex
Hydrocodone/chlorpheniramine	Capsule	Tussicaps
Hydrocodone/homatropine	Tablet	Hycodan
Hydrocodone/Homatropine	Syrup	Hydromet
Hydrocodone/homatropine	Tablet	Tussigon
Hydrocodone/ibuprofen	Tablet	Ibudone
Hydrocodone/ibuprofen	Tablet	Reprexain
Hydrocodone/ibuprofen	Tablet	Vicoprofen
Hydrocodone/pseudoephedrine	Syrup	Rezira
Hydrocodone/pseudoephedrine	Syrup	Pancof HC
Hydrocodone/pseudoephedrine/ chlorpheniramine	Syrup	Hydron PSC
Hydrocodone/pseudoephedrine/ chlorpheniramine	Syrup	Notuss-forte
Hydrocodone/pseudoephedrine/ chlorpheniramine	Liquid	Genecof HC
Hydrocodone/pseudoephedrine/ chlorpheniramine	Syrup	Zutripo
Hydromorphone	Tablet	Dilaudid
Hydromorphone	ER tablet	Exalgo
Levorphanol	Tablet	Levo-Dromoran
Meperidine	Tablet	Demerol
Meperidine	Tablet	Meperitab
Methadone	Solution, tablet	Methadose
Methadone	Tablet	Dolophine
Morphine	ER tablet	MS Contin
Morphine	Solution	Roxanol
Morphine	ER capsule	Avinza
Morphine	ER capsule	Kadian
Morphine	Tablet	MSIR
Morphine/naloxone	ER capsule	Embeda
Oxycodone	Tablet	Roxicodone
Oxycodone	ER tablet	Oxycontin
Oxycodone	Capsule	Oxy IR
Oxycodone	Solution	Eth-Oxydose
Oxycodone/APAP	Tablet	Percocet
Oxycodone/APAP	Tablet	Endocet
Oxycodone/APAP	Capsule	Tylox
Oxycodone/APAP	Solution	Roxicet
Oxycodone/APAP	Tablet	Xartemis XR
Oxycodone/aspirin	Tablet	Percodan
Oxycodone/aspirin	Tablet	Endodan
Oxycodone/ibuprofen	Tablet	Combunox
Oxymorphone	Tablet	Opana

Generic name	Dosage form	Brand name
Pentazocine/APAP	Tablet	Talacen
Pentazocine/naloxone	Tablet	Talwin NX
Tapentadol	Tablet	Nucynta
Tramadol	Tablet	Ultram
Tramadol	ODT	Rybix ODT
Tramadol	Tablet	Ryzolt
Tramadol	Capsule	Conzip
Tramadol/APAP	Tablet	Ultracet

APAP: paracetamol; ER: extended release; ODT: orally disintegrating tablet.

References

1. American Society of Addiction Medicine. Public Policy Statement: Definition of Addiction. The Short Definition of Addiction. 2011. http://www.asam.org/for-the-public/definition-of-addiction Accessed December 21, 2014.

2. McLellan AT, Lewis DC, O'Brien CP, Kleber HD. Drug dependence, a chronic medical illness: implications for treatment, insurance, and outcomes evaluation. JAMA 2000;284:1689–95.

3. Norcross JC. An eclectic definition of psychotherapy. In: What is Psychotherapy? Contemporary Perspectives. Zeig JK, Munion WM, eds. 1990. Jossey-Bass, San Francisco, CA, pp. 218–20.

4. Prochaska JO, Velicer WF. The transtheoretical model of health behavior change. Am J Health Promot 1997;12:38–48.

5. Substance Abuse and Mental Health Services Administration. Results from the 2012 National Survey on Drug Use and Health: Summary of National Findings. NSDUH Series H-46, HHS Publication No. (SMA) 13-4795. 2013. Substance Abuse and Mental Health Services Administration, Rockville, MD. http://archive.samhsa.gov/data/NSDUH/2012SummNatFindDetTables/NationalFindings/NSDUHresults2012.pdf. Accessed January 7, 2015.

6. Swendsen J, Burnstein M, Case B, Conway KP, Dierker L, He J, Merikangas KR. Use and abuse of alcohol and illicit drugs in US adolescents: results of the National Comorbidity Survey—Adolescent Supplement. Arch Gen Psychiatry 2012;69:390–8.

7. Taylor MH, Grossberg GT. The growing problem of illicit substance abuse in the elderly: a review. Prim Care Companion CNS Disord 2012;14(4):PCC.11r01320.

8. Patel KV, Guralnik JM, Dansie EJ, Turk DC. Prevalence and impact of pain among older adults in the United States: findings from the 2011 National Health and Aging Trends Study. Pain 2013;154(12):2649–57.

9. Baler R, Volkow N. Drug addiction: the neurobiology of disrupted self-control. Trends Mol Med 2006;12:559–66.

10. Volkow N, Li T-K. The neuroscience of addiction. Nat Neurosci 2005;8:1429–30.

11. Ashton CH. Protracted withdrawal from benzodiazepines: the post-withdrawal syndrome. Psychiatr Ann 1995;25:174–9.

12. Miller WR, Rollnick S. Motivational Interviewing: Preparing People for Change, 2nd ed. 2002. Guilford Press, New York.

13. Horvath AT. Enhancing motivation for treatment of addictive behavior: guidelines for the psychotherapist. Psychother Theor Res Pract Train 1993;30(3):473–80. doi: 10.1037/0033-3204.30.3.473.

14. Kadden R, Carroll K, Donovan D, Cooney N, Monti P, Abrams D, Litt M, Hester R, eds. Cognitive-Behavioral Coping Skills Therapy Manual: A Clinical Research Guide for Therapists Treating Individuals with Alcohol Abuse and Dependence. NIAA Project Match Monograph Series, vol. 3. 1995. US Department of Health and Human Services, Washington, DC.

15. Marlatt GA, Gordon JR. Relapse Prevention: Maintenance Strategies in the Treatment of Addictive Behavior. 1985. Guilford Press, New York.

16. Petry NM. Contingency management treatments: controversies and challenges. Addiction 2010;105(9):1507–9.

17. Alcoholics Anonymous, 4th ed. 2001. A.A. World Services.

18. Ries R, Roy-Byrne P, Ward NG, Donnelly P. Carbamazepine treatment for benzodiazepine withdrawal. Am J Psychiatry 1989;146, 536–7.

19. Rubio G, Bobes J, Cervera G, Terán A, Pérez M, López-Gómez V, Rejas J. Effects of pregabalin on subjective sleep disturbance symptoms during withdrawal from long-term benzodiazepine use. Eur Addict Res 2011;17(5):262–70.

20. Rickels K, Schweizer E, Garcia España F, Case G, DeMartinis N, Greenblatt D. Trazadone and valproate in patients discontinuing long-term benzodiazepine therapy: effects on withdrawal symptoms and taper outcome. Psychopharmacology (Berl) 1999;141:1–5.

21. Schweizer E, Rickels K, Case WG, Greenblatt DJ. Carbamazepine treatment in patients discontinuing long-term benzodiazepine therapy. Arch Gen Psychiatry 1991;48:448–52.

22. Hallström C, Crouch G, Robson M, Shine P. The treatment of tranquilizer dependence by propranolol. Postgrad Med J 1988;64(Suppl 2): 40–4.

23. Kraus ML, Alford DP, Kotz MM, Levounis P, Mandell TW, Meyer M, Salsitz EA, Wetterau N, Wyatt SA. Statement of the American Society of Addiction Medicine Consensus Panel on the use of buprenorphine in office-based treatment of opioid addiction. J Addict Med 2011;2:254–63.

24. O'Connor PG, Fiellin DA. Pharmacologic treatment of heroin-dependent patients. Ann Intern Med 2000;133:40–54.

25. NIDA. Bringing the full power of science to bear on drug abuse & addiction. www.drugabuse.gov/sites/default/files/addictionscience.ppt. Accessed January 7, 2015.

Resources and Further Readings

Alcoholics Anonymous.

American Society of Addiction Medicine. The ASAM Principles of Addiction Medicine. http://www.asam.org/publications/principles-of-addiction-medicine. Accessed January 5, 2015.

Chapter 3—Motivational Interviewing as a Counseling Style. 2014. http://www.ncbi.nlm.nih.gov/books/NBK64964/. Accessed January 5, 2015.

NIDA. www.drugabuse.gov/. Accessed January 5, 2015.

Substance Abuse and Mental Health Service Administration. www.samhsa.gov/. Accessed January 5, 2015.

RxDrugAbuse Solutions. 2014. wvrxabuse.org/rx-treatment.html. Accessed January 5, 2015.

Principles of Pain Management in Dentistry

3

Paul A. Moore, DMD, PHD, MPH *and Elliot V. Hersh*, DMD, MS, PHD

Introduction

Nociceptive pain is essential to maintain health. It serves to protect us from noxious stimuli and to help us avoid using injured tissues that are healing and tender. Protective reflexes that cause us to retract our hand when contacting a hot stove or to open our mouth when we bite on a kernel of popcorn are mediated through the neuropathways for pain. Because acute pain is distressing, situations that may be painful often cause anxiety and avoidance behaviors. Consequently, oral pain has dual roles in dentistry: it encourages our patients to seek dental treatment when oral diseases are present and, conversely, it causes some of our patients to avoid treatment because of the fear of pain associated with dental treatment.

The most frequently encountered pain seen in a dental office is acute inflammatory pain. Inflammatory oral pain usually has a defined etiology, such as an acute odontogenic infection or the pain and discomfort felt following surgery. Although postsurgical inflammatory pain may be severe, it is generally self-limiting and most commonly has a duration of a few days to a week. Pharmacologic management of postsurgical inflammatory pain relies on peripherally acting analgesics, such as ibuprofen, or orally administered opioid formulations containing combinations of analgesics, such as hydrocodone with acetaminophen (APAP).

Chronic pain syndromes are less commonly encountered and treated in a private dental office. These disorders are less well defined and often include a neuropathic component. When a patient presents with oral pain lasting for several months, the pharmacologic management is much more diverse owing to the musculoskeletal, vascular, and neuropathic nature of these disorders. Treatment may require peripherally acting analgesics, tricyclic antidepressants, and/or anticonvulsant medications, but it rarely requires opioid analgesics.[1]

The ADA Practical Guide to Substance Use Disorders and Safe Prescribing, First Edition. Edited by Michael O'Neil.
© 2015 American Dental Association. Published 2015 by John Wiley & Sons, Inc.

Definitions

Neuropathic Pain

Neuropathic pain is a category of pain caused by damage to the nervous system involved in bodily feelings (the somatosensory system). It is often described as a feeling of burning, tingling, or "pins and needles."

Nociceptive Pain

Nociceptive pain is a category of pain caused by activation of peripheral nerve fibers by harmful and noxious stimuli.

Neurophysiology and Neuroanatomy of Acute Inflammatory Pain

Tissue damage and noxious stimuli of peripheral tissue initiates a complex series of physiologic and biochemical events that are responsible for transmission of signals to the central nervous system (CNS) that are then interpreted as pain. These complex series of events can be divided into activities in the peripheral nervous system and events occurring within the CNS. This dichotomy was first described by Von Frey as the "perception" component of pain and the "reaction" component of pain (Figure 3.1) respectively.[2]

The perceptive component of pain includes the stimulation of specific nociceptors located on free nerve endings that recognize specific changes in the tissue, such as mechanical distortion, heat, or cold. With adequate stimulation, an "action potential" is initiated that passes along trigeminal nerve pathways to the nucleus caudalis within the brain stem. The action potentials traveling along these primary nociceptive neurons transfer this information through synapses to the spinothalamic and trigeminothalamic nerve tracts that send the information to more rostral areas of the brain. The higher brain centers provide the reactive

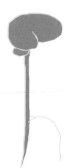

Pain Perception vs. Pain Reaction

REACTION TO PAIN
• Emotional overtones
• Activation of autonomic nervous system
• Avoidance/escape responses

PERCEPTION OF PAIN
• Nociceptor activation
• Transmission of action potential
• Includes the initial interpretation

Figure 3.1   Central and peripheral components of acute inflammatory pain.

component of noxious stimulation, where one processes the information, rapidly indicating not only the severity, duration, and location of the stimuli, but also eliciting emotional reactions, autonomic responses, and escape behaviors.

The actual pathways, neurotransmitters, and modulators for these components of pain are not very well defined for oral pain.[1,3] Nociceptors in the peripheral tissue activate two categories of pain fibers: the lightly mylenated Aδ fibers and the smaller unmyelinated C fibers (Table 3.1). The two fiber types differ in size and speed of nerve conduction. The faster Aδ fibers transmit action potentials rapidly to the brainstem to initiate reflex responses and to the cerebral cortex to initiate escape responses. Pain signals transmitted along Aδ fiber pathways are interpreted as well localized and having a sharp or bright quality. The slower transmission along C fibers is carried along more diverse neural pathways and is thought to initiate more diffuse responses, such as within the autonomic nervous system. The C fiber pathways create what has been referred to as secondary pain, which is interpreted as diffuse, dull, aching, and/or burning.[4]

Although this perception/reaction dichotomy is a quite simplistic view of the pain process, it provides a framework for understanding the classification of analgesics. The peripherally acting agents such as aspirin (acetylsalicylic acid, ASA) and ibuprofen act to

Table 3.1   Size, Conduction, Velocities, and Functions of Nerve Fibers

Type	Diameter (mμ)	Velocity (m/s)	Function
A(α)	13–22	70–120	Motor, proprioception
A(β)	8–13	40–70	Touch, kinesthesia
A(γ)	4–8	15–40	Touch, pressure
A(δ)	1–4	5–15	Pain, heat, cold
B	1–3	3–14	Autonomic
C	0.5–1	0.5–2	Pain, autonomic

limit the initiation of noxious stimulation, while the centrally acting agents such as opioids have a major role in the reactive component of pain. Research in pharmacology and neurophysiology during the last two to three decades has determined that there are many exceptions to this simple dichotomy, and this has opened the way for more sophisticated therapy of inflammatory and chronic pain.

The reaction to noxious stimulation, its transmission to the CNS, and its interpretation as pain are not a static state, and several mechanisms exist to modulate the process. The complex biochemical changes associated with inflammation can alter the sensitivity of nociceptors to tissue-damaging stimulation. Tissue is tender following an injury due to mediators of the inflammatory process. Some of the most important of these mediators are the prostaglandins, which cause free nerve endings to be more reactive to stimulation, resulting in the normal feeling of light touch being interpreted as painful or tender. Severe pain may be attenuated as a result of the release of endogenous morphine-like substances—the endorphins and enkephalins – which inhibit pain pathways via morphine receptors in the brain and spinal cord. Most recently, neurophysiologic research has focused on the plasticity of the brain and its pain pathways that may result in greater and more prolonged pain responses over time if pain is not initially managed adequately. This phenomenon is known as wind-up or central sensitization.

Orally Administered Analgesic Agents

When managing acute *inflammatory* pain in dentistry, practitioners rely on orally administered analgesic medications. Although other analgesics are presented in this chapter, the primary focus of this chapter is the agents that are most important to practicing dentists. Because this book addresses substance use disorders (SUDs) and diversion, rather than categorize agents as peripherally acting or centrally acting, we have classified the analgesics as opioids—such as morphine, hydrocodone, and oxycodone—and nonopioids—such as aspirin, APAP, and ibuprofen.

Nonopioid Analgesics

The most important and useful nonopioid analgesics in dentistry are the aniline analogue APAP and the nonsteroidal anti-inflammatory drugs (NSAIDs). Examples of analgesics in the NSAIDs category include aspirin, ibuprofen, naproxen sodium, diflunisal, ketoprofen, and diclofenac (Table 3.2). The analgesic mechanism of action common to all of the NSAIDs is their ability to limit the hyperalgesia associated with tissue trauma by inhibiting cyclooxygenase (COX) enzymes, thereby blocking the synthesis of inflammatory and hyperalgesic prostaglandins within peripheral tissues. A reduction of prostaglandin production by

Table 3.2 Commonly Administered Nonopioid Analgesics

Type	Name
Salicylic acid derivatives	
Acetylsalicylic acid	Aspirin or ASA
Diflunisal	Dolobid®
Aniline analogues	
Acetaminophen	Tylenol®, others
Nonselective prostaglandin inhibitors: over-the-counter and prescription	
Ibuprofen	Advil®, Motrin®, others
Naproxen sodium	Aleve®, Naprosyn®, Anaprox®
Nonselective prostaglandin inhibitors: prescription	
Ketoprofen	Orudis®
Diclofenac	Cataflam®, Zipsor®
Meclofenamate	Meclomen®
Etodolac	Lodine®
Ketorolac	Toradol®, SPRIX®
Selective COX-2 inhibitors	
Celecoxib	Celebrex®

NSAIDs within the CNS may also contribute to their analgesic action.[5,6]

The more commonly used NSAIDs are now discussed.

Ibuprofen

Ibuprofen is a common over-the-counter (OTC) analgesic marketed as Advil®, Motrin® IB, or Mediprin®. Prescription-strength ibuprofen is also available and marketed as Motrin®. In a survey of US oral and maxillofacial surgeons published in 2006, ibuprofen was found to be the most frequently recommended nonopioid analgesic for the management of acute pain following third molar extractions.[7] Ibuprofen and the other analgesics classified as nonselective NSAIDs have been shown to be safe and effective for treating mild to moderately severe postoperative pain and inflammation.[8]

Naproxen sodium

Naproxen sodium is another effective NSAID analgesic that is considered safe for short-term

use. It is similar to ibuprofen in its efficacy in providing relief of acute clinical pain. It has a slightly slower onset time and a longer duration of action, resulting in fewer breakthrough episodes of pain. It may be a more appropriate nonopioid analgesic for use an hour prior to surgery to prevent pain onset for the first 6–8 h after surgery. It may also be advantageous for administration in the evening to permit pain relief during sleeping hours.

> **Clinical Consideration**
>
> Patient responses to NSAIDs may vary from one type of NSAID to another. Patients not achieving adequate analgesia with a specific NSAID *may benefit* from an NSAID from a different class.

Selective COX-2 Inhibitors

Selective COX-2 inhibitors were developed in the 1990s, with several approved for use as analgesics. Their potential advantage over other NSAIDs is the selective inhibition of COX-2 enzymes, which allows the COX-1 constitutive enzymes associated with maintaining gastrointestinal health and thromboxanes that stimulate platelet aggregation to continue to function. This advantage would limit the incidence of gastrointestinal erosions, ulcers, and bleeding, a concern when taking nonselective NSAIDs for long periods of time. Unfortunately, the strategy also has resulted in a significant increase in myocardial infarctions and strokes, particularly with use of the COX-2 inhibitors rofecoxib and valdecoxib. Only one COX-2 inhibitor, celecoxib (Celebrex®) remains on the market, for use primarily in arthritis. Because other NSAIDs provide better pain relief, the use of celecoxib for the management of acute inflammatory pain is not recommended.

Acetaminophen

APAP is an effective nonopioid analgesic medication that has antipyretic activity but little anti-inflammatory activity. It is available as an OTC medication marketed under the brand names of Tylenol®, Panadol®, and Datril®. The popularity of APAP in dentistry is attributed to its relative safety, analgesic efficacy, and lack of any effect on hemostasis. A Cochrane Systematic Review of 51 randomized controlled trials found that a single dose of APAP (500 or 1000 mg) consistently provided effective postoperative pain relief for a period of about 4 h and was associated with few adverse drug reactions.[9]

In contrast to ibuprofen and other NSAIDs, APAP has limited anti-inflammatory activity and minimally inhibits platelet aggregation. Unlike traditional NSAIDs that compete with arachidonic acid during the initial enzymatic cascade that synthesizes prostaglandins, APAP may function by inactivating the COX enzymes responsible for the final catalytic reaction. Although APAP is considered to be very safe, it may not be as effective for acute inflammatory pain as a full therapeutic dose of ibuprofen or other NSAIDs.

The US Food and Drug Administration (FDA) has recently alerted practitioners and consumers about potential liver toxicity associated with excessive dosing with APAP.[10] Acute liver failure caused by unintentional consumption of excessive APAP has been reported.[11] Hepatic toxicity induced by APAP has been reported when a daily dose of 4000 mg is exceeded. To prevent excessive consumption, the FDA has requested that the dose of APAP contained in prescription opioid APAP analgesics be limited to a maximum of 325 mg. Consequently, formulations such as Vicodin HP®, which previously contained APAP 750 mg–hydrocodone 7.5 mg, have recently been reformulated to contain APAP 300 mg–hydrocodone 7.5 mg. When prescribing APAP for the management of acute postoperative pain, one must be careful to limit the dosing regimen and to avoid other APAP-containing medications to avoid potential overdose. Continuing concerns of potential hepatic toxicity has resulted in Tylenol®'s manufacturer voluntarily reducing its maximum APAP daily dose recommendation from 4000 mg to 3000 mg.

> **Clinical Consideration**
>
> Dental practitioners should review the patient's intake records for NSAIDs or APAP-containing products. Patients should also be advised not to take "extra doses" of NSAIDs or APAP, unless instructed to by the dental practitioner, to prevent possible toxicity.

Adverse Drug Reactions and Toxicities of Nonopioid Analgesics

Precautions and Contraindications

The most significant precautions and contraindications for the use of nonopioid analgesics relate to prolonged and high-dose therapy. With acute inflammation, pain management usually lasts less than 7–10 days, and serious adverse events are therefore rarely encountered. However, even low doses and short-duration exposure to some of these nonopioid analgesics may place certain patients at risk for adverse reactions.[5,12]

Toxicities associated with APAP, aspirin, and NSAIDs include renal and hepatic disease, gastrointestinal ulcers, and bleeding disorders. For patients with medical histories of these disorders, precaution is indicated. Hepatotoxicity is extremely rare and is most often associated with reports of intentional or unintentional APAP overdose. With prolonged therapy, it has been reported that older patients are at greater risk for acute liver toxicity, although this finding may be primarily due to concomitant APAP drug use in older patients.[11]

Aspirin and the NSAID analgesics have the tendency to induce gastrointestinal erosions and ulcerations, either through local irritation or through a systemic prostaglandin inhibition mechanism. Ketoprofen and naproxen sodium appear to carry a greater risk for gastrointestinal ulcerations than ibuprofen. Gastrointestinal injuries induced by NSAIDs occur twice as frequently in patients with a positive history of gastroduodenal ulcers.

Aspirin and the other NSAIDs have been reported to induce a unique intolerance reaction, with symptoms of rhinitis, uticaria, bronchial asthma, and laryngeal edema. Cross-reactivity between aspirin and other NSAIDs is possible. It has been hypothesized that an NSAID blockade of the arachidonic acid COX pathway results in increases of leukotrienes through the alternative lipoxygenase pathway. Although rare in the overall population, this intolerance reaction to aspirin may affect as many as 10–28% of adult asthmatic patients. Aspirin intolerance may also have cross-sensitivity with APAP and, therefore, should not automatically be considered a safe alternative to aspirin with these patients.

Many of the nonopioid analgesics should be avoided late in pregnancy. APAP administered in therapeutic doses is generally considered the best choice for managing acute pain during pregnancy. Aspirin, particularly when administered late in pregnancy, should be avoided because it is associated with delivery complications and postpartum hemorrhage. Chronic use of aspirin earlier in pregnancy has been associated with anemia in expectant mothers.

Aspirin and the NSAID analgesics have the common mechanism of inhibiting prostaglandin synthesis, including specific uterotropic prostaglandins. The NSAID analgesics have the capacity to inhibit contractions during labor and to prolong pregnancy. Additionally, prostaglandin inhibitors may cause constriction of the ductus arteriosus in utero, which may result in pulmonary hypertension of the newborn. The use of aspirin or any of the other NSAIDs, particularly during the third trimester of pregnancy, should be avoided.

Reye's syndrome is an acute childhood illness that causes encephalopathy and liver disease. The onset of Reye's syndrome in infants and younger children often follows respiratory viral infections. Typically, the children are recovering from influenza or varicella when the acute encephalopathic symptoms of lethargy, agitation, delirium, and seizures appear. This syndrome may be quite severe and has a significant mortality rate.

A remarkably strong association between aspirin therapy and Reye's syndrome (odds ratio of 26) has resulted in recommendations to avoid it when children have fever and flu-like symptoms. Table 3.3 lists common side effects that may be seen with nonopioid analgesics.

Drug Interactions Associated with Nonopioid Analgesics

Adverse drug interactions associated with short-term analgesic therapy are most frequently the result of altered pharmacokinetics or combined toxicities (Table 3.3). The pharmacokinetic drug interactions associated with nonopioid analgesics are usually minor and

Table 3.3 Side Effects of Nonopioid Analgesics

Adverse reactions and toxicities
  ASA intolerance/cross-sensitivity
  Pregnancy
  Reye's syndrome (aspirin only)
  Renal and hepatic toxicity
  Gastrointestinal erosions and ulcerations
  Inhibition of hemostasis
Drug interactions
  Alcohol and APAP/NSAIDs
  Antihypertensive drugs and NSAIDs
  Anticoagulant therapy and NSAIDs
  Lithium and NSAIDs
  Methotrexate and NSAIDs

and subsequently produce a greater amount of this reactive hepatotoxic metabolite.[12] Acute hepatotoxicity following short-term APAP therapy in patients who have a history of chronic alcohol consumption has occurred.[11]

Clinical Consideration

Caution should be used when prescribing NSAIDs to patients suspected of significant alcohol consumption. The deleterious effects of alcohol on the stomach may be compounded when combined with an NSAID. A conservative recommendation of separating the consumption of aspirin and alcohol by 12 h has been made.

become significant only when the concomitant drugs have small margins of safety (e.g., lithium and anticoagulant therapy). The risk of an interaction is most often clinically significant in a specific subpopulation of patients.[5,12]

Nonsteroidal Anti-inflammatory Drugs and Alcohol

The combined use of alcohol and NSAIDs significantly increases the risk of fecal blood loss associated with gastrointestinal erosions and ulcerations. Not only are NSAIDs and alcohol capable of damaging the gastric mucosa, alcohol may stimulate gastric acid secretion, thereby aggravating the gastrointestinal toxicity of NSAIDs. Hepatotoxicity is a common complication of both prolonged alcohol use and APAP overdose. APAP is primarily metabolized by conversion to inactive sulfate or glucoronide metabolites. One minor oxidative metabolite, N-acetyl-p-benzoquinone imine (NAPQI), is produced by the CYP2E1 liver isoenzyme system and is highly reactive. Normally, NAPQI is immediately detoxified by conjugation with hepatic glutathione and excreted in the urine. A patient with a history of chronic alcohol consumption may have a highly developed CYP2E1 isozyme system

- **NSAIDs and angiotensin-converting enzyme (ACE) inhibitors, diuretics, and beta-blockers.** Chronic therapy with NSAIDs has been implicated in antagonizing the blood-pressure-lowering effects of many antihypertensive agents. This antagonism has not been consistently demonstrated, particularly following short-term, low-dose analgesic therapy using the NSAIDs naproxen sodium and ibuprofen. This interaction is associated with the antihypertensive ACE inhibitors, diuretics, and beta-blockers, probably through a mechanism of antagonizing renal prostaglandin production. The calcium channel blockers do not appear to be associated with this interaction.
- **NSAIDs and anticoagulant therapy.** Hemorrhage, particularly when associated with gastrointestinal ulcers, is a serious complication of anticoagulant therapy. The combination of NSAIDs and anticoagulant therapy has been found to be significantly associated with a diagnosis of hemorrhagic peptic ulcer disease. Because of the serious possible consequences of this interaction, aspirin and NSAIDs should be avoided by patients receiving anticoagulant therapy.[12]

- **NSAIDs and aspirin.** Aspirin is used to inhibit platelet aggregation and is prescribed at low doses to prevent myocardial infarcts and strokes. In patients receiving low-dose aspirin (81 mg/day) for prophylaxis, it has been recommended that it be given 2 h before other NSAIDs used for pain and inflammation to prevent competition and causing inadequate inactivation of platelets.
- **NSAIDs and lithium.** Lithium carbonate, a psychosedative agent used for bipolar disorders, has an extremely small therapeutic index. With excessive lithium serum levels, toxicity reactions may occur, including nausea, muscle weakness, lack of coordination, seizures, and cardiac arrhythmias. The NSAIDs may decrease renal excretion of lithium and elevate the serum lithium concentrations. Although the short duration of nonopioid analgesics use for acute pain treatment would limit the likelihood of a significant pharmacokinetic drug interaction with lithium, the use of NSAIDs for even a limited period should be done cautiously.
- **NSAIDs and methotrexate.** Methotrexate, a folate antagonist, is prescribed for leukemia chemotherapy, rheumatoid arthritis, psoriasis, and bone marrow transplantation. Methotrexate's toxicities of pancytopenia, hematemesis, and acute renal failure are more likely to occur when NSAIDs are prescribed concomitantly. The increased risk for methotrexate toxicity is more likely with higher dose therapies used in cancer chemotherapy and bone marrow transplantation.

Opioid Analgesics

The term *opioid* is used to describe drugs that have pharmacologic activity similar to opium. The opioid extracts derived from the milky exudate of the poppy plant include the drugs morphine and codeine. Although the primary indication for opioids is to produce analgesia, other pharmacologic properties of these agents include sedation, euphoria, cough suppression, constipation, miosis, and respiratory depression. The opioid drugs—often referred to as the strong analgesics, the narcotics, or the centrally acting analgesics—have an important and long-standing role in medical and dental practice.

The mechanism of action for the opioid analgesics is their capacity to interact with opiate receptors found in the CNS and throughout the body. Opioid analgesics have similar molecular structures to naturally occurring endorphins. The endorphins are a group of peptide molecules that specifically bind with opiate receptors to induce their pharmacologic activity. The opioid drugs mimic these naturally occurring analgesics that are found in the body.

Of the many opioid drugs used in medicine and dentistry, dental practitioners prescribe orally administered opioids most frequently for patient convenience. The injectable opioid drugs are generally administered in hospitals and anesthesia departments. Oral opioids are easily metabolized following oral administration by the "first-pass effect," resulting in only a very small amount of the administered drug actually reaching the system circulation. Consequently, agents such as morphine and fentanyl are almost exclusively administered parenterally for acute pain. The first-pass metabolism of the orally administered agents that are commonly employed in dental practice, including codeine, hydrocodone, and oxycodone, is much more limited than that of morphine and fentanyl.

Because the opioid analgesics act at specific opiate receptors, structural alterations can create agents that bind to the receptor and initiate different degrees of activity. Analgesic agents that totally activate the opioid receptor and produce a maximal analgesic response are called agonists. Agents that bind to the receptor without initiating any intrinsic activity are referred to as antagonists. The opioids that bind to the receptor and have only partial analgesic activity are referred to as mixed

Table 3.4 **Opioid Agonists and Antagonists**

Type	Name
Single-entity opioid agonists	
Codeine	
Meperidine	Demerol®
Hydromorphone	Dilaudid®
Oxycodone	Oxycodin®
Methadone	Dolophine®
Tapentadol	Nucynta®
Fentanyl transdermal	Duragesic®
Combination opioid agonists containing APAP	
APAP with codeine	Tylenol #3®, others
APAP with hydrocodone	Vicodin®, Lorcet®, Norco®
APAP with oxycodone	Percocet®, Tylox®
APAP with tramadol	Ultracet®
APAP with pentazocine	Talwin Compound®
Opioid agonist combinations containing ibuprofen	
Ibuprofen with hydrocodone	Vicoprofen®
Ibuprofen with oxycodone	Combunox®
Other opioid agonist analgesic combinations	
APAP, caffeine, butalbital	Fioricet®
ASA, caffeine, dihydrocodeine	Synalgos-DC®
Opioid antagonists	
Naloxone	Narcan®
Naltrexone	Revia®, Depade®
Mixed opioid agonists–antagonists	
Pentazocine	Talwin®
Pentazocine–naloxone	Talwin Nx®
Nalbuphine	Nubain®
Partial agonists	
Buprenorphine	Subutex®
Buprenorphine–naloxone	Suboxone®

agonists–antagonists or partial agonists. Table 3.4 shows the types of opioid analgesics.

Clinical Consideration

Patients receiving opioids for chronic pain should not receive pure opioid antagonists (e.g., naloxone), partial agonist agents (e.g., buprenorphine) or mixed agonist–antagonist agents (e.g., nalbuphine, pentazocine) owing to their potential to induce full opioid withdrawal.

In managing acute inflammatory pain, dental practitioners generally select a full agonist with minimal first-pass metabolism. To improve the analgesic response, the selected orally administered analgesic will include a nonopioid as a component of the formulation to provide added analgesia. Consequently, the analgesic formulation of APAP with hydrocodone (Vicodin®) and the analgesic formulation of APAP with oxycodone (Percocet®) are the most frequently prescribe analgesics for the management of pain following third-molar extractions.[7] *Although opioid analgesics provide significant analgesia and are important in the management of severe inflammatory acute pain in dentistry, it is clear that the nonopioids are the most effective and most useful analgesic agents.*

Tramadol (Ultram®) is a weak opioid analgesic agent with less efficacy for inflammatory pain than ibuprofen. Tramadol is a centrally acting analgesic with very little opioid receptor activity. It may have a therapeutic advantage for treating chronic pain syndromes. It has been formulated with APAP as Ultracet®. It has limited indication in acute pain management in dentistry. In patients with a true allergy to codeine derivatives, APAP with tramadol can be employed as an alternative opioid combination drug.

Propoxyphene, found in Darvon® and Darvocet® formulations, was removed from the market in 2010 owing to its propensity to cause cardiac rhythm changes. The fentanyl transdermal patch is not appropriate for acute pain management and is reserved for the treatment of chronic pain syndromes, including cancer pain.

Clinical Consideration

A practitioner should be aware of the comparative oral dosing equivalents in dental patients as follows: ~5 mg oxycodone ≈ 10 mg hydrocodone ≈ 60 mg codeine ≈ 75 mg tramadol.

Side Effects of and Drug Interactions Associated with Opioid Analgesics

When compared with nonopioid therapy, the prescribing of opioids for pain management in dentistry carries a high incidence of side effects (Table 3.5). The most common adverse effect is nausea and vomiting. For ambulating patients, the incidence of nausea and vomiting has been reported to range from 5 to 20%. Constipation

Table 3.5   Adverse Reactions or Complications of Opioid Analgesics

Respiratory depression
CNS depression
Nausea and vomiting
Urinary retention
Constipation
Physiological dependence
Opioid abuse and addiction
Tolerance

is common and can be an unpleasant complication of opioid therapy.

With the use of parenterally administered agents and with overdosing with oral agents, the chances of respiratory depression can be significant. The mortality associated with opioid overdose is due to respiratory depression and subsequent hypoxia and cardiac arrest. With prolonged use and misuse, opioids are associated with drug tolerance and dependence. Opioid addiction is characterized by behaviors that always include a compulsion to take the drug on a continuous basis in order to experience its psychic effect and sometimes to avoid the discomfort of its absence. The phenomenon is associated with pleasure seeking. Because pharmacologic tolerance develops over time, drug-addicted patients require greater amounts of opioids to satisfy their cravings. Opioid drug dependence is associated with a high degree of cross-sensitivity, permitting substitution of one opioid with another.

Adverse reactions and drug interactions with opioids can be significant. CNS depression and associated respiratory depression can be significantly enhanced when combining opioids with alcohol, barbiturates, benzodiazepines, or other CNS depressants. Hypotension can occur when opioids are consumed concomitantly with antihypertensive alpha-adrenergic blockers. Unexpected CNS depression has been reported when opioids are administered with patients taking major psychosedatives, such as the tricyclic antidepressants, phenothiazines, and monoamine oxidase inhibitors.

Clinical considerations for patients receiving methadone or buprenorphine for opioid-based addiction treatment and patients receiving opioids for chronic nonmalignant pain will be discussed in greater detail in Chapter 4.

Medication-Assisted Therapies for Treating Drug-Dependent Patients

Several advances in opioid drug therapy have been developed in recent years and are important in the management of patients with SUD.

Methadone is an opioid receptor agonist, and its administration simply diminishes the craving and abstinence reactions associated with illicit opioid consumption. Naltrexone is an oral opioid receptor antagonist that can block opiate receptors for up to 48 h. If administered while a patient is still consuming opioids it is likely to induce withdrawal symptoms. To effectively utilize naltrexone therapy for opioid abstinence, the patient must have discontinued taking opioids for several days. Naloxone is a pure opioid antagonist that can be administered either as a nasal spray or an injection. It is the definitive treatment for an opioid overdose. Because it is an extremely safe opioid antagonist, it has been recently advocated for use by emergency medical personnel and family members to treat respiratory depression associated with opioid overdose prior to admission to an emergency department. Buprenorphine with naloxone (Suboxone®) has the capacity to decrease opioid-seeking behaviors of drug-dependent patients. When administered sublingually, it reduces opioid craving in patients who are physically dependent on opioids. The addition of a small dose of naloxone has limited activity unless the formulation is administered

parenterally. Chapters 4 and 12 will discuss clinical considerations when managing complex patients with addiction and chronic pain.

Adjunctive Drugs Used to Limit Pain in Dentistry

To avoid the side effects of and drug interactions associated with the use of opioids and to minimize the need for other systemic agents, several opioid-free alternative therapeutic approaches can be used to manage pain. Optimizing analgesia is frequently accomplished by simultaneously implementing multiple modalities of treatment. More common considerations are discussed next.

Long-Acting Local Anesthetics

Bupivacaine is a long-acting amide local anesthetic that has been thoroughly evaluated for a variety of medical and dental surgical procedures. Its long duration has a unique therapeutic value for prolonged operations, therapeutic blocks, and postoperative pain management. It has been demonstrated to be a safe and useful agent in obstetrics, ophthalmology, and orthopedics, and it is particularly well suited for the prevention of postoperative pain following abdominal, thoracic, or oral surgery. The use of long-acting local anesthetics to alleviate pain following third-molar extractions has been consistently demonstrated.[13] Patient selection for long-acting local anesthetics in endodontic and periodontal surgery is obviously more difficult. Unless at least moderate pain is anticipated, long-acting local anesthetics may not be necessary or advisable.

Dental emergencies that occur after office hours or in unequipped emergency departments can be frustrating and difficult to treat. Without the support of auxiliary dental personnel, a dental practitioner is often faced with inadequate operative support for definitive therapy. Long-acting local anesthetics provide a means of temporarily eliminating acute pain and avoiding dispensing strong analgesics until proper treatment can be provided.

Soft-tissue anesthesia and the period of painlessness following bupivacaine anesthesia is two to three times that of standard anesthetics. Mandibular blocks may last 5–8 h, and maxillary infiltration may last 3–5 h. Overall satisfaction of pain management strategy using long-acting local anesthetics requires careful patient selection and explanation. Because of possible self-mutilation of the lips, cheeks, and tongue, bupivacaine is not recommended for children younger than 12 years of age.

> **Clinical Consideration**
>
> For patients with contraindications to traditional nonopioid analgesics such as NSAIDs and who have a history of SUD, long-acting anesthetics may play a key role in postprocedure pain management.

Preemptive Analgesics

An effective strategy for limiting postoperative pain and the need for opioid analgesics is to administer a peripherally acting anti-inflammatory agent prior to surgery. Although the strategy has been demonstrated to be effective when administering APAP, the most frequently advocated approach is to use an NSAID such as ibuprofen or naproxen sodium to prevent postoperative pain.[14, 15] Because of the anti-inflammatory nature of the NSAIDs, administration of these agents prior to surgery may decrease the severity of the surgical insult, and the postoperative complications of swelling and trismus can be minimized.[16] For example, the preoperative and postoperative administration of the NSAID flurbiprofen has been shown to be more effective than the administration of APAP with oxycodone in managing postoperative pain following third-molar extractions.[17]

> **Clinical Consideration**
>
> In patients with SUD and no contraindications to NSAIDs, a preemptive strike with an NSAID is recommended to optimize postprocedure analgesia.

Corticosteroids

Postoperative pain and discomfort are frequently accompanied with significant swelling. Swelling may be particularly significant when the surgery is prolonged and when large areas of gingiva and oral mucosa are manipulated. Although edema normally occurs postoperatively and is a functional part of the healing process, healing may be compromised when it is severe. Trismus associated with swelling may inhibit adequate oral hygiene and may limit food intake. When excessive, oral and pharyngeal swelling may inhibit normal respiratory function.

Swelling following surgical procedures would similarly be expected to lessen by a preoperative NSAID such as ibuprofen. However, the anti-inflammatory effects of preoperative ibuprofen are modest at best. When the surgery is expected to produce significant swelling, a short-term therapeutic regimen of an anti-inflammatory steroid is recommended.

Glucocorticoids appear to inhibit all phases of inflammation. They block the increased capillary permeability produced by histamine and kinins and therefore decrease edema. Capillary dilatation, migration of leukocytes, and phagocytosis are all decreased. Kinin generation is also inhibited. Steroids activate the synthesis of a protein inhibitor of phospholipase A2, blocking arachidonic acid formation. Therefore, the cascade for the formation of prostaglandins, thromboxanes, prostacyclins, and leukotrienes is inhibited.

The chosen steroid—such as dexamethasone or prednisone—should have minimal mineralocorticoid effects. The drug should be administered before surgery, allowing an optimal decrease in arachidonic acid at the time of initial tissue trauma. It is preferably given in the morning, when cortisol is naturally released by the body. This schedule interferes the least with the normal adrenal system. The prescription should not exceed 6 days. Edema usually peaks in 48–72 h. Additional steroids may delay healing. A recommended regimen that meets these criteria is to administer dexamethasone 9 mg intravenously, possibly followed by 6 mg by mouth for 1 day following surgery and 3 mg by mouth for 2 days following surgery. A Medrol Pack® containing methylprednisolone (a 6-day tapering dose) is an acceptable alternative. By utilizing this approach for short-term steroids, the practitioner is optimizing the benefits while minimizing the risks.

> **Clinical Consideration**
>
> All patients with diabetes who are prescribed a steroid should be counseled about the likely glucose-increasing effects of the steroids that frequently last a few days after steroids are completed *regardless of the dose and duration*.

Guidelines for Analgesic Therapy

Orally administered analgesics are the primary therapy used to manage acute inflammatory pain in dentistry. When analgesic therapies that use a single agent are inadequate, combinations of two or more analgesic drugs have been advocated.[18] The possible advantages of using drug combinations when treating acute pain include improved analgesic efficacy, fewer adverse reactions, lower costs, adequate treatment of disorders that have multiple symptoms, improved patient adherence, and more rapid absorption.[19] The strategy of combining two analgesic agents that have distinct mechanisms of action, such as combining an opioid with a nonopioid, has been used for

many years. A common example is the analgesic formulation containing APAP combined with the opioid hydrocodone (Vicodin®). This combination is the most frequently prescribed drug in the USA.[20] Analgesic formulations containing an opioid and a peripherally acting analgesic consistently provide greater pain relief than when either agent is administered alone. In a Cochrane systematic review of 20 high-quality clinical trials, the additive pain relief that occurs when combining oxycodone with APAP was demonstrated.[21]

However, including an opioid as part of an analgesic combination formulation increases the risk of side effects such as nausea, vomiting, constipation, mental confusion, sedation, restricts the use of CNS depressants, and carries significant risk of drug misuse, abuse, and diversion. Alternative combination analgesics that do not contain opioids have been advocated as a means for avoiding the potential adverse reactions associated with opioids.

Combinations of diclofenac or ketoprofen with APAP have been evaluated and their use has been advocated for many years.[22] Various doses of ibuprofen and APAP, alone or in combination, were evaluated in a large controlled trial of pain following third-molar extractions. Subjects who received the highest dose combination of ibuprofen (400 mg–APAP 1000 mg) had significantly better pain relief during the 8 h study than subjects receiving the individual components.[23] As illustrated in Figure 3.2, additive analgesia is seen when the combination of ibuprofen and APAP was administered.[24] Combining two nonopioid analgesics appears to provide significantly greater pain relief, while avoiding the potential for side effects and abuse potential associated with nonopioid–opioid formulations such as APAP with hydrocodone (Vicodin®).

The improved analgesic efficacy seen when combining the nonopioid analgesics ibuprofen and APAP provides a therapeutic alternative to opioid-containing analgesic formulations. Prescribers may find routinely providing a

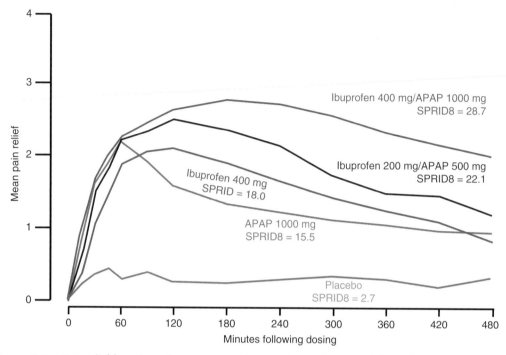

Figure 3.2   Pain relief from ibuprofen, acetaminophen, and a combination of ibuprofen with acetaminophen following third-molar extractions. Pain relief rated as 0 = none, 1 = a little, 2 = some, 3 = a lot, and 4 = complete. SPRID8 values represent the sum of pain relief/intensity differences for the total 8 h evaluation.

prescription for Vicodin® or Percocet® is not necessary; and even if an opioid combination prescription is needed, fewer pills may be necessary or a lower dose of opioid may prove sufficient.

The analgesic efficacy of an APAP with oxycodone combination or an APAP with codeine combination is not significantly better than ibuprofen or naproxen sodium. The repeated demonstration that an ibuprofen with APAP combination can provide equivalent analgesia following dental surgery without the side effects associated with opioid combinations may prove to be clinically beneficial. This nonopioid alternative to opioid-containing analgesics may be an effective strategy for preventing potential prescription drug abuse and diversion, which is a national concern associated with dispensing prescription drugs.[24] However,

it is important to limit the APAP dose to a maximum of 3000 mg/day.

The demonstration of the improved analgesic efficacy of ibuprofen with APAP combinations compared with that of the component agents provides practitioners greater flexibility when selecting analgesic therapy following dental surgery. Table 3.6 provides conservative, stepwise guidelines for acute postoperative pain management following third-molar surgery.[24] These recommendations provide valuable guidance for pain management when a practitioner has an expectation of mild, mild-to-moderate, moderate-to-severe, or severe pain. As with previous recommendations, these stepwise recommendations recognize that NSAIDs are extremely effective and remain the primary agents to use when treating most cases of postoperative dental pain.

Table 3.6 Stepwise Guidelines for Acute Pain Management

Mild pain
Ibuprofen 200–400 mg every 4–6 h: as needed for pain (p.r.n.)

Mild-to-moderate pain
Ibuprofen 400–600 mg every 6 h: fixed interval for 24 h. Then ibuprofen 400 mg q 4–6 h: p.r.n. pain

Moderate–to-severe pain
Ibuprofen 400–600 mg plus APAP 500 mg every 6 h: fixed interval for 24 h. Then ibuprofen 400 mg plus APAP 500 mg every 6 h p.r.n. pain

Severe pain
Ibuprofen 400–600 mg plus APAP 650 mg–hydrocodone 10 mg q 6 h: fixed interval for 24–48 h. Then ibuprofen 400–600 mg plus APAP 500 mg q 6 h p.r.n. pain

Additional considerations
Patients should be cautioned to avoid APAP in other medications. Maximum dose for APAP (Tylenol®) is 3000 mg/day. To avoid potential APAP toxicity, dentists should consider prescribing a rescue medication containing ibuprofen (Vicoprofen®) if patients experience breakthrough pain.
Maximum dose of ibuprofen is 2400 mg/day. Higher maximal daily doses have been reported for osteoarthritis when prescribed under the direction of a physician

Summary

Proper management of pain in dental practice requires a clear understanding of the causes of inflammatory pain and the potentially beneficial analgesics and adjunctive agents currently available. Practitioners were provided with a review of the most current information for safely and effectively preventing and treating pain encountered by dental patients. Recommendations for prescribing analgesics and analgesic combinations for all levels of pain severity were also included to guide practitioners when managing dental pain.

References

1. Hersh EV, Balusubramaniam R, Pinto A. Pharmacologic management of temporomandibular disorder. Oral Maxillofac Surg Clin N Am 2008;20:197–210.
2. Dubner R, Sessle BJ, Storey AT. The Neural Basis of Oral and Facial Function. 1978. Plenum, New York.
3. Jackson DL, Roszkowski MT, Moore PA: Management of postoperative pain. Chapter 6. In: Oral and Maxillofacial Surgery. Hersh E, Fonseca R, eds. 2000. WB Saunders, pp. 114–40.
4. Kim H, Dionne RA. Introduction to antinociceptive drugs. Chapter 19. In: Pharmacology and Therapeutics for Dentistry, 6th ed. Yagiela JA, Dowd FJ, Johnson BS, Mariotti AJ, Neidle EA, eds. 2011. Mosby, St Louis, MO.
5. Hersh EV, Desjardin PJ, Trummel CL, Cooper SA, Nonopioid analgesics, nonsteroidal anti-inflammatory drugs, and antirheumatic and antigout drugs. Chapter 21. In: Pharmacology and Therapeutics for Dentistry, 6th ed. Yagiela JA, Dowd FJ, Johnson BS, Mariotti AJ, Neidle EA, eds. 2011. Mosby Elsevier, St Louis, MO, pp. 346–8.
6. Vane JR. Inhibition of prostaglandin synthesis as a mechanism of action for aspirin like drugs. Nature 1971;231:232–5.
7. Moore PA, Nahouraii HS, Zovko J, Wisniewski SR. Dental therapeutic practice patterns in the U.S. II. Analgesics, corticosteroids, and antibiotics. Gen Dent 2006;54(3):201–7.
8. Derry CJ, Derry S, Moore RA, McQuay HJ. Single dose oral ibuprofen for acute postoperative pain in adults. Cochrane Database Syst Rev 2009;(3):CD001548.
9. Toms L, McQuay HJ, Derry S, Moore RA. Single dose oral paracetamol (acetaminophen) for postoperative pain in adults. Cochrane Database Syst Rev 2008;(4):CD004602.
10. Food and Drug Administration. MedWatch Safety Information and Adverse Event Reporting. Acetaminophen prescription products limited to 325 mg per dosage unit: Drug Safety Communication". 2011. http://www.fda.gov/Safety/MedWatch/SafetyInformation/SafetyAlertsforHumanMedicalProducts/ucm239955.htm. Accessed December 28, 2014.
11. Guggenheimer J, Moore PA. Therapeutic applications and risks associated with acetaminophen:

a review and update. J Am Dent Assoc 2011;142(12):38–44.

12. Hersh EV, Pinto A, Moore PA. Adverse drug interactions involving common prescription and over-the-counter analgesic agents. Clin Ther 2007;29(11):2477–97.

13. Moore PA. Long-acting local anesthetics: a review of clinical efficacy in dentistry. Compend Cont Dent Ed 1990;11:22–30.

14. Jackson DL, Moore PA, Hargreaves KM. Preoperative nonsteroidal anti-inflammatory medication for the prevention of postoperative dental pain. J Am Dent Assoc 1989;119:641–7.

15. Moore PA, Werther JR, Seldin E, Stevens CM. Timing of preoperative and postoperative analgesics for third molar surgery. J Am Dent Assoc 1986;113:739–44.

16. Moore PA, Brar P, Smiga ER, Costello BJ. Prevention of pain and trismus following third molar surgery: rofecoxib vs. dexamethasone. Oral Surg Oral Med Oral Pathol Oral Radiol Endod 2005;99(2):E1–7.

17. Dionne RA. Suppression of dental pain by the preoperative administration of flurbiprofen. Am J Med 1986;80(3A):41–9.

18. Moore PA, Deuben RR. Oral analgesic drug combinations. Dent Clin North Am 1984; 28:413–22.

19. Beaver WT. Combination analgesics. Am J Med 1984;77(3A):38–53.

20. Wynn RL, Meiller TF, Crossley HL. Top 200 most prescribed drugs in 2008. In: Drug Information Handbook for Dentistry, 15th ed. Wynn RL, Meiller TF, Crossley HL, eds. 2009. Lexi-Comp, Hudson, OH, pp. 2064–5.

21. Gaskell H, Derry S, Moore RA, McQuay HJ. Single dose oral oxycodone and oxycodone plus paracetamol (acetaminophen) for acute postoperative pain in adults. Cochrane Database Syst Rev 2009;(3):CD002763.

22. Hyllested M, Jones S, Pedersen JL, Kehlet H. Comparative effect of paracetamol, NSAIDs or their combination in postoperative pain management: a qualitative review. Brit J Anaesthes 2002;88(2):199–214.

23. Mehlisch DR, Aspley S, Daniels SE, Bandy DP. Comparison of the analgesic efficacy of concurrent ibuprofen and paracetamol with ibuprofen or paracetamol alone in the management of moderate-to-severe postoperative dental pain in adolescents and adults: a randomized, double-blind, placebo-controlled, parallel-group, single-dose, two-center, modified factorial study. Clin Ther 2010;32(5):882–95.

24. Moore PA, Hersh EV. Combining ibuprofen and acetaminophen for acute postoperative pain management: translating clinical research to dental practice. J Am Dent Assoc 2013;144(8):898–908.

Resources and Further Readings

National Library of Medicine Resource. Over-the-counter pain relievers. http://www.nlm.nih.gov/medlineplus/ency/article/002123.htm. Accessed December 28, 2014.

US Food and Drug Administration Resource. Drugs@FDA. FDA approved drug products. http://www.accessdata.fda.gov/scripts/cder/drugsatfda/index.cfm. Accessed December 28, 2014.

Special Pain Management Considerations: (1) Chronic Methadone, Buprenorphine, and Naltrexone Therapy; (2) Chronic Opioids for Nonmalignant Pain

Michael O'Neil, PharmD

Introduction

The management of any pain is a subjective process influenced by *at least* two major factors: the patient's perception of pain and *the prescriber's expectation of the severity of the patient's pain*. Management of acute pain with opioid analgesics in patients receiving chronic opioid therapy is significantly influenced by cross-tolerance to other opioids, misperceptions regarding the risk of opioid administration to chronic opioid patients (see Box 4.1), unrealistic treatment goals of *patients and prescribers*, and limited clinical trials detailing acute opioid pain management in opioid maintenance therapy (OMT) patients. With an increasing population, the number of patients with chronic pain conditions is increasing.[1,2] Opioid addiction and opioid overdose have reached epidemic proportions, leading to increased concerns

surrounding opioid prescribing.[3] The Drug Addiction Treatment Act of 2000 regulations

---

Box 4.1 Common Treatment Goals in the Management of Opioid Addiction

- Decrease compulsion to abuse substances or medications.
- Decrease cravings for substances or medications.
- Decrease time of "impairment."
- Decrease reckless behavior events (e.g., driving or working impaired).
- Decrease the number of "needle sharing" events.
- Decrease work absenteeism.
- Decrease healthcare associated costs.
- Return to normal functioning.
- Return to work.
- Prevent debilitating physiologic withdrawal.

The ADA Practical Guide to Substance Use Disorders and Safe Prescribing, First Edition. Edited by Michael O'Neil.
© 2015 American Dental Association. Published 2015 by John Wiley & Sons, Inc.

has increased access to buprenorphine-based treatment programs and has increased the opportunities for opioid-addicted patients to achieve recovery and successfully return to the home, work place, and community.[4]

Dental practitioners should anticipate a portion of their patient population is *likely* receiving chronic opioid maintenance treatment with methadone or buprenorphine for opioid addiction, naltrexone therapy for opioid or alcohol addiction, or receiving opioids for chronic pain (OCP) management. This chapter will provide clinical considerations for managing acute dental pain in patients receiving chronic treatment with opioids for OMT and chronic pain or naltrexone for opioid or alcohol addictions.

Definitions

Opioid Maintenance Therapy

OMT—also known as opioid substitution therapy (OST), office-based opioid treatment (OBOT), opioid replacement treatment (ORT), medication-assisted treatment (MAT), or methadone maintenance treatment (MMT) programs—is part of a comprehensive opioid addiction management strategy targeting illegal opioid abuse, the treatment of opioid addiction, and other negative social consequences. These legally prescribed medications replace illegal use of opioid medications under strict drug enforcement regulations and patient monitoring. Methadone or buprenorphine medications are prescribed in doses that help "suppress" the cravings, compulsions, and loss of control of the behavior "to abuse" opioid or opioid-like substances (also known as the symptoms of the disease). Behavior modification, environmental and social influences, as well as specific "triggers" are targeted by psychologist or psychiatrist to minimize the risk of relapse. OMT should not be confused with detoxification, which solely focuses on

the physiologic removal of a substance or medication from the body without behavior modification.[5]

For the purposes of this text, OMT will be used synonymously with OBOT, OST, ORT, MAT, or MMT terminology.

Pseudo-addiction

Pseudo-addiction is a health-care-induced condition in which health professionals misinterpret a patient's request for more medication *due to inadequate treatment* of a condition (e.g., pain, anxiety, or sedation). The patient's request for more medication is misinterpreted as "drug-seeking behavior" similar to that seen in addicts not in recovery. It is unclear how often pseudo-addiction occurs. Dental practitioners should stay vigilant for signs of drug misuse or abuse.[6]

Hyperalgesia

Hyperalgesia may be defined as a patient's increased detection or *hypersensitivity* to painful stimulus that previously was not perceived as painful without other known causes. This increased sensitivity to pain is most commonly associated with chronic opioid therapy for non-malignant pain.[7]

Cross-tolerance

Cross-tolerance is a pharmacological phenomenon that may be characterized as an *inability* to achieve a specific pharmacological effect due to prolonged exposure of a *similar* pharmacologic substance.[8] Higher doses are required to achieve the same desired pharmacological effect. Cross-tolerance is most commonly associated with the sedative, analgesic, respiratory depressant, or euphoric effects of a substance.

Interviewing the Patient: Establishing Goals of Treatment

Optimizing analgesia for dental pain actually begins during the patient interview. Reassuring the patient that the line of questioning regarding methadone, buprenorphine, or naltrexone treatment is to *optimize* pain management *as opposed to denying* pain management should be a fundamental step. For years, patients with the disease of addiction have inappropriately carried a stigma of "weak" character, criminal behavior, or distrust.[9] These misperceptions frequently create an environment of fear.[10] Patients may not be forthright about their medical treatment owing to fear of inadequate treatment of their acute pain. Perceptions of inadequate analgesia may encourage patients to exaggerate their *current* analgesic needs. Dental practitioners should verify the patient's *current* opioid maintenance medications, including doses and duration of treatment, with the patient's treatment center to optimize acute pain management. Reassuring the patient the primary goal is *adequate analgesia* may be helpful in disarming self-protecting behaviors of patients.

Working with the patient to establish specific goals for acute pain management is important to achieve successful pain management outcomes. Unrealistic or "mismatched" expectations of what "level," amount of pain, or pain score is acceptable post procedure may affect patient medication usage behaviors.[11] This is commonly seen in acute pain management practices. For example, using the visual analog scale (VAS) for pain severity of "0–10," albeit subjective, if a patient's expectation is to maintain "0" pain throughout postprocedure recovery but the dental practitioner prescribes analgesics to achieve reasonable pain control of "1–3" by VAS, the mismatch of expectations and treatment goals may inadvertently lead to behaviors associated with pseudo-addiction, patients misusing their prescription medications, or self-prescribing of leftover medications. Patient–prescriber pain treatment goals should be clarified *before* the procedure to optimize pain management and reduce unwarranted circumstances.

> **Clinical consideration**
>
> Interviewing should specifically address methadone-, buprenorphine-, naltrexone-, or opioid-based chronic pain treatment with reassurance that the questioning is to optimize acute pain management, not to deny pain treatment.

Pharmacological Treatment of Opioid Addiction

Goals of Treatment

The successful use of methadone and buprenorphine as part of a comprehensive treatment strategy for opioid addiction is well documented.[12] Addiction is a chronic, life-long brain disease characterized by symptoms of craving a substance or medication; loss of control to "not abuse"; continued use in spite of negative consequences; and frequently, but not always, relapse.[13] The disease of addiction may be further complicated by negative outcomes of addiction behaviors, such as infections from sharing needles (e.g., hepatitis, AIDS), destruction in family and work lives, and increased health-care costs.[14] Goals of pharmacological treatment primarily focus on decreasing the "cravings and compulsions" of this disease so that behavior may be optimized in such away the patient is able to return to a normal or *near normal* functioning level.[15] Although society as a whole generally evaluates successful addiction therapy terms of patients "being in recovery" or "not in recovery," it is important to understand the more global concept that *any reduction in negative behaviors or outcomes (such as needle sharing, duration of impairment, absenteeism from work, health care associated costs, etc.) should be considered, in part, as successful* treatment.[15] See Box 4.1 for treatment goals. Similar to antidepressants used in depression, oral hypoglycemic agents used in type II diabetes, or blood-pressure-lowering agents used in hypertension, pharmacological management of addiction with methadone or buprenorphine targets *signs or symptoms* of the disease while behavior modification is utilized to optimize or improve disease outcomes. Addiction is not a curative disease, but the symptomatology of addiction can be effectively managed for many patients.[16]

> **Clinical Consideration**
>
> Pharmacological therapy alone without combined counseling or behavior modification therapy offers minimal benefit, when compared with any other treatment modalities involving counseling, behavior modification, or support groups. The best treatment outcomes are associated with pharmacological management combined with counseling, behavior modification, and use of support systems.[16]

Pharmacological Considerations of Methadone and Buprenorphine

Targeting the Reward Center: Duality of Buprenorphine and Methadone

Methadone and buprenorphine are the two major pharmacologic agents used in opioid-based treatment programs. Methadone is a potent opioid analgesic agent with a characteristically long pharmacokinetic half-life that allows for once-a-day dosing in the treatment of opioid addictions.[17] The stimulation of μ receptors by methadone is associated with the analgesic effects and reduction of cravings and compulsions to abuse opioids.[18]

Buprenorphine is a potent partial μ agonist and mild κ receptor antagonist analgesic agent available in injection, sublingual, and transdermal formulations.[19,20] Sublingual formulations usually include the pure opioid antagonist naloxone. The intent of a pure opioid antagonist with a potent opioid agonist is to discourage intravenous injection of the sublingual products. When naloxone is administered orally or sublingually, minimal amounts of naloxone reach the systemic circulation due to poor absorption or first-pass effects by the liver.[21] The sublingual products are the only US Food and Drug Administration (FDA)-approved formulations for treatment of opioid addiction.[20] The high μ-receptor affinity of buprenorphine may prevent short-acting opioids with lower receptor affinity from optimally binding to the μ receptors and may induce physiologic withdrawal in patients receiving opioid agonist for long periods of time.[22]

The pharmacologic activities of methadone and buprenorphine are most commonly associated with analgesia, respiratory depression, euphoria, constipation, and sedative effects. However, both methadone and buprenorphine may stimulate receptors in the reward center of the brain to *reduce* cravings, diminish the compulsion to abuse, and regain loss of control of abuse in opioid addictions.[23] The dental practitioner must recognize that the pharmacokinetic and the pharmacodynamic profiles of methadone as well as buprenorphine are not superimposable. This is true for analgesia, respiratory depression, and stimulation of the reward pathways in the brain. *This variation in pharmacokinetics and pharmacodynamics requires different dosage regimens for the treatment of pain or suppression of symptoms of opioid addiction.* Consequently, the same variability in the pharmacokinetics and pharmacodynamics in both methadone and buprenorphine may be associated with negative consequences, such as unintentional *overdose in the opioid naive individual or individuals who lose tolerance after discontinuation of opioids, especially at high doses or in combination with other respiratory depressants.*

Clinical Consideration

OMT should not be confused with trading one addiction for another. If the major symptoms of opioid addiction (compulsion to use, loss of control to abuse, cravings, etc.) can be minimized with these medications, patients are more likely to achieve successful recovery and return to normal or near-normal functioning. When patients are compliant with their prescribed buprenorphine or methadone prescriptions, patients are not likely impaired by these medications due to tolerance to the sedative and euphoric effects of these medications.

Naltrexone

Naltrexone (Vivitrol®, Revia®) is a pharmacologic agent, FDA approved for management of patients with alcohol and opioid addiction. Pharmacologically, naltrexone works by blocking the μ receptors stimulated by opioid analgesics. The opioid antagonist effects of naltrexone have been associated with decreased abuse of opioids in opioid addiction since the euphoric effects of opioids are blocked by naltrexone. Although the exact mechanism of naltrexone is not definitely known, successful use of naltrexone for management of alcohol addiction has been associated with decreased cravings for alcohol. Naltrexone is available for daily administration under the brand name of Revia® or as a monthly depot injection (Vivitrol®). For many patients, naltrexone is an effective tool used in the management of

alcohol or opioid addiction. However, blockade of μ receptors with naltrexone makes management of acute, moderate to severe pain clinically challenging and upon ingestion or injection may induce withdrawal symptoms in patients actively using opioids. Dental practitioners are encouraged to work with the patient's naltrexone prescriber to optimize analgesia.[24]

Treating Acute Dental Pain

Evidence-based studies support nonsteroidal anti-inflammatory drugs (NSAIDs) or NSAIDs+acetaminophen (APAP) as the primary treatment for acute dental pain caused by inflammatory mediators found in bone or tissues. Use of these agents is recommended first-line therapy unless specific patient contraindications—such as renal disease, gastrointestinal bleeds, coagulation irregularities, or hypersensitivity reactions, etc.—warrant alternative or additional treatment with opioids.[25]

Evidence-based studies of acute pain in dental patients receiving OMT, chronic pain management, or naltrexone therapy are limited. Dental practitioners should clarify preferred acute pain management strategies with the patient's OMT provider or primary pain specialist whenever possible to prevent complications of combined opioid analgesic therapy or undertreatment of pain in the dental patient.

Acute Pain in Patients Receiving Opioid Maintenance Therapy

Patients with a history of opioid addiction generally fall into four categories: (1) opioid addicts in recovery in abstinence-based programs (nonpharmacological management);

(2) opioid addicts in recovery receiving OMT; (3) opioid addicts in recovery receiving naltrexone therapy; and (4) opioid addicts *still using*. While evidence-based studies are limited regarding acute pain management of dental patients with opioid addiction, there is ample evidence to support clinical considerations that are key when treating acute pain in patients with opioid addiction who are also receiving OMT.

1. Owing to the variable pharmacokinetic and pharmacodynamics characteristics of methadone and buprenorphine, dosages are different for each agent when treating pain and opioid addiction. Therefore, the dosing schedules for methadone or buprenorphine for patients receiving OMT *do not adequately control acute pain.*
2. There is sufficient evidence to suggest that patients receiving chronic opioid medications, in some instances, *may have hyperalgesia.* Hyperalgesia may be characterized as an increased sensitivity to stimulus that historically did not illicit pain without another detectable etiology other than increasing or chronic opioid dosages. This hyperalgesia is most commonly associated with high-dose opioids for chronic nonmalignant pain.
3. Patients receiving chronic opioids usually have some cross-tolerance to the sedative, euphoric, respiratory depressant, and analgesic effects of other opioids.
4. Other than anecdotal reports, there is no evidence that patients receiving methadone or buprenorphine maintenance therapy for opioid addiction and who are also prescribed opioids for acute pain *are at a greater risk of relapse of addiction* than patients in OMT *not* receiving opioids for acute pain management if monitored appropriately. *Limited information does suggest that inadequate treatment of acute pain, onset of physiologic withdrawal or anticipatory anxiety in OMT patients **may be a greater stressor for relapse.***[26]

5. Acute pain due to dental procedures or pathologic conditions such as infection is associated with an inflammatory mediated response generally limited in duration. *Most dental pain can be effectively managed with NSAIDS or NSAIDs+APAP.* If opioid therapy is warranted or true contraindications exist that prevent use of NSAIDS, the duration of treatment should be limited to the acute event.
6. Patients receiving OMT should be continued on OMT or be prescribed an *equivalent opioid* daily dosage regimen to prevent physiologic withdrawal and disruption of their opioid addiction recovery.
7. Analgesics should be scheduled around the clock during the acute pain event to optimize pain control and not simply prescribed as *needed*. Scheduling of medication prior to increased activity or known times of breakthrough pain may be beneficial. *Opioid doses should be limited in quantity and patients should be managed with NSAIDS, APAP, or combinations of both as soon as possible.*
8. Patients receiving OMT requiring opioids for acute pain should always be encouraged by their dental practitioner to optimize all of their addiction support services in the time surrounding the acute pain event. OMT patients are in treatment contracts that require strict adherence. Prescribing analgesia or sedatives that are controlled substances should always be discussed with the treatment provider and patient.
9. In the event of respiratory depression without cardiac or hemodynamic compromise, patients should receive respiratory support as opposed to reversal treatment with naloxone due to the likelihood of inducing fulminant opioid withdrawal.

Box 4.2 lists common misperceptions that should be avoided when managing acute pain in patients receiving OMT or OCP.

Box 4.2 Common Misconceptions *That Should Be Avoided* When Managing Acute Pain in Patients with Chronic Pain Conditions or Patients Receiving OMT

- Chronic opioid analgesia adequately treats acute dental pain conditions.
- Patients reporting high subjective *chronic* pain scores (e.g., 7, 8, 9, 10+ on VAS) should be demonstrating significantly *visible* signs of "clinical distress," such as tachycardia, elevated blood pressure, elevated respiratory rate, or diaphoresis.
- Chronic pain patients or opioid addicts in recovery are more likely to abuse pain medications.
- Acute pain management with opioids will cause the opioid addict in recovery to relapse.
- Patients on chronic opioid treatments for OMT or chronic pain are "drug seeking" if they complain of inadequate analgesia.

Box 4.3 lists treatment considerations for acute pain management in patients receiving OMT. The information provided in Box 4.3 should be optimized *before* prescribing opioids.

Clinical Consideration

When managing acute postprocedural dental pain or pain from limited pathological conditions such as infections, pain management goals should be to minimize or limit the pain. A goal to maintain pain scores of "0" post procedure is not a realistic goal for the dental practitioner or the patient. Mismatch in prescriber–patient pain control goals may lead to self-prescribing or patients requesting more medications due to perceived inadequate pain management.

Box 4.3 Checklist for Optimizing Pain Management in Patients Receiving OMT or Chronic Opioids for Pain Management

- Reassure the patient the intent to adequately treat pain, NOT deny treatment of pain.
- Establish specific pain management goals/expectations before the procedure (e.g., pain scores "1–3" not "0") to prevent prescriber–patient analgesia mismatch.
- Respect a patient's wishes to NOT receive or be prescribed opioid analgesics or "extra doses" if they are adamant.
- Confirm doses of buprenorphine/methadone or chronic opioid doses with the treatment facility or patient's primary pain specialist and discuss *preferred* plans of treatment with treatment providers.
- Educate and emphasize optimal nonpharmacological therapy post procedure (ice packs, oral rinses, hygiene, compliance with eating instructions, smoking discontinuation or reduction, etc.).
- Document in chart all opioids and sedatives and report information to the OMT treatment center or primary pain specialist as soon as possible.
- Consider preemptive strike with NSAID 1 h before the procedure and then *scheduled* NSAID or NSAID+APAP pain treatment around the clock and not *as needed*.
- Consider long-acting topical anesthetics like bupivacaine prior to discharge from the office.
- Use of combination analgesics with NSAIDs or APAP may add analgesia. (Caution is recommended since these agents may be contraindicated for patients with a history of renal or hepatic impairment. Doses of APAP should not exceed 3.0 g/day.)
- Do not prescribe excessive doses of medications or in quantities expected to be left over.
- Consider (with the patient's consent) that a responsible family member or friend control pain medications.
- Ideally, the OMT prescriber or the chronic pain medication prescriber should manage all pain medications.

Methadone and Buprenorphine

Currently, there are limited evidence-based studies in the outpatient management of acute dental pain in patients receiving OMT. In clinical practice, several strategies for acute pain management can be considered. For the outpatient management of acute dental pain it is usually not practical to discontinue or taper methadone owing its long pharmacokinetic half-life unless the patient is expected to be hospitalized for more than a few days. The dental practitioner should discuss with the OMT prescriber options such as addition of higher dose traditional short-acting oral opioid analgesics or combination analgesics (e.g., hydrocodone–APAP, hydrocodone–ibuprofen, oxycodone–APAP, hydromorphone) in addition to their current maintenance dose of methadone. Addition of higher dosage, short-acting opioids should be limited to the anticipated duration of acute pain. Codeine products should be avoided since they are dependent on demethylation to morphine to produce their major analgesic effects. Only about 10% of codeine is metabolized to this active form.[27] Also, many common antidepressants compete with codeine metabolism, which may reduce codeine's effectiveness.[28] In clinical practice, emergency dental events may be managed with higher traditional doses of short-acting oral opioids. Medications should be titrated daily by phone if possible to manage the acute event. The dental practitioner should document all medications administered or prescribed and notify the patient's OMT prescriber owing to potential patient contract violations such as positive urine drug screens. Another option is to have the OMT prescriber add supplemental oral methadone doses every 4–6 h for analgesia in addition to their daily OMT methadone. Minimal data exist regarding postoperative or postprocedural acute pain management in patients receiving buprenorphine.[29] Patients receiving buprenorphine for OMT may benefit by dividing the total daily dose of buprenorphine into three or four doses throughout the day to provided better analgesic coverage. Having the OMT prescriber add additional low-dose sublingual buprenorphine (e.g., 2 mg) at 4–6 h intervals is also an option.[30,31]

It is critical that the dental practitioner consult with the patient's OMT prescriber before altering the patient's OMT regimen. Adjustment of the buprenorphine by the dental practitioner is not recommended since this may put the patient at risk for depleting their opioid maintenance prescriptions before the allotted time, unintentionally creating OMT contract violations, or undertreating the patient's pain. *Additional licensure is required for practitioners to be able to prescribe buprenorphine or methadone for OMT.* Additional dosages of buprenorphine should be clearly written FOR ANALGESIA on the prescription and in the patient records to avoid confusion and unnecessary liability. In clinical practice, addition of *higher traditional dose short-acting opioids* to a patient's buprenorphine maintenance regimen may be of benefit.[30,31] *However, there are no evidence-based trials to support this.* Buprenorphine's high affinity for the μ receptor and significant patient variability in analgesic response *may* prevent optimal analgesic activity from short-acting opioids. In clinical practice, patients may be started on *higher* traditional doses of oral short-acting opioids (e.g., hydrocodone 10 mg, oxycodone 7.5 mg). Analgesia may be initiated at hydrocodone 10 mg total dose every 4–6 h. The patient should follow up in 24 h by phone for evaluation and dosage titration. Dental practitioners should anticipate likely inadequate analgesia in some of these patients that should not be confused with pseudo-addiction. Dosages should be titrated based on individual pain responses and goals of analgesia therapy. Frequently, initial analgesia may be beneficial but the duration of analgesia does not last. Dosing intervals may need to be shortened to *every 4 h*. Patients usually have developed tolerance to the respiratory depressant, sedative, and euphoric effects of chronic opioids. As previously mentioned, patients requiring treatment for acute pain while receiving methadone or buprenorphine as part of OMT have not been shown to be at an increased risk for addiction relapse in any evidence-based studies after they have received acute pain treatment with *other opioids*. In the event of emergency dental treatment, the patient's OMT treatment provider should be notified as soon as possible. Box 4.4 lists strategies that may be considered in patients receiving OMT.[30,31]

Clinical Consideration

Patients receiving chronic opioid agonist (e.g., morphine, methadone, oxycodone, hydrocodone) for pain should not be prescribed an opioid agonist, antagonist (pentazocine, butorphanol, nalbuphine), or partial agonist (buprenorphine) owing to the potential to cause opioid withdrawal.

The Active Opioid Addict

Although the acute management of dental pain in opioid addicts in OMT may be very labor intensive due to the necessity of multiple communications with the patient and OMT treatment team, necessary chart documentation, as well as patient monitoring, acute pain management of the opioid addict *not in recovery* poses different treatment challenges. Regardless of the opioid abused (e.g., heroin, oxycodone, hydromorphone, buprenorphine), it is impossible to predict the amount of analgesic or respiratory tolerance the patient will experience. Additional clinical challenges present when the patient is prescribed or dispensed opioids for acute moderate to severe postprocedural pain: How can the patient be prevented from using or abusing all the medications at once risking possible overdose and how can the dental practitioner ensure reasonable analgesia after the procedure? When the

Box 4.4   Acute Pain Management Strategies in Patients Receiving OMT[a] in the Outpatient Setting[30–32]

Buprenorphine

- Patients receiving buprenorphine for OMT may benefit by dividing the total daily dose of buprenorphine into three or four doses throughout the day to provide better *analgesic* coverage.[b]
- In addition to the daily buprenorphine maintenance dose, low-dose buprenorphine (e.g., 2 mg sublingual) at 4–6 h intervals specifically for acute pain management may be considered.
- In addition to the patient's daily buprenorphine regimen, addition of *higher* traditional short-acting opioid agonist or combination products (hydrocodone 10 mg–APAP, hydrocodone 10 mg–ibuprofen, oxycodone 7.5 mg–APAP products, etc.) may be prescribed. Patients should be titrated to desired postprocedural analgesic goals. Follow-up phone calls in 24 h are recommended to optimize dosage titration.[c]

Methadone

- In addition to the patient's daily methadone regimen, addition of *higher* dose traditional short-acting opioid agonist or combination products (hydrocodone, hydrocodone–ibuprofen oxycodone–APAP, oxycodone–ibuprofen products, etc.) may be prescribed. Patients should be titrated to desired postprocedural analgesic goals. Follow-up phone calls in 24 h are recommended to optimize dosage titration.[c]

[a]Adapted in part from Ref. 31.
[b]In addition to the daily methadone dose for OMT, supplementation of additional methadone for analgesia *by the methadone OMT prescriber* at 4–6 h intervals may be beneficial.
[c]Dosage adjustments of the patient's buprenorphine or methadone dosage for acute pain management should only be done under consultation with the patient's OMT provider. State regulations and the patient's health/dental insurance may impose restrictions of sublingual buprenorphine for analgesia. *With the exception of buprenorphine in buprenorphine patients,* μ-receptor agonist/antagonists, such as pentazocine, butorphanol, or nalbuphine, should be avoided owing to induction of physiologic opioid withdrawal.

patient's acute pain is controlled during the procedure, presenting the patient with the opportunity to receive help for SUD should be considered. Items in Box 4.3 should be optimized whenever possible. Additional considerations for management of these patients are listed in Box 4.5.

Acute Pain Management in Patients Receiving Naltrexone Therapy

Patients receiving *daily* naltrexone therapy should have their naltrexone discontinued, ideally 72 h before any planned surgical or interventional procedures where opioids may be necessary for management of moderate to severe acute pain.[33] Considerations to optimize analgesia in these patients should include items listed in Box 4.6. Patients receiving depot

---

Clinical Consideration

In clinical practice, the short office dental procedure time prevents optimal titration and monitoring for efficacy and toxicity of opioids for urgency/emergency dental procedures in OMT patients, active opioid addicts, and treatment of chronic nonmalignant pain. Use of traditional *starting doses* of short-acting opioids may be considered and titrated cautiously by the dental practitioner with very specific treatment goals. A 24 h postprocedure follow-up call to or from the patient is helpful in titrating doses on postprocedure day 1 (see Box 4.4).

Clinical Consideration

Patients should be asked about depot naltrexone therapy even if it is not reported on their office intake form. Patients frequently dismiss this information either intentionally or unintentionally since it is not part of their daily medication list.

Box 4.5   Additional Considerations for Active Addicts Requiring Acute Pain Management

- After adequate analgesia has been achieved, the dental practitioner should encourage the patient to receive SUD treatment and should be prepared with address and phone numbers of local treatment options.
- To minimize the risk of misuse or abuse of the total prescription at once, the prescriber may write more than one prescription but limit the prescription to a 24–48 h supply.
- Writing specific hour dosing schedules may benefit some patients.
- The dental practitioner can have the patient sign an opioid treatment agreement warning the patient that loss, theft, or overutilization of opioid medication may result in discontinuing of treatment.

Box 4.6   Considerations for Acute Pain Management in Patients Receiving Naltrexone

- Discontinue daily naltrexone 72 h before the procedure.
- Reassure the patient the intent to adequately treat pain, NOT deny treatment of pain.
- Establish specific postprocedure pain management goals/expectations *before* the procedure (e.g., pain scores "1–3" not "0").
- Educate and emphasize optimal nonpharmacological therapy post procedure (ice packs, oral rinses, hygiene, compliance with eating instructions, etc.).
- Consider preemptive strike with NSAIDs and then scheduled NSAID therapy.
- Consider long-acting topical anesthetics like bupivacaine prior to discharge from the office.
- Use of combination analgesics with NSAIDs+ APAP may add additional analgesia. (Caution is recommended since these agents may be contraindicated for patients with a history of renal or hepatic impairment.)

naltrexone therapy pose a clinical dilemma. High doses of opioids are required to overcome the μ-receptor blockade by naltrexone. When patients are not responsive to nonopioid treatment options and opioids are clinically necessary, higher opioid doses should be expected. These patients require continuous monitoring for possible respiratory depression and oversedation at an appropriate treatment facility due to increased doses of opioids that are necessary to overcome naltrexone μ-receptor blockade and achieve adequate analgesia.[34]

Acute Pain Management in Patients Receiving Opioids for Chronic Pain

Patients receiving treatment with OCP that require acute dental pain management have similar considerations as patients receiving OMT. Like OMT patients, these patients have usually developed tolerance to the sedative, respiratory depressant, euphoric, and analgesic effects of opioids. OCP therapy may be further complicated by hyperalgesia. *The clinical phenomena of hyperalgesia and analgesic tolerance may be misinterpreted as drug-seeking behavior due to the patient's inadequate analgesic response to traditional opioid dosing regimens.* OCP patients are commonly maintained on extended-release, sustained-released, or delayed-release opioids for oral administration or opioid transdermal delivery systems. Box 4.3 lists acute pain management strategies that should be optimized prior to administering outpatient opioids. OCP patients may require higher dosages of traditional short-acting opioid dosages *in combination with shorter dosing intervals* (3–4 h compared with 4–6 h) to achieve optimal pain control. *Prescribing of opioids should be limited to treating the acute event.* Whenever possible, dental practitioners should have the prescriber of the patient's OCP prescribe additional opioid

analgesia since they are likely more familiar with the patient's tolerance and other opioid dosing considerations. In the event of urgency or emergency treatment where the OCP provider is not available, considerations in Box 4.3 should be optimized. In addition to patient's chronic opioid medications, short-acting oral opioids may be administered at traditional doses and titrated accordingly. It should be anticipated that these patients are likely to have higher analgesic requirements that may require a shorter dosing interval (every 3–4 h versus 4–6 h) as well as increased doses. *Patient follow-up by phone 24 h post procedure is suggested to optimize dosing in these patients.*

> **Clinical Consideration**
>
> For complex oral surgery cases requiring hospital admission, dental practitioners should consult anesthesiology services for treatment plans *regarding pre-, intra-, and postprocedure* pain management. Complications occurring post procedures frequently involve inadequate analgesia after the anesthesia service has signed off on the patient's case.

Summary

Acute pain management in patients with chronic conditions such as nonmalignant pain, opioid addiction, or alcohol addiction is a clinical challenge for dental practitioners. Misperceptions surrounding effective analgesia in these patients may create an environment of mistrust that leads to inadequate analgesia. Clinical conditions such as tolerance and hyperalgesia must be understood and anticipated by dental practitioners when treating patients receiving chronic opioid therapy for pain or OMT. Dental practitioners have the ethical obligation to treat acute pain reasonably regardless of other underlying psychiatric diagnosis or pathology. Starting with the patient interview, acute pain management can be optimized with reassurance to the patient, collaboration with the patient primary OMT or pain specialist, and a comprehensive treatment strategy.

References

1. Smith M, Davis MA, Stano M, Whedon JM. Aging baby boomers and the rising cost of chronic back pain: secular trend analysis of longitudinal Medical Expenditures Panel Survey data for years 2000 to 2007. J Manipulative Physiol Ther 2013;36(1): 2–11.

2. Hanks-Bell M, Halvey K, Paice J. Pain assessment and management in aging. Online J Issues Nurs 2004;9(3). www.nursingworld.org/MainMenu Categories/ANAMarketplace/ANAPeriodicals/ OJIN/TableofContents/Volume92004/No3Sept0 4/ArticlePreviousTopic/PainAssessmentandMa nagementinAging.aspx. Accessed December 29, 2014.

3. CDC Grand Rounds: prescription drug overdoses—a U.S. epidemic. Morb Mort Wkly Rep 2012;61(1);10–13.

4. SAMHSA. Drug Addiction Treatment Act of 2000. http://www.buprenorphine.samhsa.gov/fulllaw .html. Accessed December 29, 2014.

5. American Society of Addiction Medicine. Office-based opioid agonist treatment (OBOT). http://www.asam.org/advocacy/find-a-policy- statement/view-policy-statement/public-policy -statements/2011/12/15/office-based-opioid-ag onist-treatment-(obot). Accessed December 29, 2014.

6. Colleau SM, Joranson DE. Tolerance, physical dependence and addiction: definitions, clinical relevance and misconceptions. Cancer Pain Release 1998;11(3). http://www.whocancerpain. wisc.edu/index?q=node/245. Accessed December 29, 2014.

7. Lee M, Silverman SM, Hansen H, Patel VB, Manchikanti L. A comprehensive review of opioid-induced hyperalgesia. Pain Physician 2011;14(2):145–61.

8. SAMHSA CSAT SBIRT Glossary. http://www. dhcs.ca.gov/services/medi-cal/Documents/SBI _glossary.pdf. Accessed December 29, 2014.

9. Alcohol Rehab. Stigma of addiction. http:// alcoholrehab.com/addiction-articles/stigma-of- addiction/. Accessed December 29, 2014.

10. HCP Live. Myths and misconceptions surrounding addiction in chronic pain patients treated with opioid analgesics. October 11, 2011. http://www.hcplive.com/publications/pain-ma nagement/2011/september-2011/Myths-and-Mi sconceptions-Surrounding-Addiction-in-Chronic -Pain-Patients-Treated-with-Opioid-Analgesics. Accessed December 29, 2014.

11. Prater CD, Zylstra RG, Miller KE. Successful pain management for the recovering addicted patient. Prim Care Companion J Clin Psychiatry 2002;4(4):125–31.

12. National Institutes of Health. Effective medical treatment of opiate addiction. NIH Consensus Statement Online 1997;15(6):1–38. http:// consensus.nih.gov/1997/1998treatopiateaddictio n108html.htm. Accessed December 29, 2014.

13. American Society of Addiction Medicine. Definition of addiction. http://www.asam.org/for-the- public/definition-of-addiction. Accessed December 29, 2014.

14. Behavioral Health Coordinating Committee, Prescription Drug Abuse Subcommittee, US Department of Health and Human Services. Addressing prescription drug abuse in the United States: current activities and future opportunities. 2013. http://www.cdc.gov/HomeandRecreationalSafe ty/pdf/HHS_Prescription_Drug_Abuse_Report _09.2013.pdf. Accessed December 29, 2014.

15. CDC, Department of Health and Human Services. Substance abuse treatment for injection drug users: a strategy with many benefits. http://www.cdc.gov/idu/facts/TreatmentFin.p df. Accessed December 29, 2014.

16. McGovern MP, Carroll KM. Evidence-based practices for substance use disorders. Psychiatr Clin N Am 2003;26:991–1010.

17. Gutstein H, Akil H. Opioid analgesics. In: Goodman & Gilman's the Pharmacological Basis of Therapeutics, 11th ed. Brunton L, Lazo L, Parker K, eds. 2005. McGraw-Hill, New York, pp. 547–590.

18. NIH, National Institute on Drug Abuse. Drug-Facts: treatment approaches for drug addiction. http://www.drugabuse.gov/publications/drug facts/treatment-approaches-drug-addiction. Accessed December 29, 2104.

19. US National Library of Medicine, DailyMed. Buprenorphine hydrochloride—buprenorphine hydrochloride injection, solution [Hospira, Inc.]. http://dailymed.nlm.nih.gov/dailymed/drugInfo.cfm?setid=23aa1bb3-cecf-4e62-29bb-48488bb66fc3. Accessed December 29, 2014.

20. Buprenorphine.Drugdex.Micromedex. Accessed August, 2014.

21. Mendelson J, Fernandez E, Welm S, Upton RA, Chin BA, Jones RT. Bioavailability of oral and sublingual buprenorphine and naloxone tablets (abstract PI-113). Clin Pharmacol Ther 2001;69(2):P29.

22. Product Information: SUBOXONE oral sublingual tablets, buprenorphine HCl naloxone HCl dihydrate oral sublingual tablets. 2006. Reckitt Benckiser Pharmaceuticals, Inc., Richmond, VA.

23. Bart G. Maintenance medication for opiate addiction: the foundation of recovery. J Addict Dis 2012;31(3):207–25.

24. Naltrexone.Drugdex.Micromedex. Accessed August, 2014.

25. Hersh EV, Kane WT, O'Neil MG, Kenna GA, Katz NP, Golubic S, Moore PA. Prescribing recommendations for the treatment of acute pain in dentistry. Compend Contin Educ Dent 2011;32(3): 22–30.

26. Savage SR. Principles of pain treatment in the addicted patient. In: Principles of Addiction Medicine, 2nd ed. Graham AW, Schultz TK, Wilford BB, eds. 1998. American Society of Addiction Medicine, Chevy Chase, MD, pp. 919–44.

27. Gutstein H, Akil H. Opioid analgesics. In: Goodman & Gilman's the Pharmacological Basis of Therapeutics, 11th ed. Brunton L, Lazo L, Parker K, eds. 2005. McGraw-Hill, New York, p. 566.

28. Michalets EL. Update: clinically significant cytochrome P-450 drug interactions. Pharmacotherapy 1998;18(1):84–112.

29. Kornfeld H, Manfredi L. Effectiveness of full agonist opioids in patients stabilized on buprenorphine undergoing major surgery: a case series. Am J Ther 2010;17(5):523–8. doi: 10.1097/MJT.0b013e3181be0804.

30. Alford DP. Management of acute and chronic pain. Chapter 11. In: Handbook of Office-Based Buprenorphine Treatment of Opioid Dependence. Renner JA, Levounis P, eds. 2010. American Psychiatric Publishing, Arlington, VA, pp. 213–25.

31. Alford DP, Compton P, Samet JH. Acute pain management for patients receiving maintenance methadone or buprenorphine therapy. Ann Intern Med 2006;144(2):127–34.

32. Ries RK, Fiellin DA, Miller SC, Saitz R, eds. The ASAM Principles of Addiction Medicine, 5th ed. 2014. Lippincott Williams and Wilkins.

33. Revia package insert. http://www.accessdata.fda.gov/drugsatfda_docs/label/2013/018932s017lbl.pdf. Accessed December 29, 2014.

34. Vivitrol package insert. http://www.accessdata.fda.gov/drugsatfda_docs/label/2010/021897s015lbl.pdf. Accessed December 29, 2014.

Sedation and Anxiolysis

5

Matthew Cooke, DDS, MD, MPH

Introduction

Dental practitioners who provide sedation or anesthesia to patients with substance use disorders (SUDs) are urged to be current in their knowledge of pharmacology, including content related to drugs of abuse. They must recognize indications and contraindications to the delivery of sedation and anesthesia medications, including epinephrine-containing local anesthetics for patients with SUDs both active and in remission.[1] The acutely intoxicated patient and the chronic abuser may present in ways that mimic other organic processes or obscure the presentation of concurrent medical issues.[2] These patients present significant challenges for dental practitioners providing sedation- and anesthesia-related services. Management of pain and anxiety is the goal with safety as the first priority. All decisions must be made considering risk versus benefit. Dental practitioners are obligated to use safe prescribing practices. This chapter will provide recommendations to aid the dental practitioner and dental hygienist in managing pain and anxiety and

modifying behavior to safely complete dental procedures in patients with SUDs.

Definitions

There have been many definitions of sedation in dentistry used over the years. Recent documents defining sedation and anesthesia are from the American Dental Association (ADA) House of Delegates Meeting in 2007.[3,4] Clinical standards for sedation in dentistry parallel the 2002 guidelines established by the American Society of Anesthesiology (ASA).[5] The American Academy of Pediatric Dentistry (AAPD) and the American Academy of Pediatrics (AAP) also maintain guidelines for sedation of the pediatric patient, defined as any patient under the age of 21.[6]

The following definitions for levels of sedation are excerpted from the ADA, AAPD, and AAP guidelines:[3-6]

- **Minimal Sedation.** (Old terminology "anxiolysis") a drug-induced state during which

The ADA Practical Guide to Substance Use Disorders and Safe Prescribing, First Edition. Edited by Michael O'Neil.
© 2015 American Dental Association. Published 2015 by John Wiley & Sons, Inc.

patients respond normally to verbal commands. Although cognitive function and coordination may be impaired, ventilatory and cardiovascular functions are unaffected.

- **Moderate Sedation.** (Old terminology "conscious sedation" or "sedation/analgesia") a drug-induced depression of consciousness during which patients respond purposefully to verbal commands (e.g., "open your eyes" either alone or accompanied by light tactile stimulation such as a light tap on the shoulder or face, not a sternal rub). For older patients, this level of sedation implies an interactive state; for younger patients, age-appropriate behaviors (e.g., crying) occur and are expected.

Note: "In accord with this particular definition, the drug(s) and/or techniques used should carry a margin of safety wide enough to render loss of consciousness unlikely. Repeated dosing of an agent before the effects of previous dosing can be fully appreciated may result in a greater alteration of the state of consciousness than is the intent of the dental practitioner. Further, patients whose only response is reflex withdrawal from repeated painful stimuli would not be considered to be in a state of moderate sedation".[7]

- **Deep Sedation.** A drug-induced depression of consciousness during which patients cannot be easily aroused but respond purposefully after repeated verbal or painful stimulation. The ability to independently maintain ventilatory function may be impaired. Patients may require assistance in maintaining a patent airway, and spontaneous ventilation may be inadequate. Cardiovascular function is usually maintained. A state of deep sedation may be accompanied by partial or complete loss of protective reflexes.
- **General Anesthesia.** A drug-induced loss of consciousness during which patients are not arousable even by painful stimulation.

The ability to independently maintain ventilatory function is often impaired. Patients often require assistance in maintaining a patent airway, and positive pressure ventilation may be required because of depressed spontaneous ventilation or drug-induced depression of neuromuscular function. Cardiovascular function may be impaired.

Spectrum of Anesthesia and Sedation

Arthur Guedel, MD, introduced the concept of anesthetic signs and stages (Figure 5.1). His early work studied diethyl ether for general anesthesia. He observed four distinct stages as patients were administered increasing quantities of inhaled ether. The stages represent a continuum or spectrum from which no sedation becomes general anesthesia.[9]

In stage 1, or the analgesia phase, consciousness is not lost. Stage 2 is the excitatory phase. Between stages 2 and 3 consciousness is lost. Stage 3 is defined as the surgical anesthesia stage. **Dental practitioners who have not been trained in the use of deep sedation and general anesthesia need to limit their practice to stage 1, the analgesia phase.**

Although Guedel's original classification still has merit, it has been modified and adapted to include new drugs and techniques. Dental practitioners must understand that as drugs are given they produce an effect along a "spectrum of pain and anxiety control".[7] Drugs administered via different routes will, also, produce various levels of sedation or anesthesia.

Figure 5.2 shows the spectrum of "pain and anxiety control." At the left there is no sedation or anesthesia. Moving right, there are levels of conscious sedation up to the vertical bar. The bar represents loss of consciousness. To the right of the bar is deep sedation/general anesthesia. Although an experienced provider may not need a graphic representation to help

Stage	Muscle tone	Breathing	Eye movement
1 Analgesia	Normal	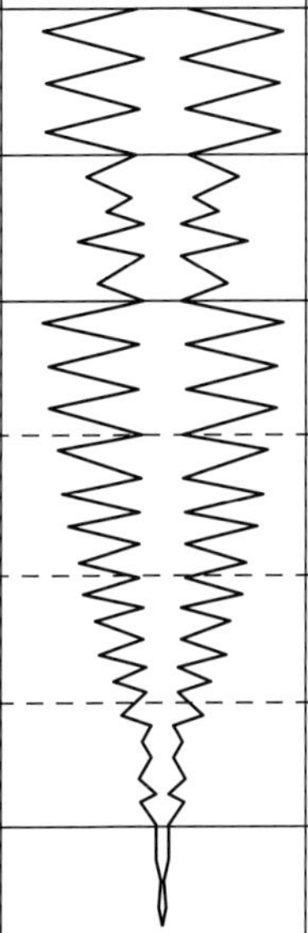	Slight
2 Excitement	Normal to markedly increased		Moderate
3	Slightly relaxed		Slight
	Moderately relaxed		None
	Markedly relaxed		None
	Markedly relaxed		None
4 Respiratory paralysis	Flaccid		None

Surgical anesthesia

Figure 5.1   Graphic illustration of Guedel's early work.[8]

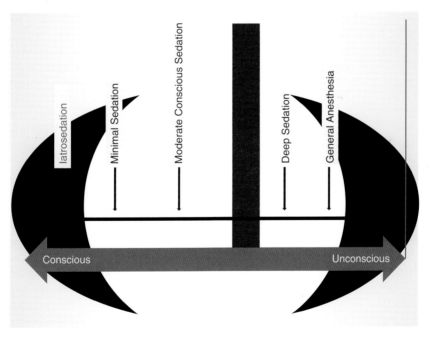

Figure 5.2   The spectrum of pain and anxiety control.

determine level of sedation or anesthesia, a classification system is necessary. The dental practitioner must understand where they are on the spectrum and its relationship to where they want to be.

Sedation without the use of drugs is termed iatrosedation. Techniques include acupressure, acupuncture, biofeedback, electronic dental anesthesia, and hypnosis.[7] These modalities may be an alternative to traditional sedation and/or general anesthesia for patients with SUD. However, for the purposes of this chapter, the focus is on the use of pharmacotherapy to obtain a desired outcome.

Communication is paramount to success. There is no substitute for good verbal and nonverbal communication, which is developmentally age appropriate, and nonjudgmental. Good communication alleviates fear and anxiety, allowing treatment to proceed in a "normal" fashion.[7] Traditional behavior management/guidance, such as distraction, tell–show–do, guided imagery, topical anesthesia, and hypnosis, may reduce the need for or depth of pharmacologic sedation.[6,10] *Patients with an SUD, both active and in remission, benefit from effective communication.* Good communication will facilitate moderate levels of sedation with agents that have less addictive properties.

Rescue

"Rescue" is an essential concept for safe sedation. Because sedation and anesthesia are a continuum, a provider must be able to recover a patient from unintended entry to a more profound level of central nervous system (CNS) depression.[5–7,11] In an effort to reduce morbidity and mortality, the ASA guidelines include and stress the concept of rescue during the administration of sedation by "non-anesthesiologists":[5]

Because sedation is a continuum, it is not always possible to predict how an individual patient will respond. Hence, practitioners intending to produce a given level of sedation should be able to rescue patients whose level of sedation become deeper than initially intended. Individuals administering Moderate Sedation/Analgesia (Conscious Sedation) should be able to rescue patients who enter a state of deep sedation/analgesia, while those administering deep sedation/analgesia should be able to rescue patients who enter a state of general anesthesia.[5]

Preoperative Evaluation

Dental treatment can have profound effects on both the physical and psychological "well-being" of patients with SUD. Prior to dental treatment (with or without sedation) patients should have a complete physical and psychological assessment to evaluate risk. This assessment allows the dental practitioner to determine whether a patient will tolerate a procedure and/or determine whether an alternative modality is needed. Medical and psychological histories should guide the dental practitioner in choosing a treatment modality. The evaluation should include a medical history questionnaire, physical examination, and a discussion with the patient, parent, and/or care giver. For the patient with SUD, extra time and attention should be spent on understanding the magnitude of their disease. With information collected, the dental practitioner can establish a physical status classification and determine risk factors. Medical consults can be obtained as needed .[7]

A preoperative consult/evaluation with a physician is not medical clearance. The purpose is to evaluate a patient's *current* medical and physical status and make recommendations concerning management of risk factors over the entire perioperative period. The goal in the preoperative phase is medical optimization, in which strategies are developed to reduce risk and improve outcome.[12,13]

Physical Status Classification

The ASA uses a physical classification system for estimating medical risk for patients receiving general anesthesia for a surgical procedure:[14]

Class 1: A healthy patient (no physiologic, physical or psychological abnormalities).

Class 2: A patient with mild systemic disease without limitation of daily activities (i.e., controlled asthma; controlled hypertension).

Class 3: A patient with severe systemic disease that limits activity but is not incapacitating (i.e., uncontrolled hypertension; uncontrolled diabetes).

Class 4: A patient with incapacitating systemic disease that is a constant threat to life.

Class 5: A moribund patient not expected to survive 24 h without the operation.

Class 6: A brain-dead patient whose organs are being removed for donor purposes.

If the procedure to be performed is an emergency an "E" is added to this classification system (e.g., ASA PS 2 E). In the outpatient medical and dental settings classes 5 and 6 have been eliminated.[14]

The system was adopted in 1962. It has remained virtually unchanged and has since been adopted for evaluation of medical risk associated with all surgical procedures regardless of anesthetic technique.[15,16]

Patients who are ASA PS 1 and 2 are generally considered appropriate candidates for minimal, moderate, or deep sedation in the dental office.[6] Individuals in classes 3 and 4 require individual consideration, particularly for moderate and deep sedation.[6,17] Dental practitioners are encouraged to consult with appropriate subspecialties when necessary for patients at increased risk. The ultimate responsibility and liability rest with the dental practitioner, who decides to treat or not treat. Special attention should be given to patients with a history of SUD or chronic pain. Consultation with

the provider responsible for the patient's "treatment contract" is essential to avoid unnecessary contract violations by the patient or to potentially provoke cravings of substances of abuse. Limitations to this system may include, but are not limited to, the following:

1. No consideration for age.
2. No consideration of pregnancy.
3. Limited psychiatric considerations.
4. Minimal information regarding patients with SUD.

Dental practitioners are encouraged to be familiar with this classification system prior to treating complex patients. (See the Resources and Further Readings section.)

Clinical Consideration

Most outpatients presenting with SUD will be classified as ASA class 1 or 2. It is recommended that dental practitioners treating patients with classifications of ASA 2 or higher consider consultation with a dental anesthesiologist.

Sedation

Because of patient extremes in responsiveness and acceptance to various modalities, the goals and outcomes for sedation of a patient with an SUD will vary depending upon a host of factors. Sedation of patients with SUD disorders for the delivery of oral health care is uniquely challenging. A sedation plan should maximize benefit and minimize associated risks for adverse outcomes.

Once pharmacosedation is planned, the dental practitioner must consider which agents to use and how to administer. Choosing a method for delivery will vary depending on desired level of sedation. Patients with SUD provide a challenge, because *some will require additional agents to obtain a desired affect due to tolerance and others will require less due to concurrent organic illness, such as hepatic dysfunction.* Therefore, dose and route of delivery must be part of the sedation plan.

Clinical Considerations

The ideal sedation should:

1. Be safe.
2. Be easy to administer.
3. Have rapid and reliable onset.
4. Alleviate pain and anxiety.
5. Have minimal undesirable side effects.
6. Be reversible.
7. Have limited potential to provoke "cravings."

The following routes are available for delivery of drugs to a patient with SUD:

1. Oral/rectal
2. Topical
3. Intranasal
4. Inhalational
5. Subcutaneous
6. Intramuscular (IM)
7. Intravenous (IV)
8. Inter-arterial
9. Intrathecal (in spinal fluid)
10. Transdermal (through epidermis).

Oral and rectal sedation are referred to as enteral sedation. The drug is absorbed from the gastrointestinal tract. After absorption, it enters the enterohepatic circulation and is released to the systemic circulation. This is different from all other routes of delivery in which drug absorption occurs directly into the systemic circulation (parenteral sedation).

The most popular route used for sedation in dentistry is the oral route. Advantages over the parenteral routes include acceptance by patients, low cost, ease of administration, decreased incidence of adverse reaction, and no equipment needed for delivery.[7] However, oral sedation does have some significant disadvantages, such as reliance on patient compliance, a prolonged latent period, erratic and incomplete absorption from the gastrointestinal tract, inability to titrate, inability to lighten or deepen sedation as needed, and a prolonged duration of action. *With oral sedation, adding more medicine after the initial dose is not recommended.*

Drugs administered topically are more readily absorbed from nonkeratinized skin. Topical applications of drugs in dentistry are usually limited to local anesthetics. They are highly effective at relieving pain associated with intraoral injections of local anesthesia.[18]

Intranasal administration has become increasingly popular in pediatric dentistry. It is easily administered to resistant, uncooperative, or pre-cooperative patients.[7,19–21] Although there is brief discomfort with administration, direct absorption into the systemic circulation makes the drug rapidly bioavailable. Midazolam, a water-soluble benzodiazepine, is the most commonly used drug via the intranasal route.[7,19–22] The mucosal atomization device (MAD™) is the preferred method for nasal administration. Compared with oral sedation, there is reduced time to onset and total time spent in the office.

Inhalational administration of drugs occurs when gaseous agents pass from the nose or mouth to the trachea and lungs into the cardiovascular system. There are a variety of agents available for inhalational sedation and anesthesia. In dentistry, nitrous oxide–oxygen sedation is the main drug used for inhalation sedation.[7,23] It is easily titrated to effect, with minimal side effects or complications. Disadvantages of nitrous oxide are that it is not a potent anesthetic, so there may be failure. Also, a delivery system is required with a failsafe, and scavenging system. The equipment must be calibrated annually and there needs to be adequate office ventilation to prevent chronic exposure to those administering the sedation. Other more potent inhalation agents include sevoflurane, isoflurane, desflurane, and halothane. These agents are used in the induction and maintenance of general anesthesia.[7]

Subcutaneous injection is administration of a drug beneath the skin into the subcutaneous tissue. Rate of absorption is directly proportional to the vasculature in the area of injection. Slow rates of absorption limit its usefulness in dentistry.

The intramuscular route directly administers the drug into the muscle. This parenteral technique allows for quick onset with rapid maximal clinical effect. The disadvantages include prolonged deep sedation, injury to tissues at the site of injection, and overdose. Intramuscular administration is often unpredictable, and there is no mechanism for titration to effect. Ketamine, a dissociative anesthetic, is the most commonly used drug via the intramuscular route and is often used for sedation and induction of the uncooperative patient.[24]

Intravascular drug administration represents the most effective, predictable method of delivery for adequate sedation of most patients.[7] Advantages include rapid onset with short duration of latency, and a shortened recovery period. However, complications at the site of venipuncture and risk for overdose are disadvantages. IV injections may often be difficult to obtain on patients with SUDs. Many drugs given via the IV route do not have reversals; therefore, the dental practitioner must be prepared to manage deeper sedation and other complications, such as allergic reactions, that may not be seen with other, less effective modes of delivery.[7]

A variety of drugs are available for sedation and anesthesia of the patient with an SUD. These primarily include inhalation sedation/anesthesia, benzodiazepines, sedative hypnotics, antihistamines, alpha agonists, and analgesics. Table 5.1 lists available drugs for sedation.

The sedation/anesthetic regimen for patients with an SUD should carry a high therapeutic index with a wide safety margin and a low probability for abuse. It should be

Table 5.1 Drugs Available for Sedation and Anesthesia of the Patient with SUD

Alpha agonists	**Anticholinergics**
Clonidine	Atropine
Dexmedetomidine	Scopolamine
	Glycopyrrolate
Antihistamines	**Barbiturates**
Hydroxyzine	Methohexital
Diphenhydramine	Sodium thiopental
Promethazine	
Benzodiazepines	**Dissociative anesthetics**
Diazepam	Ketamine[a]
Midazolam	
Lorazepam	
Triazolam	
Hypnotics	**Opioid agonists**
Chloral hydrate	Fentanyl
	Morphine
	Meperidine
	Alfentanil,[a] Sufentanil,[a]
	Remifentanil[a]
Non-narcotic analgesics	**Other**
Acetaminophen	Propofol[a]
Ketorolac	

[a]Not recommended for use in IV moderate sedation without anesthesia training.

modified based on the substance of abuse and account for patients' physical, developmental, mental, sensory, behavioral, cognitive, or emotional impairments. Selection of the fewest number of drugs paired with the goal of the procedure are essential for safe practice.[25–30] This means that if a painful procedure was planned, an analgesic would be the drug of choice. If the procedure is more diagnostic, a sedative may be used. Combinations of different classes are often used. However, when three or more agents are used together the potential for an adverse outcome increases.[5,31] Paradoxical reactions, the opposite of the desired outcome, are more frequent in patients with an SUD.[32]

Medications Available for Sedation of Patients with Substance Use Disorder

Nitrous Oxide–Oxygen Sedation

Short-term exposure to nitrous oxide induces sedation, euphoria, giddiness, elation, and a general sense of well-being. The pharmacological mechanism of action of nitrous oxide is not fully understood. Nitrous oxide modulates a broad range of ligand-gated ion channels, with moderate activity on the *N*-methyl-D-aspartate (NMDA) receptor. The sedation/anesthetic, hallucinogenic, and euphoriant effects are likely caused by inhibition of NMDA-mediated currents.[33–35] The analgesic effects of nitrous oxide are linked to endogenous opioids and the noradrenergic systems. Additionally, nitrous oxide may imitate nitric oxide in the CNS to provide analgesic and anxiolytic properties.[33–35]

Nitrous oxide is the least potent of the inhalation anesthetics, but in dentistry it is the most frequently used.[7] The MAC (minimum alveolar concentration of an agent that prevents movement in 50% of patients to a surgical incision) for nitrous oxide is 105%. It is difficult to reach this level unless administered under hyperbaric conditions.[7] However, Guadel's stage 2, delirium, can be reached if nitrous oxide is not properly administered.[8,9] Nitrous oxide may be administered alone or in combination with other agents.

There are relatively few absolute contraindications to nitrous oxide as long as the percentage of oxygen administered is not allowed to go below 21% that of ambient air, which is unlikely because of built in fail-safe mechanisms.[36] *Relative* contraindications to nitrous oxide include:[7]

- patients with compulsive personalities;
- claustrophobic patients;
- children with severe behavioral issues;
- personality disorders;
- upper respiratory tract infections (URIs);
- chronic obstructive pulmonary disease;
- pregnancy;
- neutropenia (e.g., patients with HIV absolute neutrophil count <200);
- pneumothorax;
- middle-ear/sinus disease.

Perhaps, nitrous oxide may be a safe choice for sedation for some patients with a drug-related SUD. Nitrous oxide has been used as an effective and safe treatment for alcohol withdrawal and has been shown to reduce the use of potentially addictive sedative medications, such as benzodiazepines.[37] The potential for stimulating cravings in patients with similar pharmacological agents is a danger for any patient with an SUD.

> ### Clinical Consideration
>
> Anecdotally, alcoholics in recovery have reported significant return of "cravings" after receiving nitrous oxide. Additionally, patients with a known history of inhalant abuse should specifically be asked about abusing nitrous oxide.

The fundamental principles for appropriate administration of nitrous oxide–oxygen sedation are as follows:[36]

- Be enthusiastic and confident that the experience will be positive.
- Have confidence in nitrous oxide and what it can do. Also, be knowledgeable about the limits.
- Recognize that patients in your care represent the best opportunity you have to express genuine care and concern.
- Informed consent must be obtained for each patient before nitrous oxide–oxygen administration.

- Practice titration.
- The procedure begins and ends with 100% oxygen.
- The patient should not be left alone.
- Accurately document all procedures, reactions, complications, and so on in patient's record.
- Place patient in comfortable position before administration.
- Inform the patient to ask for assistance at any time in the procedure if needed.
- If nitrous oxide is to be used at the next appointment, recommend that they not have a large meal prior to their appointment.

Titrate to the level of sedation that is determined by patient comfort and relaxation. There is no percentage for sedation for a given experience or patient. There is also no pre-set LPM (liters per minute) of nitrous oxide/oxygen. The percentage of nitrous oxide/oxygen given to a patient or experience will not reflect the amount necessary for any other experience. The goal is to keep the patient relaxed and comfortable.[36]

Emergence from nitrous oxide is the mirror image of induction; the patient should return to their original emotional state. Terminate nitrous oxide flow; continue delivering 100% oxygen during the final minutes of the procedure. This begins the postoperative oxygenation phase of 3–5 min. Following the 3–5 min period, the patient should be recovered from the pharmacological effects.[38]

Nitrous oxide–oxygen sedation may be used to augment other modalities of sedation and anesthesia. This can add a degree of safety because the patient is getting a minimum of 30% oxygen, which is greater than the 21% of room air. However, some states do not allow polypharmacy, so augmentation may not be an option. Box 5.1 lists potential adverse effects of nitrous oxide therapy.

> **Box 5.1   Potential Adverse Effects of Nitrous Oxide–Oxygen Therapy**
>
> - Diffusion hypoxia
> - Nausea/vomiting
> - Postprocedure memory "fogginess"
> - Coordination–balance impairment

The Benzodiazepines

The benzodiazepines have become the most popular and widely used sedatives in dentistry. Benzodiazepines bind the GABA-A receptor and inhibit CNS function, mainly in the thalamus and limbic systems, the area of the brain responsible for emotion and behavior. Benzodiazepines are reversible with flumazenil and have a wide safety margin (therapeutic dose to toxic dose), making them desirable for sedation in dentistry. Table 5.2 shows available benzodiazepines used in anxiolysis and sedation for dentistry. The doses represent estimated values for average healthy adult patients and are based on a wide range of patient responses to blood levels of the drug. *Pediatric dosing is usually adjusted downward and based on weight (mg/kg) for a desired level of sedation.*

Midazolam (Dormicum® or Versed®), a short-acting water-soluble benzodiazepine, is perhaps the most popular, versatile agent. It is often referred to as the mainstay of moderate sedation in dentistry.[39,40] This agent causes sedation with antegrade amnesia and has a relatively short half-life, which can be reversed.[41–43]

Midazolam's routes of administration are as follows:

1. IM—not well accepted and should be reserved for difficult patients; peaks in 15 min.
2. IV—venous access required. Smaller therapeutic index. Caution when used with opioids for premedication owing to its blunting of hypoxic ventilator drive.

Table 5.2   **Benzodiazepines[7]**

Generic name	Brand name	Class	Availability (mg)	Concentration (mg/mL)	Average dose (mg)
Oral moderate sedation					
Alprazolam	Xanax	AA	0.25, 0.5, 1		0.25–0.5
Chlordiazepoxide	Librium	AA	5, 10, 25		10
Diazepam	Valium	AA	2, 5, 10		10
Lorazepam	Ativan	SH AA	0.5, 1, 2		2–4
Midazolam	Dormicum	SH	15		15–30
Triazolam	Halcion	SH	0.25, 0.5		0.25–0.5
Intravenous moderate sedation					
Diazepam	Valium			5	10–12
Lorazepam	Ativan			2	2–4
Midazolam	Versed			1	2.5–7.5

AA: anti-anxiety; SH: sedative–hypnotic.

3. Oral—most popular pediatric route but difficult to mask bitter taste. Optimal separation from parents in 30–45 min. Dose: 0.5 mg/kg up to total of 20 mg maximum.
4. Rectal—most often use in diaper-age patients over age of 12 months. Maximum plasma level is in 19–29 min. Disadvantage is variation in absorption and sometimes causing defecation.
5. Nasal—acidic solution that burns. May be poor absorption in cases of URI with increased nasal secretions. Sedation occurs in 7–10 min.
6. Oral transmucosal—effective, but not good in young or noncompliant children because of bitter taste.

Benzodiazepines frequently induce sedation; however, paradoxical disinhibition has been observed.[44] These reactions are described as increased talkativeness, emotional release, hostility, impulsivity excitement, and excessive movement. Paradoxical reactions may occur in some patients with SUD when compared with other groups. Most paradoxical reactions are idiosyncratic.[44] However, there is evidence to suggest these reactions may occur secondary to a genetic link, history of alcohol abuse, or psychological disturbances.[44–46] Box 5.2 lists common adverse effects seen with benzodiazepines.

Box 5.2   Common Adverse Effects Seen with Benzodiazepines

- Oversedation
- Mild postprocedure amnesia
- Hypotension (IV administration)
- Respiratory depression
- Drowsiness
- Coordination–balance difficulties
- Paradoxical reactions

Clinical Consideration

Benzodiazepines should be used cautiously in patients with a history of alcohol or barbiturate addiction since the pharmacologic pathways for these agents *may* overlap and intense "cravings" may be provoked.

Flumazenil, or Romazicon®, is the reversal agent for benzodiazepines. Given via IV bolus, 0.2 mg (4–20 µg/kg) at rate of 0.2 mg/min, it is titrated to effect. The dental practitioners may repeat at 20 min intervals, if needed.[43] Lack of patient response after cumulative doses of above implies that the major cause of sedation is unlikely to be benzodiazepines.[7] Sublingual administration of flumazenil is extremely controversial. Few studies have been performed to evaluate its efficacy.[47] If multiple fluid boluses are given under the tongue it could cause the tongue to swell and obstruct the airway.[47]

Clinical Considerations

Practitioners should be aware that the half-life of flumazenil is generally shorter than the benzodiazepine that has been administered or taken by patients. Patients should be evaluated frequently for "relapse" of sedation or respiratory depression.

Caution should also be used when administering flumazenil to patients receiving chronic benzodiazepines, since complete reversal may induce significant withdrawal symptoms and possible seizures.

Opioids

Opioids produce analgesia, sedation, anxiolysis, and respiratory depression. Clinically, opioids are used as strong analgesics, for the relief of moderate to severe pain.[7] Opioid analgesics are divided into three categories: (1) opioid agonists, (2) opioid agonist–antagonist, and (3) opioid antagonists. Opioid agonists interact with the receptor (µ, κ, σ, and δ) and produce a physiologic change.[48,49] Opioid antagonists when bound produce no pharmacologic effect. Mixed agents produce characteristics of both. The receptor activated will determine the physiologic effect, which may include analgesia, sedation, euphoria, dysphoria, and respiratory depression.[49]

A number of opioid agonists are used for sedation (moderate and deep) in dentistry. Meperidine (Demerol®) was one of the commonly used opioids in dentistry. It has been replaced by newer, safer agents like fentanyl and morphine, which have fewer side effects.[7] Meperidine's anticholinergic properties caused increased heart rate, decreased secretions, and localized histamine release.[50] These properties are not seen with the newer agents.

Morphine is the gold standard, by which other opioid agonists are compared for strength. Morphine's relatively long duration of action makes it less desirable for outpatient dental surgery under sedation or anesthesia. However, fentanyl, 100 times more potent than morphine, is the opioid of choice owing to its rapid onset and short duration of action.[51] Analgesia and sedation are often immediate with IV fentanyl, with maximum effect seen in approximately 2–3 min.[51]

Relative contraindications to use of opioid agonists include: patients under the age of 2, pregnant patients, recent history of head trauma or CNS-related pathology, and monoamine oxidase inhibitors within past 14 days. Caution must be used in patients with renal or liver dysfunction. Decreased metabolism and clearance could result in opioid overdose.[7] Opioids also cause respiratory depression and stiff chest syndrome, which may result in hypoventilation and hypoxia. *Dental practitioners must be prepared to administer positive-pressure ventilation if they are using opioids for sedation.*

Opioids are reversed with a pure opioid antagonist, naloxone hydrochloride.[48] IV administration should result in rapid improvement of respiratory depression, and reversal of the sedative effects. Naloxone's duration of action is about 20–30 min; therefore, resedation is possible if long-acting agonists were used. Reversals should be administered with care to persons with known or suspected physical dependence on opioids. Abrupt or complete reversal may result in "acute abstinence syndrome."[7]

Opioid use and abuse is on the rise. Over the last several decades, self-reported lifetime use of heroin and nonmedical use of prescription opioids have increased.[2] Increased availability of highly addictive prescription opioids, which are readily available, make this a frequently abused drug.[2] When the SUD is opioid related, patients may present with increased tolerance, in withdrawal, or with other side effects/complications (such as hepatic dysfunction); see Box 5.3. Users of opioids are at increased risk for drug overdose, drug dependence, and mental health disorders. This group also has increased risk for developing blood-borne viral infections, either through sharing of injection equipment or unsafe sexual activities performed under the influence.[2] Common adverse effects of opioids are listed in Box 5.4.

Box 5.3   Signs of Opioid Withdrawal

- Elevated resting heart rate
- Diaphoresis (not accounted for by ambient temperature or activity)
- Restlessness (frequent shifting or extraneous movements)
- Mydriasis (greater than expected given ambient light)
- Bone or joint pain
- Rhinorrhea or lacrimation (not accounted for by cold symptoms or allergy)
- Nausea, vomiting, or diarrhea
- Tremor of outstretched hand
- Yawning
- Anxiety or irritability
- Piloerection

Box 5.4   Common Adverse Effects of Opioids

- Sedation
- Dry mouth
- Constipation
- Dizziness
- Hypotension (IV administration)
- Confusion

Chronic Pain or Opioid-Based Maintenance Programs

Methadone (Dolophine®), levo-α-acetyl-methadol (LAAM; ORLMM®), and buprenorphine (Buprenex®, Suboxone®) are opioids used for the treatment of opioid addictions. Methadone, available in oral solution, tablet, and injectable forms, is primarily used for narcotic addiction and chronic pain management.[7] Methadone maintenance helps relieve narcotic craving, suppress abstinence syndrome, and blocks the euphoric effects associated with opiates.[52] Buprenorphine is a semisynthetic opioid approved in 2002 for narcotic addiction. Like methadone and LAAM, it has a long half-life, but with less respiratory depression improving its safety profile and decreasing risk for fatal overdose.[2]

The chronic opioid abuser may present similarly to the chronic pain patient who has developed tolerance to opioids. *Dental practitioners may assume a 20–30% increase in opioids needed compared with the opiate naive patient.*[2] Dental practitioners should take advantage of cross-tolerance of receptors among the various opioid agents. Another strategy for dealing with tolerance is by adding nonopioid analgesics such as intravenous nonsteroidal anti-inflammatory drugs (ketorolac), centrally acting μ agonists (tramadol,) or α agonists (clonidine or dexmedetomidine). See Table 5.3. The NMDA inhibitor ketamine has also been shown to decrease chronic pain and be a useful adjunct in opiate-tolerant patients.[2] Management of acute pain in the chronic opioid pain patient or in patients in opioid maintenance programs for addiction is discussed in more detail in Chapters 3 and 4.

Ketamine

Ketamine hydrochloride, a dissociative anesthetic, is a noncompetitive NMDA receptor antagonist.[53] Patients appear awake, but unaware of, or dissociated from the

Table 5.3 Adjuvant Therapy for Opioid Abusers[2]

Ketamine	0.1–0.5 mg/kg IV bolus pre-incision followed by 0.1–0.5 mg/(kg h) infusion
Clonidine	0.3 µg/kg IV bolus pre-incision followed by 0.3 µg/(kg h) infusion
Ketorolac (Toradol)	30 mg IV every 6 h as needed[a]
Acetaminophen (Tylenol® or Ofirmev®)	PO or IV 650 mg every 4–6 h as needed[b]
Pregabalin (Lyrica®)	75–150 mg PO twice daily or 50–100 mg PO three times daily

[a]Nonsteroidal anti-inflammatory drugs increase risk for bleeding (decision to use must be made with surgical team).
[b]Do not exceed maximum daily dose; reduce dose if acetaminophen-containing opioid analgesics are also administered.

environment.[54] It is commonly used with pediatric anesthesia and older patients with developmental disorders. Routinely it is given with benzodiazepines to provide amnesia, and analgesia. Ketamine produces little to no respiratory depression, compared with benzodiazepines and opioids. However, it increases heart rate, blood pressure, and intracranial pressure and causes nystagmus and an incompetent gag reflex. Copious secretions are a result of ketamine administration and must be aggressively managed to prevent laryngospasm.[54] Many experts believe dental practitioners untrained in anesthesia should not administer ketamine.[7] There is no reversal agent for ketamine; therefore, the dental practitioner must be prepared to manage the patient and their level of sedation. Different states have different guidelines for the use of ketamine for sedation in the dental office.

Ketamine has emerged as a club drug, referred to as "special k" or "vitamin k."[55] Ketamine produces effects similar to phencyclidine (PCP). Individuals describe their experience with ketamine, also known as the "K-hole," as profound distortions in or complete loss of bodily awareness, with sensations of floating or falling, euphoria, and total loss of time perception.[55] Common adverse effects of ketamine are listed in Box 5.5.

Box 5.5 Common Adverse Effects of Ketamine

- Emergence reactions
- Increased salivation
- Fasciculations
- Hypotension
- Tachycardia

Propofol

Propofol is a non-benzodiazepine, non-barbiturate anesthetic, originally designed as an induction agent for general anesthesia.[56] It induces sleep through potentiation of the GABA receptor slowing the channel's closing time.[58] Propofol has received interest in outpatient venues because of its sedation properties.[58,59] When given at subhypnotic doses, it produces excellent sedation with minimal respiratory depression and a short recovery period. Propofol is not recommended in pediatric patients and should only be administered by dental practitioners with anesthesia training.[56] Common adverse effects of propofol are listed in Box 5.6.

Box 5.6 Common Adverse Effects of Propofol

- Hypotension
- Nausea
- Discolored urine
- Phlebitis
- Respiratory depression

Table 5.4	**H1 Antagonist Dosing (Adult Dosing)**
Diphenhydramine (Benadryl®)	20–50 mg PO, IV, IM (5 mg/(kg/day))
Hydroxyzine	25–50 mg PO 1 h prior to treatment (1 mg/(kg/day))

Antihistamines

Histamine (H1) blockers are used in the treatment of allergic reactions, drying of secretions, and mild anxiolysis/sedation (see Table 5.4). A side effect of the histamines is CNS depression or sedation (see Box 5.7).[60] Antihistamines carry a wide therapeutic window and high margin of safety, making them popular in sedation dentistry.[7] Hydroxyzine, a diphenylethane, is perhaps the most widely used antihistamine in pediatric dentistry.[61,62] It is used as a solo agent for management of patients with mild to moderate fear. Combinations of hydroxyzine and other drugs, such as meperidine and midazolam, are used for patients who require deeper levels of sedation.[63] Fatal overdose with antihistamines is extremely uncommon, and withdrawal from long-term use is not reported. Research shows that patients who chronically use generation H1 antihistamines may develop tolerance to the sedation produced by these drugs.[60]

Box 5.7   Common Adverse Effects of H1 Antagonists

- Anticholinergic (dry eyes, urinary retention, dry mouth, constipation)
- Sedation
- Confusion in geriatric patients

Antihistamines, like benzodiazepines, cause paradoxical reactions in young children, elderly adults with genetic predisposition, alcoholics, and individuals with psychiatric and/or personality disorders.[44] Patients with SUDs are at higher risk for the development of comorbid psychiatric conditions, which predispose to idiosyncratic reactions.[32] Therefore, management of the psychiatric illness may reduce the severity of the paradoxical reaction.

Alpha Agonists

Precedex®, or dexmedetomidine, is an α_2 agonist indicated for sedation. Because dexmedetomidine exerts its effects via the α_2-adrenoceptor, it has a different mechanism of action than its GABA-mimetics such as propofol or benzodiazepines.[64] The sedative effects of dexmedetomidine are mediated by subtype A of the α_2 adrenergic receptor, a G-protein-coupled receptor. Activation in the brain and spinal cord inhibits neuronal firing, causing hypotension, bradycardia, sedation, and analgesia. The presynaptic receptor inhibits the release of norepinephrine, terminating the propagation of pain signals. Postsynaptic activation of α_2 receptors inhibits sympathetic activity, which decreases blood pressure and heart rate. The highest densities of α_2 receptors are in the locus coeruleus, the predominant noradrenergic nucleus in the brain and an important modulator of vigilance. The hypnotic and sedative effects of α_2-adrenoceptor activation have been attributed to this site in the CNS.[65] Studies show the level of sedation with dexmedetomidine was comparable to that of midazolam and better than lorazepam.[66] It was also shown to have less delirium and tachycardia.[67] Another study appreciated dexmedetomidine for treatment of symptoms of distress intractable pain, agitation, and delirium.[68] In addition, dexmedetomidine is being used for patients with cocaine intoxication and overdose treating the deleterious cardiovascular effects.[69] Dexmedetomidine may offer a new paradigm in the pharmacologic management of patients with SUD. Further studies are warranted in patients with SUD.

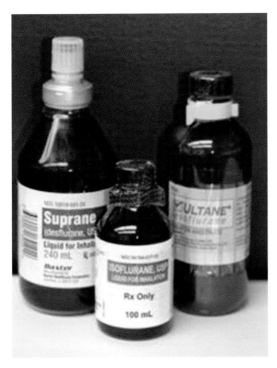

Figure 5.3 Inhalation anesthetics.

Inhalation Anesthetics and Neuromuscular Blocking Drugs

Inhalation anesthetics are the most frequent producers of general anesthesia.[7] The ideal agent should provide smooth induction and maintenance of general anesthesia, and be nontoxic to the organ systems. Sevoflurane, isoflurane, and desflurane are the mainstay of inhalation anesthetics (Figure 5.3).

Inhalation Agents

Muscle relaxants or neuromuscular blocking drugs provide skeletal muscle relaxation to facilitate tracheal intubation and mechanical ventilation.[7] There are two types of muscle relaxants: depolarizing muscle relaxants (succinylcholine) and nondepolarizing muscle

relaxants (e.g., atracurium, vecuronium, rocuronium, pancuronium). All neuromuscular blocking agents impair respiratory function and cause apnea; therefore, the dental practitioner must have training in general anesthesia. *General anesthesia provides optimal operating conditions. Patients with SUD who have extensive dental needs may benefit from a gas anesthetic either as an outpatient or in a hospital setting.*

Local Anesthetics

Local anesthetic agents should be administered with caution to patients with SUD. Local anesthetics are cardiac depressants and may cause CNS excitation or depression.[6] Therefore, it is paramount not to exceed the maximum allowable safe dosage.[6,70,71] Biotransformation of amide-type local anesthetics (articaine, bupivacaine, lidocaine, mepivacaine, prilocaine) is more complex than the ester type (cocaine, tetracaine, procaine, benzocaine).[72] Pseudocholinesterases in the plasma hydrolyze ester local anesthetics. Amides' primary site of biotransformation is the liver. Therefore, amide metabolism is significantly dependent upon liver function and hepatic perfusion. Patients with poor liver function (cirrhosis, severe hepatitis) and decreased hepatic perfusion (hypotension, congestive heart failure) may be unable to metabolize amide local anesthetics at a "normal" rate. Significant liver dysfunction and heart failure are "relative contraindications to the administration of amide local anesthetics."[71] Articaine, an amide local anesthetic, contains an additional ester group allowing it to be metabolized in the blood by the enzyme plasma cholinesterase, similar to ester anesthetics. The half-life of articaine is 20–30 min.[73] Because articaine can be hydrolyzed in the blood, the risk for overdose or intoxication is significantly less when compared with other amide-type local anesthetics.[72] Box 5.8 lists adverse reactions and complications with local anesthetics.

> **Box 5.8   Common Adverse Reactions or Complications to Local Anesthetics**
>
> - Hypersensitivity reactions
> - Vascular administration
> - Injection-site pain post procedure

> **Clinical Consideration**
>
> It is recommended that the dental practitioners calculate the dose (mg/kg) of local anesthetics prior to administration and administer slowly and with frequent aspiration to avoid possible intravascular injection.

The Concept of Balanced Anesthesia

Balanced anesthesia is a concept designed to allow dental practitioners to minimize risk and maximize comfort and safety. A balanced protocol requires individual assessment of the patient and the procedure. Balanced technique often uses concurrent mixtures of small amounts of several agents to summate in the desired level of sedation.

Monitoring and Documentation

Studies show that routine application of minimal monitors enable the detection of subtle physiologic changes, which permit measures to be taken before there is a catastrophic event.[74] A national standard now exists for intraoperative monitoring. As a rule of thumb, the deeper the sedation the more monitors should be used.

The following are excerpts from the AAPD and AAP guidelines on monitoring sedation.[6]

- **Moderate Conscious Sedation**
  Baseline. Before administration of sedative medications, a baseline determination

of vitals should be documented, for patients who are noncooperative or are very upset, this may not be possible, and a note should be written to document behavior.

During the Procedure. The dental practitioners should document the name, route, site, time of administration, and dosage of all drugs administered. There shall be continuous monitoring of oxygen saturation and heart rate and intermittent recording of respiratory rate and blood pressure; these should be recorded on a time-based record. Restraining devices should be checked to prevent airway obstruction or chest restriction. A functioning suction apparatus must be present.

After the Procedure. The patient who has received moderate sedation must be observed in a suitably equipped recovery facility (e.g., the facility must have functioning suction apparatus as well the capacity to deliver more than 90% oxygen and positive-pressure ventilation). The patient's vital signs should be recorded at specific intervals, until the patient meets discharge criteria or has completely returned to baseline status.

> **Clinical Consideration**
>
> If reversal agents have been used the patient will require a longer period of observation, because duration of the drugs administered may exceed the duration of the antagonist, which could lead to resedation or respiratory depression.

- **Deep Sedation.** The monitoring shall include all parameters as for moderate sedation. A competent provider shall observe the patient continuously. Vital signs, including oxygen saturation and heart rate, must be documented in a time-based record. Precordial stethoscope or capnography is encouraged for patients difficult to observe.[75,76]

Emergencies

The standards of care for sedation-related emergencies are the same as for any medical emergency. Recognition and action are the key steps to address the issue. Dental practitioners who treat using local anesthesia alone see syncope as a medical emergency. Dental practitioners who administer moderate sedation occasionally experience unconsciousness or apnea and should be prepared to treat the patient seamlessly. Deep sedation and general anesthesia render the patient unconscious, so apnea is a routine occurrence and would not be considered an emergency. What may be an emergency to one provider may be a normal occurrence to another.[7] Risk versus benefit analysis specific for the patient with SUD may help prevent medical emergencies. Dental practitioners should have a comfortable relationship with the patient and their medical providers, use familiar drugs and techniques, limit the use to patients who require them, have a comprehensive preop evaluation, and use continuous monitoring all in an effort to minimize sedation-related events. An emergency system should be in place with trained personnel who can follow the protocol. *High-risk patients should be managed in a hospital setting.*[6]

The selection of emergency drugs and an armamentarium should be based on the training and background of the dental practitioner who is responsible for its use. It is vital that the dental practitioner is familiar with indications, contraindications, dosages, and method of administration of emergency drugs and be able to correctly operate any available equipment.

Potential emergency situations include:[7]

1. Overdose.
2. Allergic reactions.
3. Hypotension/hypertension.
4. Cardiac arrhythmias.
5. Angina pectoris/acute myocardial infarction.
6. Airway obstruction.
7. Laryngospasm.
8. Foreign body aspiration.
9. Hyperventilation.
10. Respiratory depression.
11. Seizures.
12. Hypoglycemia.
13. Syncope.
14. Accidental induction of full opioid or alcohol withdrawal.

Once an emergency has been identified, it is important that everyone remain calm, assess the situation, and follow the PABCs[7]:

P: position—always position patient appropriately.

A: airway—assess to see if patient's airway is patent.

B: breathing—determine if patient is breathing.

C: circulation—check to see if there is a pulse.

D: definitive care—may include activation of emergency medical services and establishing IV access.

E: electricity—assess need.

Clinical Consideration

Respiratory events are a common cause of sedation-related emergencies in pediatric patients with normal cardiac function. Therefore, the dentist must have airway management skills and be proficient with positive-pressure ventilation (bag–valve–mask) with 100% oxygen. When airway issues are not addressed, the respiratory event could result in cardiac arrest.

Special Considerations

The ADA has a policy statement on The Provision of Dental Treatment for Patients with Substance Use Disorder.[1] The section in the fourth edition of the Diagnostic and Statistical Manual of Mental Disorders dealing with SUD describes 11 designated classes of pharmacological agents of abuse and dependence: alcohol, amphetamines or similarly acting agents, caffeine, cannabis, cocaine, hallucinogens, inhalants, nicotine, opioids, PCP or similar agents, and sedatives/hypnotics/anxiolytics.[77] Each substance provides a unique clinical challenge for the dental practitioner who must treat patients who are abusing these substances. Chapter 6 discusses individual substances of abuse in greater detail.

Alcohol dependence is a physiological dependence resulting in tolerance and/or withdrawal symptoms, such as tremor, weakness, sweating, and delirium tremens.[77,78] Patients with alcohol dependence are predisposed to liver disease. The first stage of liver disease is fatty liver, followed by acute or chronic hepatitis, and finally cirrhosis.[77,78] A cirrhotic liver is unable to perform normal function, such as metabolism of drugs, production of clotting factors (II, VII, IX, X), synthesis of bile, glycemic control, and detoxification.

The goal prior to treatment is optimization. For the recovered alcoholic there is a tight balance between too little and too much. Excess medications with addictive potential could provoke cravings for alcohol.[79]

Cannabis or marijuana is believed to be the most commonly used illegal drug in the USA.[80] However, a few states now allow medical use and recreational use of marijuana. Marijuana increases levels of the neurotransmitter dopamine, which creates the good feelings or "high" associated with its use. Smoking cannabis has been linked to cardiovascular disease. Studies show patients who use marijuana are at increased risk for atrial fibrillation, increased heart rate, and postural hypotension.[81] Older patients have reported angina after use due to cardiovascular changes, which lead to lack of oxygenated blood in cardiac muscle.[82] Using marijuana may also contribute to changes in the brain that have been associated with schizophrenia.[83]

Cocaine, the second most commonly used illicit drug in the USA, is an addictive stimulant.[80] Users often "binge." This is when cocaine is used repeatedly and at increasingly higher doses, leading to increased irritability, restlessness, panic attacks, and paranoia—even a full-blown psychosis, where the individual loses touch with reality and experiences auditory hallucinations.[84] Acute overdose with cocaine manifests itself as excitement, restlessness, confusion, tremor hypertension, tachycardia, tachypnea, nausea, vomiting, abdominal pain, and mydriasis.[71] Cocaine blocks the reuptake of norepinephrine and dopamine, causing increased catecholamines. Low doses of cocaine have been associated with vasoconstriction of coronary arteries.[85]

> **Clinical Consideration**
>
> Dental treatment should be postponed for a minimum of 6–24 h after the use of cocaine.[71] Use of epinephrine-containing vasoconstrictors is contraindicated for the cocaine abuser.[86]

Summary

Dental practitioners have many modalities to control pain and anxiety in patients with SUD. The method of choice should be based on risk versus benefit, the provider's comfort level and training, and the patient's needs. The challenge for patients with SUD is keeping a balance between enough and too much. This is accomplished by choosing agents that will not exacerbate the disorder or lead to relapse. There is no one correct method for each patient or provider. No panacea exists, nor is one technique going to work for every patient with SUD. Therefore, having multiple options for sedation will decrease risk of failure.

Disclaimer

This chapter is not intended to make you proficient in sedation for the patient with SUD. Information presented is based on *Guidelines* from the AAPD, ADA, AAP, and the ASA. Practitioners are required to know state guidelines before administering any type of sedation.

References

1. American Dental Association. Statement on Provision of Dental Treatment for Patients with Substance Use Disorders. 2005. http://www.ada.org/en/about-the-ada/ada-positions-policies-and-statements/provision-of-dental-treatment-for-patients-with-substance-abuse. Accessed December 30, 2014.

2. Bryson EO. The anesthetic implications of illicit opioid use. Int Anesthesiol Clin 2011;49(1):67–78.

3. American Dental Association, Council on Dental Education. Guidelines for the use of sedation and general anesthesia by dentists. 2012. http://www.ada.org/~/media/ADA/About%20the%20ADA/Files/anesthesia_use_guidelines.ashx. Accessed January 1, 2015.

4. American Dental Association, Council on Dental Education. Guidelines for teaching pain control and sedation in dentist and dental students. 2007. http://www.ada.org/~/media/ADA/Member%20Center/FIles/anxiety_guidelines.ashx. Accessed January 1, 2015.

5. American Society of Anesthesiologists Task Force on Sedation and Analgesia by Non-Anesthesiologists. Practice guidelines for sedation and analgesia by non-anesthesiologists. Anesthesiology 2002;96:1004–17.

6. American Academy of Pediatric Dentistry. Guidelines for Monitoring and Management of Pediatric Patients During and After Sedation for Diagnostic and Therapeutic Procedures. Pediatr Dent 2007–2008;29(7 Reference Manual):134–51.

7. Malamed, SF. Sedation: A Guide to Patient Management, 5th ed. 2010. Mosby Elsevier, St Louis, MO.

8. Harrison-Calmes S. Arthur Guedel, M.D., and the eye signs of anesthesia. Am Soc Anesthesiol Newsletter 2002;66(9):17–19.

9. Douglas BL. A re-evaluation of Guedel's stages of anesthesia: with particular reference to the ambulatory dental patient. J Am Dent Soc Anesthesiol 1958;5(1):11–14.

10. Kennedy RM, Luchman JD. The "ouchless emergency department." Getting closer: advances in decreasing distress during painful procedures in the emergency department. Pediatr Clin North Am 1999;46;1215–47.

11. Coté CJ, Notterman DS, Karl HW, Weinberg JA, McCloskey C. Adverse sedation events in pediatrics: a critical incident analysis of contributory factors. Pediatrics 2000;105:805–14.

12. Fleisher LA, Beckman JA, Brown KA, Calkins H, Chaikof EL, Fleischman KE, Freeman WK, Froehlich JB, Kasper EK, Kersten JR, Riegel B, Robb JF. ACC/AHA 2007 Guidelines on Perioperative Cardiovascular Evaluation and Care for Noncardiac Surgery: Executive Summary. Circulation 2007;116:1971–96.

13. Eagle KA, Berger PB, Calkins H, Chaitman BR, Ewy GA, Fleischmann KE, Fleisher LA, Froehlich JB, Gusberg RJ, Leppo JA, Ryan T, Schlant RC, Winters WL, Jr, Gibbons RJ, Antman EM, Alpert, JS Faxon DP, Fuster V, Gregoratos G, Jacobs AK, Hiratzka LF, Russell RO. Circulation 2002;105:1257–67.

14. American Society of Anesthesiologists. New classification of physical status. Anesthesiology 1963;24:111.

15. Fleisher LA. Risk of anesthesia. In: Miller's Anesthesia, 6th ed. Miller RD, Fleisher LA, Johns RA, eds. 2005. Elsevier/Churchill Livingstone, Philadelphia, PA, pp. 893–925.

16. Lagasse RS. Anesthesia safety: model of myth? A review of published literature and analysis of current original data. Anesthesiology 2002;97:1609–17.

17. Malviya S, Voepel-Lewis T, Tait AR. Adverse events and risk factors associated with the sedation of children by non-anesthesiologist. Anesth Analg 1997;85:1207–13.

18. Carr MP, Horton JE. Clinical evaluation and comparison of 2 topical anesthetics for pain caused by needle sticks and scaling and root planing. J Periodontol 2001;72(4):479–84.

19. Fukota O, Braham RL, Yanase H, Atsumi N, Kurosu K. The sedative effect of intranasal midazolam administration in the dental treatment of patients with mental disabilities. Part 1 the effect of 0.2 mg/kg dose. J Clin Pediatr Dent 1993;17(4):231–7.

20. Fuks AB, Kaufman E, Ram D, Hovav S, Shapira J. Assessment of two doses of intranasal midazolam for sedation of pediatric dental patients. Pediatr Dent 1994;16(4):301–5.

21. Lam C, Udin RD, Malamed SF, Good DL, Forrest JL. Midazolam premedication in children: a pilot study comparing intramuscular and intranasal administration. Anesth Prog 2005;52(2):56–61.

22. Walbergh EJ, Wills RJ, Eckhert J. Plasma concentrations of midazolam in children following intranasal administration. Anesthesiology 1991;74:233–5.

23. Jastak JT, Donaldson D. Nitrous oxide. Anesth Prog 1991;38(4–5);142–53.

24. Sinner B. Graf BM. Ketamine. Handb Exp Pharmacol 2008;(182):313–3.

25. Mace SE, Barata IA, Cravero JP, Dalsey WC, Godwin SA, Kennedy RM, Malley KC, Moss RL, Sacchetti AD, Warden CR, Wears RL. Clinical policy: evidence-based approach to pharmacologic agents used in pediatric sedation and analgesia in the emergency department. Ann Emerg Med 2004;44:342–77.

26. Deshpande JK, Tobias JD, eds. The Pediatric Pain Handbook. 1996. Mosby, St Louis, MO.

27. Alcaino EA. Conscious sedation in paediatric dentistry: current philosophies and techniques. Ann R Australas Coll Dent Surg 2000;15:206–10.

28. Yaster M, Krane EJ, Kaplan RF, Cote CJ, Lappe DG, eds. Pediatric Pain Management and Sedation Handbook. 1997. Mosby, St Louis, MO.

29. Cravero CH, Notterman DS, Karl HW, Weinberg JA, McCloskey C. Review of pediatric sedation. Anesth Analg 2004;99:1355–64.

30. Krauss B, Green SM. Procedural sedation and analgesia in children. Lancet 2006;367:766–80.

31. Mitchell AA, Louik C, Lacouture P, Slone D, Goldman P, Shapiro S. Risks to children from computed tomographic scan premedication. JAMA 1982;247:2385–8.

32. Antochi R, Stavarkaki C, Emery PC. Psychopharmacological treatments in persons with dual diagnosis of psychiatric disorders and developmental disabilities. Postgrad Med J 2003;79:139–46.

33. Yamakura T, Harris RA. Effects of gaseous anaesthetics nitrous oxide and xenon on ligand-gated ion channels. Comparison with isoflurane and ethanol. Anesthesiology 2000;93(4):1095–101.

34. Mennerick S, Jevtovic-Todorovic V, Todorovic SM, Shen W, Olney JW, Zorumski CF. Effect of nitrous oxide on excitatory and inhibitory synaptic transmission in hippocampal cultures. J Neurosci 1998;18(23):9716–26.

35. Emmanouil DE, Quock RM. Advances in Understanding the actions of nitrous oxide. Anesth Prog 2007;54(1):9–18.

36. Clark MS, Brunick AL. Handbook of Nitrous Oxide and Oxygen Sedation, 3rd ed. 2008. Mosby, St Louis, MO.

37. Gillman MA, Lichtigfeld FJ. Enlarged double-blind randomised trial of benzodiazepines against psychotropic analgesic nitrous oxide for alcohol withdrawal. Addict Behav 2004;29(6):1183–7.

38. Jastak JT, Orendruff D. Recovery from nitrous sedation. Anesth Prog 1975;22:113–6.

39. Parnis SJ, Foate JA, van der Walt JH, Short T, Crowe CE. Oral midazolam is an effective premedication for children having day-care anaesthesia. Anaesth Intensive Care 1992;20:9–14.

40. Feld LH, Negus JB, White PF. Oral midazolam preanesthetic drug in pediatric outpatients. Anesthesiology 1990;73:831–4.

41. Conner JT, Katz RL, Pagano RR, Graham CW. RO 21-3981 for intravenous surgical premedication, and induction of general anesthesia. Anesth Analg 1978;57:1–5.

42. Hennesy MJ, Kirby KC, Montgomery IM. Comparison of the amnesic effects of midazolam and diazepam. Psychopharmacology 1991;103:545–50.

43. Longmire AW, Seger DL. Topics in clinical pharmacology: flumazenil, a benzodiazepine antagonist. Am J Med Sci 1993;306:49–52.

44. Mancuso CE, Tanzi MG, Gabay M. Paradoxical reactions to benzodiazepines: literature review and treatment options. Pharmacotherapy 2004;24(9):1177–85.

45. Weinbroum AA, Szold O, Ogorek D, Flasishon R. The midazolam-induced paradox phenomenon is reversible by flumazenil: epidemiology, patient characteristics and review of the literature. Eur J Anaesthesiol 2001;18:789–97.

46. Short TG, Forrest P, Galletly DC. Paradoxical reactions to benzodiazepines: a genetically determined phenomenon? Anaesth Intens Care 1987;15:330–45.

47. Hosaka, K, Jackson D, Pickrell JE, Heima M, Milgrom P. Flumazenil reversal of sublingual triazolam: a randomized controlled clinical trial. J Am Dent Assoc 2009;140(5):559–66.

48. Martin WR. Naloxone. Ann Intern Med 1976;85:765–8.

49. Phillips WJ. Central nervous system pain receptors. In: Anesthesiology Review. Faust RJ, ed. 1991. Churchill Livingstone, New York.

50. Pallasch TJ. Clinical Drug Therapy in Dental Practice. 1973. Lea & Febiger, Philadelphia, PA.

51. Wedell D, Hersh EV. A review of the opioid analgesics, fentanyl, alfentanil and sufentanil. Compendium 1991;12:184–7.

52. Joseph H, Stancliff S, Langrod J. Methadone maintenance treatment (MMT): a review of historical and clinical issues. Mt Sinai J Med 2000; 67(5–6):347–64.

53. Reich DL, Silvay G. Ketamine: an update on the first twenty-five years of clinical experience. Can J Anaesth 1989;36:186–97.

54. Haas DA, Harper DG. Ketamine: a review of its pharmacologic properties and use in ambulatory anesthesia. Anesth Prog 1992;39:61–8.

55. Jansen K. Ketamine: Dreams and Realities. 2001. Multidisciplinary Association for Psychedelic Studies, Sarasota, FL, p. 55.

56. Diprivan. Drug Package Insert. 1992. Stuart Pharmaceuticals, Wilmington, DE.

57. Trapani G, Altomare C, Liso G, Sanna E, Biggio G. Propofol in anesthesia. Mechanism of action, structure–activity relationships, and drug delivery. Curr Med Chem 2000;7(2):249–71.

58. MacKenzie N, Grant IS. Propofol for intravenous sedation. Anaesthesia 1987;42:3–6.

59. MacKenzie N. Grant IS. Propofol infusion for sedation in the intensive care unit. Br Med J (Clin Res Ed) 1987;294:774.

60. Richardson GS, Roehrs TA, Rosenthal L, Koshorek G, Roth T. Tolerance to daytime sedative effects of H1 antihistamines. J Clin Psychopharmacol 2002;22(5):511–15.

61. Wright GZ, Chiasson RC. Current premedicating trends in pedodontics. ASDC J Dent Child 1973;40:185–7.

62. Wright GZ, Chiasson RC. The use of sedation drugs by Canadian pediatric dentists. Pediatr Dent 1987;9:308–11.

63. Torres-Pérez J, Tapia-García I, Rosales-Berber MA, Hernández-Sierra JF, Pozos-Guillén Ade J. Comparison of three conscious sedation regimens for pediatric dental patients. J Clin Pediatr Dent 2007;31(3):183–6.

64. Precedex. Drug Package Insert. 2012. Hospira, Inc: Lake Forest, IL.

65. Gertler R, Brown HC, Mitchell, DH, Silvius EN. Dexmedetomidine: a novel sedative-analgesic agent. Proc (Bayl Univ Med Cent) 2001;14(1):13–21.

66. Riker RR, Shehabi Y, Bokesch PM, Ceraso D, Wisemandle W, Koura F, Whitten P, Margolis BD, Byrne DW, Ely EW, Rocha MG. Dexmedetomidine vs Midazolam for sedation of critically ill patients: a randomized trial. JAMA 2009;301(5):489–99.

67. Pandharipande PP, Pun BT, Herr DL, Maze M, Girard TD, Miller RR, Shintani AK, Thompson JL Jackson JC, Deppen SA, Stiles RA, Dittus RS, Bernard GR, Ely EW. Effect of sedation with dexmedetomidine vs lorazepam on acute brain dysfunction in mechanically ventilated patients: the MENDS randomized controlled trial. JAMA 2007;298(22):2644–53.

68. Jackson KC, Wang Z, Wohlt P, Fine PG. Dexmedetomidine a novel analgesic with palliative medicine potential. J Pain Palliat Care Pharmacother 2006;20(2):23–7.

69. Menon DV, Wang Z, Fadel PJ, Arbique D, Leonard D, Li JL, Victor RG, Vongpatanasin W. Central sympatholysis as a novel countermeasure for cocaine-induced sympathetic activation and vasoconstriction in humans. J Am Coll Cardiol 2007;50(7):626–33.

70. Yagiela JA, Dowd FJ, Neidle EA. Local anesthetics. In: Pharmacology and Therapeutics for Dentistry. 2004. Elsevier Health Science, pp. 251–70.

71. Malamed SF. Local anesthetic considerations in dental specialties. In: Handbook of Local Anesthesia, 5th ed. 2004. Mosby, St Louis, MO, pp. 269, 274–5.

72. Moore PA, Hersh EV. Local anesthetics: pharmacology and toxicity. Dent Clin North Am 2010;54(4):587–99.

73. Oertel R, Ebert U, Rahn R, Kirch W. Clinical pharmacokinetics of articaine. Clin Pharmacokinet 1997;33(6):417–25.

74. Emergency Care Research Institute. Death during general anesthesia: technology-related, due to human error, or unavoidable? An ECRI technology assessment. J Health Care Technol 1985; 1:155–75.

75. Standards for basic intra-operative monitoring. ASA Newsletter 1986;50:13–15.

76. Hart LS, Berns SD, Houck CS Boenning DS. The value of end-tidal CO_2 monitoring when

comparing three methods of conscious sedation for children undergoing painful procedure in the emergency department. Pediatr Emerg Care 1997;13:189–93.

77. Diagnostic and Statistical Manual of Mental Disorders, 4th ed. 2000. American Psychiatric Publishing, Arlington, VA.

78. Friedlander AH, Marder SR, Pisegna JR, Yagiela JA. Alcohol abuse and dependence: psychopathology, medical management and dental implications. J Am Dent Assoc. 2003;134:731–40.

79. Lindroth JE, Herren MC, Falace DA. The management of acute dental pain in the recovering alcoholic. Oral Surg Oral Med Oral Pathol Oral Radiol Endod 2003;95(4):432–6.

80. Hughes, A, Sathe, N, Spagnola, K. State estimates of substance use from the 2005–2006 National Surveys on Drug Use and Health. DHHS Publication No. SMA 08-4311, NSDUH Series H-33. 2008. Substance Abuse and Mental Health Services Administration, Office of Applied Studies, Rockville, MD.

81. Korantzopoulos P, Liu T, Papaioannides D, Li G, Goudevenos JA. Atrial fibrillation and marijuana smoking. Int J Clin Pract 2008;62(2): 308–13.

82. Friedlander AH, Norman DC. Geriatric alcoholism: pathophysiology and dental implications. J Am Dent Assoc 2006;137:330–8.

83. Paul M. Marijuana users have abnormal brain structure and poor memory. Drug abuse appears to foster brain changes that resemble schizophrenia. 2013. Northwestern University. http://www.northwestern.edu/newscenter/stories/2013/12/marijuana-users-have-abnormal-brain-structure–poor-memory.html. Accessed December 31, 2014.

84. National Institute on Drug Abuse. Cocaine. 2013. http://www.drugabuse.gov/drugs-abuse/cocaine. Accessed January 9, 2015.

85. Lange RA, Cigarroa RG, Yancy CW, Jr, Willard JE, Popma JJ, Sills MN, McBride W, Kim AS, Hillis LD. Cocaine-induced coronary-artery vasoconstriction. N Engl J Med 1989;321:1557–62.

86. Maloney W. The significance of illicit drug use to dental practice. Webmed Central Dent Drug Abuse 2010;1(7):WMC00455.

Resources and Further Readings

ADA. Statement on the Use of Opioids in the Treatment of Dental Pain. http://www.ada.org/en/about-the-ada/ada-positions-policies-and-statements/statement-on-opioids-dental-pain. Accessed January 1, 2015.

ADA. Statement on Alcoholism and Other Substance Use Disorders. http://www.ada.org/en/about-the-ada/ada-positions-policies-and-statements/alcoholism-and-substance-use-disorders. Accessed January 1, 2015.

ADA. Statement on Provision of Dental Treatment for Patients with Substance Use Disorders. http://www.ada.org/en/about-the-ada/ada-positions-policies-and-statements/provision-of-dental-treatment-for-patients-with-substance-abuse. Accessed January 1, 2015.

dentalcare.com. Designing a Comprehensive Health History. http://www.dentalcare.com/en-US/dental-education/continuing-education/ce76/ce76.aspx?ModuleName=coursecontent&PartID=5&SectionID=-1. Accessed January 1, 2015.

DHEd. ASA Physical Status Classification System (for Dental Patient Care). http://www.dhed.net/ASA_Physical_Status_Classification_SYSTEM.html. Accessed January 1, 2015.

Common Substances and Medications of Abuse

William J. Maloney, DDS and George F. Raymond, DDS

Introduction

Substance use disorder (SUD) has a significant impact on the practice of dentistry regardless of the age or socioeconomic status of the patient population. There is a wide range of dental-related problems associated with SUD. Dental practitioners must be able to evaluate the causal link between an individual's SUD and both educate the patient as to the detrimental effects of substance abuse and misuse and provide appropriate dental therapies to combat its dental and oral effects. Additionally, certain modifications to dental procedures must, at times, be made in order to ensure the safe and effective treatment of both pain and dental/oral disease in patients with SUD. In order to provide safe and effective dental care, a thorough and complete medical history must be taken. Dental professionals should provide patients with education, interventions, and referrals when SUD is suspected.

Definitions

Drug Misuse

Drug misuse is defined as taking a prescription or over-the-counter (OTC) medication for nonprescribed purposes, in excessive doses, at shorter intervals than prescribed or recommended or for reasons other than the original intent of the prescription. Examples include doubling the dosage, shortening dosing intervals, or treating disorders for which the medication was not prescribed.

Opiates and Opioids

Opiates refer to natural substances derived from the poppy plant. Opioids function in a similar manner to opiates but are either synthetic or partially synthetic derivatives of opiates.

The ADA Practical Guide to Substance Use Disorders and Safe Prescribing, First Edition. Edited by Michael O'Neil.
© 2015 American Dental Association. Published 2015 by John Wiley & Sons, Inc.

For the purpose of this text, the term opioid will be used interchangeably for opiate.

Prescription Drug Abuse

Prescription drug abuse is the intentional use of a medication without a prescription in a way other than as prescribed, as well as for the experience or feeling that it can cause.[1]

Substance Abuse

Substance abuse is a maladaptive pattern of chemical use (e.g., alcohol, medications, marijuana, cocaine, solvents, etc.) leading to clinically significant impairment or distress, as manifested by one (or more) of the following, occurring within a 12-month period:

- Recurrent chemical use resulting in a failure to fulfill major role obligations at work, school, or home
- Recurrent chemical use in situations in which it is physically hazardous
- Recurrent chemically-related legal problems
- Continued chemical use despite having persistent or recurrent social or interpersonal problems caused by or exacerbated by the effects of the chemical.[2]

Substance Use Disorder

In May 2013, The American Psychiatric Association redefined terminology previously used in the Diagnostic and Statistical Manual of Mental Disorders Text Revision (DSM-IV-TR) guidelines regarding diagnostic classifications of Substance Dependence and Substance Abuse Disorders. SUD in Diagnostic and Statistical Manual of Mental Disorders DSM-5 combines the DSM-IV-TR categories of substance abuse, substance dependence, and addiction disorders into a single disorder measured on a continuum from mild to severe. Nearly all SUDs are diagnosed based on the same overarching criteria. In this overarching disorder, the criteria have

not only been combined but strengthened. Whereas a diagnosis of substance abuse previously required only one symptom, mild SUD in DSM-5 requires two to three symptoms from a list of 11 (see Box 6.1).[3]

> **Box 6.1   SUD Symptoms List[3]**
>
> - Taking the substance in larger amounts or for longer than you meant to take it.
> - Wanting to cut down or stop using the substance but not managing to be successful.
> - Spending a lot of time getting, using, or recovering from use of the substance.
> - Cravings and urges to use the substance.
> - Not managing to do what you should at work, home, or school because of substance use.
> - Continuing to use, even when it causes problems in relationships.
> - Giving up important social, occupational, or recreational activities because of substance use.
> - Using substances again and again, even when it puts you in danger.
> - Continuing to use, even when you know you have a physical or psychological problem that could have been caused or made worse by the substance.
> - Needing more of the substance to get the effect you want (tolerance).
> - Development of withdrawal symptoms, which can be relieved by taking more of the substance.

Tolerance

Tolerance is a state in which either an organism no longer responds to a drug or a higher dose of the drug is required to achieve the same effect.[4]

Visual Analog Pain Scale

The visual analog pain scale (VAPS) is a 10 cm baseline scale containing the words "no pain" on the far left of the line and "pain as bad as it could possibly be" on the far right of the line. This tool enables the patient to make a mark in order to visually indicate the level of pain which they are experiencing.[5]

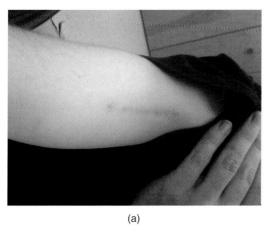

(a)

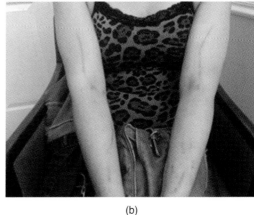

(b)

Figure 6.1 Intravenous track marks.

For the purposes of this book, the terms psychological or psychiatric dependency, addiction, and substance use disorder will be used interchangeably.

The psychological and social aspects of various substances of abuse are nearly the same.

For the purposes of this book the terms chemical, medication, drug, substance, chemical substance, or illicit substances will be used interchangeably. Differences are only likely to occur based on federal and state classifications or medically accepted use.

Signs and Symptoms of Substance Use Disorder

Individuals with SUD may exhibit certain signs and symptoms. It is important to note that solely because an individual exhibits one or more of the symptoms of drug use, it does not definitely mean that they are misusing or abusing drugs. The symptoms may be due to mental issues, a result of a medical condition, or appropriately prescribed medications. Common signs include a change in the individual's physical appearance, behavior, personality, or attitude. Physical signs or symptoms of substance abuse include unusual laziness, change in appetite, unusual body odors, needle marks (Figure 6.1),

or deterioration in the individual's general appearance and cleanliness. Other behavioral signs are frequently present. These include an unexplained need for money, secretive behavior, paranoia, and a lack of motivation.[6] For dental practitioners who see patients who are previously unknown and only for a brief amount of time, lifestyle changes or appearance changes are usually unknown. More telling signs or behaviors may be more clinically relevant to dental practitioners and will be mentioned later with each class of abused substances where clinically relevant.

Clinical Consideration

Dental practitioners are often concerned about ruining the doctor–patient relationship when asking about SUD. Beginning the interview with statements such as "I want to ask you a few personal questions. My intent is to optimize your dental treatment not judge you or deny treatment." Or, "I have a couple of questions I need to ask to make sure there are not any life-threatening drug interactions with your dental treatment. Regardless of your answers, my intent is not to judge you, deny you treatment, or to notify law enforcement."

Putting the patient's mind at ease before you start treatment can be a very effective tool.

Common Substances of Abuse

Stimulants

Stimulants are generally characterized as causing increased energy, wakefulness, focus, or physiological functioning. Illicit stimulants refer to traditional "street drugs," such as methamphetamine or cocaine. Illicit stimulants can be very addictive. Some signs and symptoms of the use of illicit stimulants include racing of the heart, increase in energy, elevated mood, euphoria, insomnia, weight loss, loss of appetite, increase in sexual activity, and participation in criminal activity.[7] Commonly used stimulants are discussed in depth in the following subsections. Table 6.1 lists individual and summary information for stimulants that are commonly abused, patients' physical examination findings, and treatment considerations.

Methamphetamine

Methamphetamine's relatively low financial cost and ease of producing in the community using simple chemistry skills, coupled with its long "high," makes this stimulant very popular among abusers. The high period is characterized by an increased sense of well-being, increased energy levels, heightened libido, and appetite suppression.[8,9] Methamphetamine causes dopamine and norepinephrine to be released into the synapse in the prefrontal cortex, the nucleus accumbens, and the striatum.[10] Methamphetamine is used by snorting, injecting, or smoking/inhaling the powder. Various toxic and corrosive ingredients are used in methamphetamine's manufacturing process. These include iodine, red phosphorus, ether, anhydrous ammonia, hydrochloric acid, and pseudoephedrine. The typical pattern of decay in methamphetamine users can be seen in the buccal smooth surfaces of the teeth and the interproximal surfaces of anterior teeth.[11–13]

Methamphetamine users have higher rates of dental disease than the general population.[14]

Users who inject methamphetamine actually have a higher rate of dental disease than those who either smoke or inhale it.[14] This may be due in part to the severity of addiction, although this has not been confirmed. Dental manifestations of methamphetamine use have been referred to as "meth mouth."[15,16] The characteristic dental appearance of individuals with meth mouth has been described as blackened, rotting, stained, or crumbling teeth.[14,17] The dental effects of methamphetamine can be particularly severe due, in part, to the drug's pharmacological effects and its duration of action, which may be up to 24 h.[18,19] Xerostomia, clenching of the teeth,[20] and occlusal wear are also common dental findings in these individuals. In addition, methamphetamine users often consume large quantities of acidic soft drinks, which contributes to dental caries and tooth erosion. Careful attention must be given to the methamphetamine user's periodontal condition, as methamphetamine reduces blood flow to the periodontal structures.[21] The application of topical fluorides, the management of xerostomic conditions, and use of occlusal guards are strongly recommended. It is prudent for dental practitioners to consult with the patient's physician prior to prescribing any analgesics,[22] and caution must be exercised when administering nitrous oxide. The methamphetamine user is at an increased risk for myocardial infarction, cerebrovascular accidents, hypertension, and cardiac dysrhythmias.[23–27] Therefore, local anesthetics and retraction cords *without* vasoconstrictors should be utilized (see Tables 6.1 and 6.2).

Cocaine

Cocaine is an addictive stimulant made from the leaves of the coca plant native to South America. Cocaine can be inhaled through the nose, smoked in the form of "crack," or injected. The duration of cocaine's pleasurable effects can last up to 30 min, depending on its route of administration. Cocaine's effects are caused

Table 6.1 Clinical Findings and Treatment Considerations of Commonly Abused Substances

Abused substances	Psychiatric signs and symptoms	Dental findings	Other physical examination findings	Treatment considerations[a]
Methamphetamine, synthetic cathinones ("bath salts"), and prescription stimulants	• Euphoria • Hyperactivity • Paranoia • Dissociation • Insomnia	• Xerostomia • Black rotting teeth • Occlusal wear • Mass caries • Bruxism • Nasal septal necrosis • Powder in nares • Clear mucus discharge from nostrils	• Formication/picking • Track marks • Open or scabbed skin lesions • Cachexia • Burnt fingers • Profound weight loss • Tachycardia • Skin abscess	• Avoid injection or use of local epinephrine products • Occlusive guards • Xerostomia treatment products • Topical fluoride treatments • Avoid treatment at least 24 h from last "use" if possible
Cocaine	• Euphoria • Paranoia • Dissociation • Insomnia	• Xerostomia • Occlusal wear • Mass caries • Bruxism	• Open or scabbed skin lesions • Track marks • Nasal septal necrosis • Powder in nares • Profound weight loss • Dilated pupils • Tachycardia • Skin abscess	• Avoid injection or use of local epinephrine products • Occlusive guards • Xerostomia treatment products • Topical fluoride treatments • Avoid treatment at least 12 h from last "use" if possible
Lysergic acid diethylamide (LSD), phencyclidine (PCP), mescaline	• Euphoria • Hyperactivity • Dissociation • Insomnia • Paranoia • Agitation • Delusions • Hallucinations • Panic reactions	• Xerostomia • Occlusal wear • Mass caries • Bruxism	• Dilated pupils • Slurred speech • Confusion • Tachycardia	• Xerostomia treatment products • Occlusal guards • Topical fluoride treatments • Avoid treatment at least 12 h from last "use" if possible

(continued)

Table 6.1 (Continued)

Abused substances	Psychiatric signs and symptoms	Dental findings	Other physical examination findings	Treatment considerations[a]
3,4-Methylenedioxy-methamphetamine (MDMA)	• Psychotic episodes • Depression • Impulsive behavior • Panic reactions • Dissociation • Euphoria	• Jaw-clenching • Jaw soreness • Xerostomia • Occlusal wear • Mass caries • Bruxism	• Dehydration • Dilated pupils • Excessive sweating • Tachycardia	• Avoid injection or use of local epinephrine products • Occlusive guards • Xerostomia treatment products • Topical fluoride treatments • Avoid treatment at least 24 h from last "use" if possible
Heroin, opium, and prescription opioids	• Euphoria • Sedation • Dissociation • Delusions • Hallucinations • Slurred speech • Track marks	• Xerostomia • Occlusal wear • Mass caries • Bruxism	• Track marks (Figure 6.1) • Skin erosions • Staph sores over skin • Dilated/pinpoint pupils • Goose flesh • Piloerection • Yawning • Formification	• Xerostomia treatment products • Occlusal guards • Topical fluoride treatments • Avoid treatment at least 12 h from last "use" if possible • Evaluate patients for recent treatment with naltrexone for opioid addiction (especially IM products) to optimize analgesia
Solvents/paints	• Euphoria • Hyperactivity • Dissociation • Insomnia • Paranoia • Tachycardia • Agitation • Delusions • Hallucinations • Panic reactions	• Paint residue around nose, mouth, teeth, tongue • Redness or irritation around nose, mouth, teeth	• Confusion • Lethargy • Memory lapses • Strong odor of solvents or paints • Tachycardia • Slurred speech	• Delay treatments at least 12 h when possible

Abused substances	Psychiatric signs and symptoms	Dental findings	Other physical examination findings	Treatment considerations[a]
Marijuana and δ-9-tetrahydrocannabinol (THC) (including synthetics)	• Euphoria • Hyperactivity • Dissociation • Tachycardia • Paranoia • Delusions • Hallucinations	• Xerostomia • Gingivitis • Alveolar bone loss • Gingival leukoplakia • Gingivitis • Increased caries	• Poor coordination • Irritated conjunctiva	• Avoid injection or use of local epinephrine products • Occlusive guards • Xerostomia treatment products • Occlusal guards • Topical fluoride treatments • Avoid treatment at least 12 h from last acute event
Alcohol (ethyl alcohol or ethanol)	• Euphoria • Hyperactivity • Loss of inhibition • Excessive talking • Poor gait • Slurred speech • Overt odor of alcohol • Nystagmus • Confusion • Coagulopathies • Sedation	• Angular cheilitis • Jaundice • Overt smell of alcohol • Bilateral parotid swelling • Red nose • Spider petechiae on nose	• Confusion • Lethargy • Memory lapses • Slurred speech • Poor coordination • Poor balance • Nystagmus	• Caution with local (e.g., lidocaine) or systemic anesthetics in patients with end-stage liver disease • Patients could be receiving naltrexone that can block effects of opioids

[a]In all patients with suspected SUD, counseling or treatment referrals to specialist involved with substance abuse is recommended. Patients with known or suspected intravenous (IV) drug abuse should also be referred to a medical practitioner for acquired immunodeficiency syndrome (AIDS) and hepatitis testing.

Table 6.2   Dental Considerations for "Active" Methamphetamine Abusers

Signs/symptoms	Routes of administration	Common dental findings	Special dental treatment
• Euphoria • Hyperactivity • Paranoia • Dissociation • Tachycardia • Insomnia • Profound weight loss • Track marks	• IV • Inhalation • Snorting	• Severe xerostomia • Black rotting teeth • Occlusal wear • Mass caries • Bruxism	• Avoid injection or topical epinephrine products • Occlusive guards • Xerostomia treatment products • Topical fluoride treatments • Avoid treatment at least 24 h from last "use" if possible

by its actions on the brain's limbic system. There is an initial buildup of the neurochemical dopamine, which gives rise to euphoria.[28] Cocaine blocks uptake by neuronal plasma membrane transporters for dopamine, serotonin, and norepinephrine.[29] Some signs of cocaine abuse include hyperactivity, euphoria, dilated pupils, xerostomia, irritability, and weight loss.[6]

There are a plethora of dental effects from cocaine use. They include gingival lesions, an increased rate of periodontal disease, bruxism, an increased rate of tooth decay, cervical abrasions, excessive hemorrhage after tooth extraction, occlusal wear, and corrosion of dental restorations.[30–36] The tarnishing of gold crowns is seen in crack users due to a decrease in salivary pH.[30] Cervical abrasions are thought to be due to excessive and vigorous toothbrushing.[37] Additionally, there are many intraoral/craniofacial manifestations of cocaine abuse of which dental practitioners must be aware. They include erosive lichen planus, oral candida infections, halitosis, nasal necrosis, angular cheilitis, headaches, xerostomia, and oral ulcers.[30–36,38] There are many modifications to treatment that are deemed necessary in treating cocaine-using dental patients. The primary cause of concern is the vasoconstriction activity of cocaine. The use of local anesthetics with epinephrine or retraction cords, which

are impregnated with epinephrine, may place an individual who has recently used cocaine at an increased medical risk during dental treatment. Therefore, dental treatment should be postponed at least 12–24 h after cocaine use[39] (see Tables 6.1 and 6.3).

Khat

Khat, or qat, is a leafy shrub that originated in Ethiopia. Khat leaves are found on the *Catha edulis* plant and are very popular in Yemeni and Somali societies. Khat produces euphoria, stimulation, and alertness. It has a natural amphetamine known as cathinone. Khat leaves are either chewed or stored in the mouth between the molars and the cheek.[40] Khat is second only to marijuana in total pounds seized throughout the USA by US customs agents.[41] Its use is associated with Middle Eastern or Mediterranean cultures. There are many dental and oral manifestations of khat use. Khat chewing appears to be associated with periodontal loss and gingival recession at the site of chewing. The development of mucosal white lesions and dark pigmentation can occur due to chemical and mechanical irritation.[42] Oral ulcers, gingival bleeding, an oral burning sensation, difficulty in swallowing, and difficulty in opening the mouth have also been noted in users of khat[43] (see Table 6.4).

Table 6.3   Dental Considerations for "Active" Cocaine Abusers

Signs/symptoms	Routes of administration	Common dental findings	Special dental treatment
• Euphoria • Paranoia • Dissociation • Tachycardia • Insomnia • Profound weight loss • Dilated pupils • Track marks	• IV • Inhalation • Snorting	• Severe xerostomia • Occlusal wear • Mass caries • Bruxism	• Avoid injection or topical epinephrine products • Occlusive guards • Xerostomia treatment products • Topical fluoride treatments • Avoid treatment at least 12 h from last "use" if possible

Synthetic Cathinones

Synthetic cathinones are often referred to as "bath salts" and are a family of drugs that may contain one or more synthetic chemicals structurally related to cathinones or other amphetamines. This white or brown crystalline powder should not be confused with legitimate products meant to be used for bathing purposes, as the legitimate products have no psychoactive properties. Synthetic cathinones are derivatives of a naturally occurring β-ketone amphetamine analogue, which is found in the leaves of the *Catha edulis* plant.[44] Systemic effects of synthetic cathinones include euphoria, increased sex drive, paranoia, bizarre behavior, muscle rigidity, hyperthermia, hypertension, dysrhythmia, and agitation. Deaths have also been reported.[45] Dental practitioners should be aware of the adverse cardiac and neurological effects in synthetic cathinone abusers (see Tables 6.1 and 6.5).

> **Clinical Consideration**
>
> Dental practitioners should avoid using epinephrine-containing products with active stimulant abusers owing to possible additive effects of the stimulant–epinephrine combination that may lead to cardiac distress or hypertension.

Hallucinogens

Hallucinogens are produced from various plants and mushrooms. Hallucinogens make up the largest and most pharmacologically

Table 6.4   Dental Considerations for "Active" Khat Abusers

Signs/ symptoms	Routes of administration	Common dental findings	Special dental treatment
• Euphoria • Hyperactivity • Dissociation • Tachycardia • Insomnia	• Inhalation • Snorting • Oral (chewing) • Buccal	• Xerostomia • Occlusal wear • Mass caries • Bruxism	• Avoid injection or topical epinephrine products • Occlusive guards • Xerostomia treatment products • Topical fluoride treatments • Avoid treatment at least 24 hours from last "use" if possible

Table 6.5   Dental Considerations for Active "Synthetic Cathinones" Abusers

Signs/ symptoms	Routes of administration	Common dental findings	Special dental treatment
• Euphoria • Hyperactivity • Dissociation • Tachycardia • Insomnia • Paranoia • Tachycardia • Agitation • Delusions • Hallucinations	• Inhalation • Snorting • Oral • Rectal • Injection	• Xerostomia • Occlusal wear • Mass caries • Bruxism	• Avoid injection or topical epinephrine products • Occlusive guards • Xerostomia treatment products • Topical fluoride treatments • Avoid treatment at least 24 h from last "use" if possible

diverse group of abused substances. Their effects vary greatly among different people at different times and with different doses. Hallucinogens are known to activate 5-HT2A receptors in the brain that are normally triggered by serotonin. Some signs that an individual is using a hallucinogen include dilated pupils, bizarre behavior, hallucinations, mood swings, slurred speech, and confusion.[6]

Oral lesions specifically related to LSD, mescaline, PCP, psilocybin, and MDMA are generally rare or difficult to clinically diagnose due to multiple factors, including the method of abuse, drying of the mouth or pH changes from smoking, topical irritation due to the specific substance, abuse of multiple substances, or concurrent diseases (see Table 6.6).

Lysergic Acid Diethylamide, Mescaline, Phencyclidine

LSD, mescaline (peyote), and PCP are the most common hallucinogens. The use of hallucinogens does not generally result in physiologic withdrawal symptoms. The effects of these hallucinogens may last between 1 and 12 h. It is important for dental professionals to be cognizant of the fact that users might exhibit extreme excitement, bizarre behavior, or a panic reaction.[46] LSD is the most available

hallucinogen. The route of administration of LSD is usually oral, buccal, or sublingual, but it can also be inhaled, transdermally applied, and injected. It is usually found absorbed into tiny papers known as "blotters," and it can be found in a pure liquid form or absorbed into food or sugar cubes.[47] The onset of action of LSD is within 10 min following IV administration. After oral ingestion, effects are felt within 30 min. These effects from LSD can last up to 8 h[48] (see Tables 6.1 and 6.6).

Psilocybin

Psilocybin is a hallucinogen that is obtained from various mushrooms that are grown in subtropical and tropical climates. Psilocybin is usually taken orally or smoked, and onset of effects occurs within 20 min of ingestion. These effects may last up to 6 h (see Table 6.6).

3,4-Methylenedioxymethamphetamine

MDMA, most commonly known as "ecstasy," is a drug of abuse that is used by many young individuals in urban areas as part of the "rave" or nightclub scene. It is an illegal designer drug sometimes referred to as the "love drug." MDMA is both a stimulant and a mild calming substance.[49] It is a powerful releaser of serotonin, an indolamine neurotransmitter. To a lesser degree, MDMA is also a

Table 6.6   Dental Considerations for "Active" Hallucinogen Abusers

Signs/ symptoms	Routes of administration[a]	Common dental findings	Special dental treatment
• Euphoria • Hyperactivity • Dissociation • Tachycardia • Insomnia • Paranoia • Tachycardia • Agitation • Delusions • Hallucinations • Slurred speech • Panic reactions	• Inhalation • Snorting • Oral • Rectal • Injection • Sublingual	• Xerostomia • Occlusal wear • Mass caries • Bruxism	• Xerostomia treatment products • Occlusal guards • Topical fluoride treatments • Avoid treatment at least 12 h from last "'use" if possible

[a]Routes of administration vary significantly and are substance specific.

releaser of dopamine, a neurotransmitter, into the nervous system.[50–54] MDMA's neurochemical actions result in the user having certain psychoactive properties[50–54] and in experiencing a relaxed, euphoric state, increased empathy, and a loss of inhibitions.[50–54] Dental practitioners must not only be concerned with the physical effects of MDMA but also its behavioral aspects, which might interfere with the delivery of dental care. Psychotic episodes, depression, impulsive behavior, and panic disorders have been reported in individuals using MDMA.[55] The dental effects of MDMA are numerous. Users often experience jaw-clenching and jaw soreness. This leads to increased wear of the molars and premolars. MDMA abuse is associated with dehydration, which can result in the consumption of a large number of carbonated or acidic beverages. The dental effects are enamel erosion and an increase in tooth decay.[56]

Dental practitioners must also be concerned about the occurrence of nausea and vomiting, which is common after using MDMA.[57] The stomach acids increase tooth erosion, necessitating that dental practitioners consider the use of various fluoride applications to control the rate of tooth decay and hypersensitivity. Occlusal guards are also indicated in individuals who exhibit signs of occlusal wear. Substances containing alcohol should be avoided, as xerostomia is a common side effect of MDMA use. Systemic effects of MDMA use include sleep problems, memory loss, nausea, blurred vision, rapid eye movement, fainting, muscle breakdown, heart failure, kidney failure, and skin rash.

MDMA can last for up to 16 h in the user's body. It has other pharmacological properties similar to stimulants. Dental considerations for MDMA abusers should also include precautions listed for stimulants (see Box 6.2 and Tables 6.1 and 6.6).

Box 6.2   Systemic Effects of MDMA[50,53,54,58–62]

- Hyperthermia
- Increased heart rate
- Cardiac arrhythmias
- Renal failure
- Intracranial hemorrhage
- Increased activation of hypothalamic–pituitary–adrenal axis
- Suppression of circulating lymphocyte numbers

Salvia divinorum

Salvia divinorum is a perennial herb in the mint family that is native to the Sierra Mazateca region of Mexico. Its hallucinogenic effects are due to an ingredient known as salvinorin A, which is a powerful κ opioid receptor agonist. *S. divinorum* can be smoked, chewed, or brewed in teas. When chewed, the leaf and juice are kept in the cheek area, with absorption occurring across the lining of the buccal mucosa.[63] The high achieved by the abuser is sometimes characterized as a very spiritual experience. Its use is associated with Native American cultures in the southwest or in young teens experimenting with hallucinogens. Abusers of *S. divinorum* may have oral mucosal changes similar to those associated with chewing tobacco (see Table 6.6).[64]

> **Clinical Consideration**
>
> With the exception of MDMA, the duration of effect of hallucinogens is usually a few hours. Clinical detection of abuse is often very difficult.

Opioids: Heroin and Opium

Heroin and opium are highly addictive illicit drugs. Opium, the dried extract from the poppy plant, contains several alkaloids, including heroin, morphine, and codeine, while heroin is processed from morphine.[65] Effects of opium are similar to heroin, although it is predominately smoked versus injected and generally less available in the USA than heroin. Traditionally, heroin abuse has been more commonly found in large metropolitan areas than in rural areas. The strict regulation of prescription opioids and the high street "cost" of prescription opioids have created an explosive surge of heroin abuse throughout all communities. The "cheaper" heroin products, increased heroin availability, and "better high"

from heroin have also been associated with the surge of heroin abuse.

Heroin undergoes rapid deacetylation to 6-acetylmorphine (6-AM) and, subsequently, morphine. Both 6-AM and morphine are active metabolites.[66] The most common mode of heroin use is IV administration. Recently, sniffing and smoking have become very popular routes of administration.[67] Heroin binds to the endogenous opiate receptors, which are located throughout the body and, unlike morphine, can cross the blood–brain barrier very easily.[68] The initial effects of heroin, when injected, are felt within minutes.

The dental/oral effects of heroin use include periodontitis, increased risk of caries, bruxism,[69] oral fungal and viral infections,[70] poor oral hygiene, anxiety surrounding dental treatment, and hyperpigmentation of the tongue[71] (Figures 6.2, 6.3, and 6.4). The increase in dental caries is thought to be due to the user's intense craving for sweets.[72–76] Central nervous system (CNS) depressants, such as benzodiazepines, sedative hypnotics, general anesthetics, barbiturates, MAO inhibitors, antihistamines, and tricyclic antidepressants, have the ability to produce respiratory depression, hypotension, coma, and profound sedation in heroin users.[77] Heroin users may have

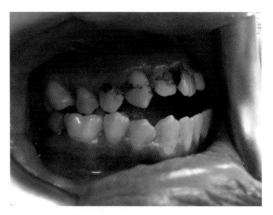

Figure 6.2 The dentition of a recovering heroin abuser. These individuals often exhibit a high rate of dental caries.

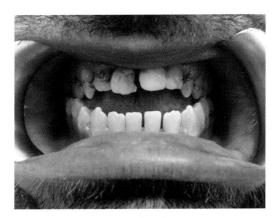

Figure 6.3   An individualized preventive regimen is of paramount importance. Regular recall visits and various fluoride therapies should be included.

developed a tolerance to the effects of CNS-depressant drugs, which may pose a problem in the dental setting in circumstances in which certain anesthetic agents are usually utilized. An individualized preventive regimen[78] should be implemented, with the possible inclusion of various fluoride products, sialagogues, bite splints, dietary advice, regular recall appointments, and antifungal medications (see Table 6.1).

Physiologic withdrawal for most heroin addicts is predictable. Classic signs include

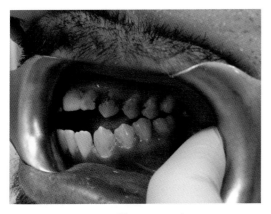

Figure 6.4   Poor oral hygiene and anxiousness surrounding dental treatment is common among illicit drug abusers.

severe nausea, vomiting, diarrhea, piloerection, "goose bumps," diaphoresis, dilated pupils, and yawning. Many patients may receive chronic treatment with naltrexone to decrease the cravings for opioids (see Tables 6.1 and 6.7). Dental practitioners should be aware of naltrexone products and the potential for blocking necessary analgesia. This information is discussed in greater detail in Chapter 4.

> **Clinical Consideration**
>
> Unless otherwise clinically indicated, dental procedures should be postponed until withdrawal symptoms are appropriately managed due to increased risk of complications.

Inhalants

Inhalant abuse refers to the deliberate inhalation or sniffing of various products for the purpose of achieving a high. The common street term for inhalant abuse is known as "huffing." These products are usually legal and accessible as they have very commonplace intended uses. When misused, they can be extremely dangerous and addictive. There are more than 1400 products that are potentially dangerous inhalants.[79] Inhalants, with the exception of nitrites, are depressants and act on the central nervous system (CNS).[80–82] Dental practitioners must be aware of the possibility of liver damage in these individuals. The liver damage is the result of the accumulation of fatty tissue. A severe rash, known as "glue-sniffer's rash," may develop around the nose and mouth. The physical effects of inhalant abuse resemble those of alcohol intoxication. The high period is very short and is usually followed by a period of lethargy and depression.[83,84]

Solvents, Paints, and Aerosols

Volatile solvents are liquids that vaporize at room temperature. Examples include paint

Table 6.7   Dental Considerations for "Active" Heroin/Opium Abusers

Signs/symptoms	Routes of administration[a]	Common dental findings	Special dental treatment
• Euphoria • Sedation • Dissociation • Dilated/pinpoint pupils • Delusions • Hallucinations • Slurred speech • Track marks	• Inhalation • Snorting • Injection	• Xerostomia • Occlusal wear • Mass caries • Bruxism	• Xerostomia treatment products • Occlusal guards • Topical fluoride treatments • Avoid treatment at least 12 h from last "use" if possible • Evaluate patients for recent treatment with naltrexone for opioid addiction (especially IM products) to optimize analgesia

[a]Routes of administration vary significantly and are substance specific.

thinners, gasoline, lighter fluids, correction fluids, glues, and felt-tip marker fluids. Aerosols are sprays that contain propellants and solvents. Examples include spray paints, hair sprays, and fabric protector sprays. Gases such as butane and propane are also subject to abuse.

The various modes of administration of inhalants can lead to oral anomalies that dental practitioners may encounter. Some abusers soak rags with inhalants (such as gasoline, toluene, or turpentine) and place them in their mouth. Other administration techniques include spraying paints into a plastic or paper bag and then inhaling the contents of the bag. Abusers using this method frequently may have paint residue or "rings" around their nose or mouth or chemical irritation rings from the paints or solvents. Abusers of spray paints generally prefer gold- or silver-colored paints (owing to slight chemical alterations necessary in producing these colors) that may produce a better perceived high. This can lead to various oral and dental sequelae. See Tables 6.1 and 6.8 for clinical findings of various inhalant abuses.

Nitrous Oxide

Nitrous oxide is used safely in many dental practices throughout the world to aid in the control of patient pain and anxiety. However, it has been misused by many individuals who are seemingly unaware of its potentially devastating effects. The mechanism of action of nitrous oxide involves the stimulation of the neuronal release of endogenous opioid peptide or dynorphins.[85] The recreational inhalation of nitrous oxide has also become popular. Easily purchased canisters of nitrous oxide known as "whip-its" are being abused, particularly by teens. Abusers of nitrous oxide may suffer from impairment of the nervous system, uncontrolled muscle movement, and a depletion of vitamin B12. Since nitrous oxide displaces oxygen in the bloodstream, misuse can lead to a loss of consciousness, brain damage, and death. It is imperative that all individuals in the dental office who might have access to nitrous oxide receive education on the dangers of nitrous oxide misuse. It is also imperative that all nitrous oxide be secured safely to prevent it from being used for nondental purposes.

Nitrites

Nitrites such as isoamyl, isobutyl, and cyclohexyl are used primarily as sexual enhancers and are commonly referred to as "poppers." Unlike other inhalants, nitrites do not act directly on the CNS. They relax the muscles and produce vasodilation. Owing to the relatively short duration of effect, as well as the social circumstances in which these agents are abused,

Table 6.8   Dental Considerations for "Active" Inhalant Abusers

Signs/ symptoms	Routes of administration[a]	Common dental findings	Special dental treatment
• Euphoria • Confusion • Dissociation • Paranoia • Delusions • Hallucinations • Slurred speech • Memory lapses • Strong odor of solvents	• Inhalation	• Paint residue around nose, mouth, teeth, and tongue • Redness or irritation around nose, mouth, and teeth	• Delay treatments at least 12 h when possible

[a]Routes of administration vary significantly and are substance specific.

dental practitioners are not likely to deal with any direct consequences of these agents.

> **Clinical Consideration**
>
> Huffing *generally* occurs in two unique populations: (1) adolescent or teens experimenting with their peers or (2) adults with limited financial means. Because these substances are literally available all over the household, detection of abuse can be very difficult.

Central Nervous System Depressants

CNS depressants may be defined as substances that induce decreased brain activity or brain function, anxiolysis, sedation, and sleep. CNS depressants are frequently classified as sedatives. Many substances have both stimulant and depressant effects, depending on several factors, including the specific receptors activated in various parts of the brain, concentration of the substance in the brain, and activity of metabolic by-products. For the purposes of this book, CNS depressants include substances abused to intentionally cause anxiolysis, decrease inhibition, increase sedation, or induce sleep. These agents generally may

reduce the heart rate and breathing and can be very dangerous or even fatal, especially when mixed with other depressant-like substances such as opioids and alcohol.[86] Cross-tolerance to other CNS depressants may also occur.

> **Clinical Consideration**
>
> Abusers of a CNS depressant may be clinically very difficult to detect. However, individuals who seem "resistant" to traditional dosages of sedative or analgesic medications should be suspected of a possible SUD.

Alcohol (Ethyl Alcohol or Ethanol)

Each year, there are approximately 88,000 deaths attributable to excessive alcohol ingestion in the USA.[87] These numbers indicate the extent of moderate-to-severe drinking throughout the country. Regardless of the type of practice or locality, there is a strong chance a provider will treat a patient with alcohol dependency and/or encounter an actively intoxicated patient. Recently, there have been instances where large amounts of alcohol are mixed with high-energy drinks. This can lead to a masking effect where the caffeine interferes with the perceived intoxication. Essentially, the stimulant effects of caffeine counteract the sedative effects

Table 6.9   Stages of Alcohol Withdrawal Symptoms

Stage	Onset	Signs/symptoms
1	6–10 h	Tremors, agitation, anxiety, tachycardia
2	24 h	Hallucinations
3	6–48 h	Seizures
4	2–5 days	Autonomic hyperactivity, global confusion

Clinical Consideration

Dental practitioners should be aware of naltrexone products that are used to decrease cravings of alcohol or opioids, and their potential for blocking necessary analgesia. This information is discussed in greater detail in Chapter 4.

of alcohol.[88] The consumption of alcohol can produce intoxication and, with repeated use, tolerance and dependence. Alcohol affects endogenous opiates and several neurotransmitters in the brain, including γ-amino butyric acid (GABA), glutamate, and dopamine.[89] Patients who regularly use alcohol and experience a period of cessation could experience alcohol withdrawal symptoms[90] (see Table 6.9). An additional concern with this population is Wernicke–Korsakoff syndrome, which may be characterized by nystagmus, gait, ataxia, and confusion. This altered mental state is a result of a decrease in thiamine, and it can be treated medically when noticed; however, it could be fatal if overlooked.[91]

In addition to these complications, patients who are intoxicated may also have coagulopathies, hepatic deficiencies, malnutrition, and behavioral hindrances. Since lidocaine and other medications routinely used by the oral health-care provider are metabolized via the liver, patients with cirrhosis and other hepatic maladies require special attention with regard to this fact. Various indicators may be available to dental practitioners that indicate a patient is intoxicated, including the odor of alcohol, difficulty in gait, slurring of speech, erratic behavior, and sedation (see Tables 6.1, 6.9, and 6.10). Patients who are acutely intoxicated should be clinically stabilized prior to initiating treatment with anesthetics or analgesics.

γ-Hydroxybutyrate

γ-Hydroxybutyrate (GHB) is found as an odorless, colorless liquid; a pill; or a white powder. It is also known as "liquid x" or "cherry meth," among many other slang terms. GHB affects brain chemistry by increasing the levels of dopamine. GHB is very easily manufactured at home, as it only has two structural components. Particular concern in the dental environment should be given to the tachycardic effects that are experienced during GHB withdrawal and the extremely dangerous effects of combining GHB with alcohol or other CNS depressants. Systemic effects of GHB use include drowsiness, dizziness, slow heart rate, nausea, loss of consciousness, seizures, coma, possible death, and loss of memory while being under the influence of GHB.[92] Detection of GHB abuse is extremely difficult.

Marijuana and Other δ-9-Tetrahydrocannabinol Derivatives

Marijuana and Hashish

Marijuana is a mix of shredded flowers, stems, seeds, and leaves of the *Cannabis sativa* plant.[93] Marijuana is well known throughout the world by its popular street names of "grass," "pot," "weed," and "Mary Jane."[94,95] Hashish generally refers to the condensed oil or compressed plant that contains concentrated THC, the main active chemical in marijuana or hashish. Owing to the commercial availability, as well as the high quality, of marijuana being produced in North America, the demand for hashish is low.

Table 6.10   Dental Considerations for "Active" Alcohol Abusers

Signs/symptoms	Routes of administration[a]	Common dental findings	Special dental treatment
• Euphoria • Hyperactivity • Loss of inhibition • Excessive talking • Poor gait • Slurred speech • Overt odor of alcohol • Nystagmus • Confusion • Coagulopathies • Sedation	• Oral • Rectal • Inhalation • Vaginal	• Angular cheilitis • Jaundice • Overt smell of alcohol • Bilateral parotid swelling • Red nose • Spider petechiae on nose	• Caution with local (e.g., lidocaine) or systemic anesthetics in patients with end-stage liver disease • Patients could be receiving naltrexone that can block effects of opioids

[a]Routes of administration vary significantly and are substance specific.

When THC is inhaled, psychotropic effects set in within minutes and its maximum effect is reached within 15–30 min. The effect generally tapers off within 2–3 h.[96] The psychoactive properties of THC are mediated by THC interacting primarily with CB_1 cannabinoid receptors in a large number of areas of the brain.[97] Signs of THC use include glassy, red eyes; loud and inappropriate laughter followed by sleepiness; a sweet burnt odor; loss of interest and/or motivation; and weight gain or loss.[6] Dental practitioners need to take certain precautions and make modifications to dental treatment to ensure the well-being of the patient in the dental environment. Rees suggested all patients who are categorized as being heavy marijuana users should be advised to refrain from its use for at least 1 week prior to their dental appointment.[46] Clinically, significant cardiovascular effects of cannabis usually subside within a few hours.

Cannabis toxicity has been associated with tachycardia. The use of epinephrine could *potentially* precipitate a life-threatening incident, such as acute psychiatric behaviors and peripheral vasodilation. This condition may be enhanced in anxious patients.[46] Any substances containing alcohol should also be avoided in patients who use marijuana, as xerostomia

is a manifestation of marijuana smoking. Other dental/oral manifestations include gingivitis, alveolar bone loss, gingival leukoplakia, gingivitis, gingival hyperplasia,[98,99] oral papillomas,[100,101] hyperplastic gingiva,[102] uvulitis,[103,104] tongue carcinoma,[105] and an increased risk of dental caries[106] (see Tables 6.1 and 6.11).

Clinical Consideration

The consideration for avoiding epinephrine in patients *acutely intoxicated* from cannabis products is potentiation of cardiovascular effects similar to that seen with stimulants.

Synthetic Cannabinoids

Recently, the use of synthetic cannabinoids has become popular. They are often referred to as "spice" or "K2." Synthetic cannabinoids were first reported in the USA in December 2008 when a shipment of spice was seized and analyzed by US Customs and Border Protection in Dayton, Ohio. Synthetic cannabinoids are usually smoked, although they may also be ingested orally. They act on the same cell

Table 6.11   Dental Considerations for "Active" Marijuana and Hashish Abusers/Users

Signs/symptoms	Routes of administration	Common dental findings	Special dental treatment
• Euphoria • Hyperactivity • Dissociation • Tachycardia • Paranoia • Delusions • Hallucinations	• Inhalation • Oral • Rectal	• Xerostomia • Gingivitis • Alveolar bone loss • Gingival leukoplakia • Gingivitis • Increased caries	• Avoid injection or topical epinephrine products • Xerostomia treatment products • Topical fluoride treatments • Avoid treatment at least 24 h from last "use" for patients demonstrating possible cannabis toxicity

receptors as THC and can cause myocardial ischemia, increased heart rate, increased blood pressure, CNS disturbances, agitation, vomiting, and confusion. These synthetic derivatives are usually more potent than traditionally grown marijuana and frequently cause unpredictable behaviors that require hospitalization. Since these substances are commonly smoked, the deleterious dental effects seen with tobacco-related products are common. Alteration of the chemical structures of these agents may enhance all pharmacological effects seen with THC products. The oral manifestations are similar to traditional cannabis agents. Clinical considerations for dental treatment are the same for cannabis patients (see Tables 6.1 and 6.11).

Clinical Consideration

In reality, patients reporting having smoked or ingested synthetic marijuana or bath salts have no idea what actual drug or drug quantity has actually been ingested. Toxicology screens are very limited in providing additional helpful information. Dental practitioners should expect "combinations" of these agents in an acutely intoxicated patient reporting abuse of these substances.

Prescription Medications

Prescription drug overdose has quickly become a common cause of death in the USA. The sources of these medications have been attributed to sharing from friends and family, leftover prescriptions, or criminal activity. Dental practitioners have become a common target for patients with SUD or drug-related criminal behavior (see Chapter 8). Indiscriminate prescribing of prescription drugs is becoming a major focus of state dental boards. Dental practitioners must be aware of current drugs or combinations of drugs that may be abused by patients in order to protect themselves, the community, and the patient. Prescription medications may be broken down into groups of controlled substances and *noncontrolled substances*. Controlled substances are regulated by the federal Drug Enforcement Agency (DEA) and are further categorized into five different subgroups based on their potential for abuse and recognized medical use in the USA (see Box 6.3). Specific state pharmacy boards or other state boards also categorize medications into various subgroups based on the potential for abuse. Noncontrolled substances are generally recognized as having limited risk for abuse

> **Box 6.3   Federally Controlled Substance Schedules[107]**
>
> **Schedule I Controlled Substances**
> Substances in this schedule have no currently accepted medical use in the USA, a lack of accepted safety for use under medical supervision, and a high potential for abuse. Examples include heroin, LSD, marijuana (cannabis), mescaline, and MDMA ("ecstasy").
>
> **Schedule II Controlled Substances**
> Substances in this schedule have a high potential for abuse, which may lead to severe psychological or physical dependence. Examples for Schedule II include hydromorphone (Dilaudid®), methadone (Dolophine®), meperidine (Demerol®), oxycodone (Oxycontin®, Percocet®), hydrocodone (Zohydro®), fentanyl (Sublimaze®, Duragesic®), amphetamine (Dexedrine®, Adderall®), methamphetamine (Desoxyn®), methylphenidate (Ritalin®), and pure codeine.
>
> **Schedule III Controlled Substances**
> Substances in this schedule have less potential for abuse than substances in Schedules I or II, and abuse may lead to moderate or low physical dependence or high psychological dependence. Examples for Schedule III include combination products containing not more than 90 mg of codeine per dosage unit (Tylenol with Codeine®), and buprenorphine (Suboxone®), benzphetamine (Didrex®), phendimetrazine, ketamine, and anabolic steroids such as Depo®-Testosterone.
>
> **Schedule IV Controlled Substances**
> Substances in this schedule have a low potential for abuse relative to substances in Schedule III. Examples for this schedule include alprazolam (Xanax®), carisoprodol (Soma®), clonazepam (Klonopin®), clorazepate (Tranxene®), diazepam (Valium®), lorazepam (Ativan®), and tramadol (Ultracet®).
>
> **Schedule V Controlled Substances**
> Substances in this schedule have a low potential for abuse relative to substances listed in Schedule IV and consist primarily of preparations containing limited quantities of certain narcotics. Examples for this schedule include cough-suppressant preparations containing not more than 200 mg of codeine per 100 mL or per 100 g (Robitussin AC®, Phenergan with Codeine®).

and are approved for medical purposes. These substances include medications like antibiotics, antihypertensives, muscle relaxants, or antipsychotics.

Opioids

Opioids are the most commonly abused of all prescription drugs in the USA. They are misused and abused for their analgesic, euphoric, or stimulatory effects. A substance abuser's "opioid of choice" is usually based on desired effect, the medication's potency, the quantity available, the purchasing cost, and ease of abuse (e.g., tamperproof formulation).

> **Clinical Consideration**
>
> Pain management is a special consideration when the dental practitioner encounters an opioid-abusing patient experiencing dental pain. The patient must receive adequate and timely relief of pain. The first thing the dental practitioner must do is determine the pathological etiology of the patient's pain. In doing so, the dental practitioner must remember that the ultimate relief or *minimizing of pain* in the addicted patient *must be the same as in the nonaddicted individual.* (See Chapters 3 and 4 for analgesic considerations.)

Hydrocodone and Oxycodone (Schedule II)

Hydrocodone is the most commonly prescribed opioid in the USA. There were nearly 140 million prescriptions for hydrocodone products in 2011.[108,109] This medication is often prescribed by dental providers to control moderate to moderately severe pain. Hydrocodone binds to the μ-opioid receptor in the CNS to produce its primary effect of an analgesic. Hydrocodone is demethylated by the cytochrome P450 2D6 (P4502D6) into the active metabolite hydromorphone.[110,111]

It is imperative to evaluate each patient's risk of abuse versus treatment of pain (see Chapters 4 and 8). It may be helpful to utilize a VAPS to establish a baseline of perceived pain and to reassess the pain levels at follow-up visits. A patient's expectation may be to have instantaneous relief of pain. This may not be possible depending on the particular clinical situation. A VAPS may help demonstrate an improvement of pain as the treatment or postoperative period progresses. The use of an opioid risk tool assessment can also be utilized as an adjunct to gauge the risk of abuse by the patient.

Possible contraindications to the use of any opioids may include alcoholism and current use or a history of drug addiction.[110,111] However, emergency conditions may warrant limited opioid use in patients. Dental practitioners must be concerned about drug interactions in individuals misusing opioids in order to avoid CNS depression. Use of narcotic analgesics, alcohol, antianxiety agents, and other CNS depressants could lead to respiratory failure in the dental setting. Dental practitioners may also encounter difficulty in obtaining the desired degree of analgesia or sedation due to cross-tolerance. Bleeding can be a concern due to liver damage or failure as a result of a prolonged period of opioid abuse.

Oxycodone is a μ-opioid agonist that has been used clinically since 1916.[112] At higher doses, oxycodone will act on δ and κ receptors.

Box 6.4 Adverse Effects of Opioid Abuse

- Constipation
- Nausea
- Sedation
- Respiratory Depression
- Vomiting
- Dizziness
- Miosis
- Pruritus

This medication is used in the dental setting to treat moderate to severe pain. It is metabolized via cytochrome P450 and the CYP3A enzymatic pathway into its active metabolites: noroxycodone and oxymorphone. Noroxycodone has been shown to be the most abundant metabolite in circulation after administration of oxycodone to patients.[113] Pharmacokinetic studies have shown variability in behavior and toxic risks.[114] These studies have indicated that people who exhibit this polymorphism of the P450 pathway are more prone to the "abuse potential" of opioids. The effects of oxycodone,[115] such as analgesia, miosis, constipation, sedation, dizziness, vomiting, depression, tolerance, physical dependence, and respiratory depression, mimic other opioids (see Box 6.4 and Table 6.12). There have also been some reports of hyperalgesia due to long-term oxycodone use.[116] The routes of administration in patients who abuse this medication can be oral, snorting, injection, or smoking. Miosis (pinpoint pupils) is a classic sign of opioid use, but it is not pathognomonic since other disorders could potentially be the cause. However, it is a strong indicator that warrants further investigation while interviewing the patient. Marked mydriasis with hypoxia may be seen in oxycodone or hydrocodone overdoses.[117] Oxycodone should be used with caution in geriatric patients and patients with kidney or liver disease since these disorders may slow the clearance of the drug. Interactions with other medications have the potential to

Table 6.12   Dental Considerations for "Active" Opioid Abusers

Signs/symptoms	Routes of administration	Common dental findings	Special dental treatment
• Euphoria • Sedation • Dissociation • Dilated/pinpoint pupils • Slurred speech • Track marks • Excessive energy • Paranoia • Goose flesh • Piloerection • Excessive yawning	• Inhalation • Snorting • Injection • Oral	• Xerostomia • Mass caries • Occlusal wear • Red inflamed nostrils • Powder in nostrils • Nasal septal damage	• Xerostomia treatment products • Topical fluoride treatments • Avoid treatment at least 12 h from last "use" if possible • Bite splints • Occlusal guards

lead to respiratory depression (see Box 6.5 and Table 6.1). When hydrocodone or oxycodone are considered, it should be for short-term use, and they should be prescribed only after assessing the patient's potential for abuse.

Box 6.5   Potentially Clinically Significant Drug Interactions with Oxycodone or Hydrocodone Products

- Fluconazole hydrocodone or oxycodone products
- Azithromycin oxycodone products
- Rifampin oxycodone or hydrocodone products

Hydrocodone and oxycodone in pure form are both Schedule II controlled substances. When hydrocodone was combined in DEA-defined proportions of aspirin, acetaminophen, or ibuprofen it was *historically* classified as a Schedule III agent. Classifying controlled substances as Schedule III as opposed to Schedule II allows for refills as well as phone-in prescriptions and prescription renewals. When the Controlled Substance Act was implemented in 1970, the presumption was that combination of hydrocodone with aspirin,

acetaminophen, or ibuprofen would be prohibitive to patient abuse. Clinical experience has clearly demonstrated that the acetaminophen, aspirin, or ibuprofen quantities combined with hydrocodone or oxycodone have minimal, if any, impact on the quantity of these agents abused by a patient with an SUD. Federal regulations were established in 2014 to make *all* hydrocodone combination products Schedule II substances. Table 6.13 list popular combination oxycodone/hydrocodone products.

Certain drugs that are used routinely in dentistry can affect the removal of oxycodone and hydrocodone from the body. They include macrolide antibiotics, azole antifungals, and rifamycins. Drug interactions with oxycodone or hydrocodone could have a very dangerous effect, causing respiratory depression. Dental practitioners must be aware of clinically significant drug interactions with common agents prescribed *and dispensed* from the dental office (see Box 6.5). Reformulated OxyContin® (Oxycodone-HCL controlled release) tablets became available in the USA in August 2010. Originally, the formulation of OxyContin® utilized a delivery system that did not incorporate inherent resistance to crushing and dissolving the medication for illicit use.[118] Although patients can still take an overprescribed amount

Table 6.13   Examples of Hydrocodone and Oxycodone Products

Oxycodone with aspirin	Percodan®, Endodan®, Roxiprin®
Oxycodone with ibuprofen	Combunox®
Oxycodone with acetaminophen	Percocet®, Endocet®
Hydrocodone with aspirin	Damason-P®, Lortab ASA®, Azdone®, Alor 5/500®
Hydrocodone with ibuprofen	Vicoprofen®, Reprexain®, Ibudone®
Hydrocodone with acetaminophen	Norco®, Vicodin®, Lortab®

orally, this new formulation promotes abuse by deterring patients from snorting or injecting the medication. When patients with a history of abuse have been questioned about their choice of opioids, abusers preferred oxycodone to other opioids.[119] As a general rule, long-acting opioid agents such as OxyContin® should never be prescribed for acute pain by dental practitioners.

Morphine (Schedule II)

Morphine is an opioid pain reliever. It acts on the CNS to relieve pain and has a high potential for abuse. Signs and symptoms of morphine abuse that dental practitioners must be concerned about are shallow breathing, oversedation, and low blood pressure. Proper management of pain and anxiety in the chronic opioid abuser is often difficult to achieve due to cross-tolerance. Increased rates of caries, xerostomia, mucosal infections, and periodontal disease are also prevalent in these individuals. IV morphine is a preferred agent for in-office administration to manage moderate to severe pain when rapid systemic analgesia is warranted.

Hydromorphone/Oxymorphone (Schedule II)

Hydromorphone (Dilaudid®) and oxymorphone (Opana®) are potent opioid analgesics. They have a high abuse and dependence potential and are commonly abused in rural and suburban areas.[120] Many individuals who

are originally prescribed these medications for legitimate purposes develop physical dependence and addiction. Xerostomia is a key adverse event related to its use.[121]

Fentanyl (Schedule II)

Fentanyl is a drug that has an action similar to that of other opioids. It is available in multiple forms, including transdermal patch, lozenge, dissolvable film, tablet, nasal spray, and injection. There have been recent documented incidences of fentanyl overdoses. This drug is often mixed with heroin or cocaine, which results in many deleterious effects, such as euphoria, addiction, drowsiness, respiratory depression, coma, nausea, loss of consciousness, confusion, sedation, and constipation.[122] Oral transmucosal fentanyl citrate (OTFC) is a lollipop form of fentanyl that contains 2 g of sugar.[123] A causal relationship between the sugar content of OTFC and advanced tooth decay has been proposed.[124]

Methadone (Schedule II)

In 1972 the US Food and Drug Administration approved methadone (Dolophine®) for the treatment of individuals addicted to opioids. Methadone is a synthetic opioid and can be used as an analgesic. It is frequently a drug of choice in opioid maintenance therapy programs since it is a synthetic long-acting agonist to the same receptor as heroin and morphine. Methadone deters cravings while blocking the euphoric effects of heroin to establish abstinence.[125] Methadone meets two key components for maintenance treatment: high systemic bioavailability when given orally and a long half-life. Methadone is metabolized by the liver and is excreted in urine and feces.[126] Those participating in a methadone maintenance treatment (MMT) program have an average therapeutic dose of 60–120 mg of methadone per day. Dental treatment should be postponed if the patient appears to have recently abused or misused methadone. Patient appointments should be structured around their methadone schedule and kept to short periods to enable optimal cooperation and patient safety. Methadone can mask some of the pain a patient is experiencing due to its analgesic effect. *However, it should not be assumed that MMT provides adequate analgesia for acute dental pain.* This is discussed in more detail in Chapter 4.

The pharmacokinetic properties, analgesic pharmacodynamics, and respiratory pharmacodynamics of methadone are extremely complicated and vary significantly between patients. The use of methadone for analgesia in dentistry has limited use (*if any*) in the management of acute pain unless under consultation with the prescriber responsible for the patient's MMT contract. Often, the patient on MMT will present with dental issues that are long-standing and severe. This is usually a combination of their former lifestyle, diet, and possibly dental phobias. At times, this cohort of patients may place unrealistic demands upon dental providers. It is imperative to establish a treatment plan and thoroughly explain the risks, benefits, and alternatives to the patient. A clear estimation of the amount of time and visits treatment will take is also helpful. Clarifying if patients are in MMT contracts is important to help protect the patient from contract violations.

There are multiple caries risks that present with a methadone patient. Oral findings include xerostomia and bruxism from the years of drug abuse and poor diet. This population may combat xerostomia and sugar cravings by consuming large amounts of cariogenic drinks. Also, they may ingest large amounts of water as they journey on to a drug-free life. This attempt to cope with xerostomia should be addressed, since water is a poor substitute for saliva due to the lack of necessary ions, buffering capacity, lubricating mucins, and protective proteins.[127]

When an MMT patient presents to the dental practitioner with a genuine interest in oral rehabilitation, there are a few key issues that the provider should consider. Many of these patients have dental phobias that need to be dealt with, as well as lifestyle changes. Areas such as nutritional counseling and oral hygiene instruction should be discussed. The issue of pain control is a potential dilemma in this group because of tolerance and the history of SUD. Using a VAPS can be considered to establish a baseline and help educate the patient about the expectation of relief of pain as the treatment progresses. The use of opioid pain medications should only be used in cases when all other drugs have failed and there is a clear pathogenic reason for the pain for which the patient is actively seeking treatment or there is a true contraindication to traditional nonsteroidal anti-inflammatory drugs (NSAIDs). This is discussed in more detail in Chapter 4.

Codeine (Schedule II, III, or V)

Codeine is an analgesic that has great variation in its pharmacokinetics among different individuals. It is considered to be a weak opioid. Codeine requires metabolism to morphine for its analgesic effects. Codeine is often combined therapeutically with acetaminophen or NSAIDs. Liver toxicity, gastric hemorrhage,[128] tolerance, and drug dependence are associated with its long-term use.[129] Traditionally, codeine has been a commonly prescribed analgesic by dental practitioners. However, due to poor gastrointestinal tolerance and variation in patient responses to analgesia, hydrocodone products are more frequently prescribed. Abuse of codeine parallels other Schedule II and III opioids.

Buprenorphine (Schedule III)

Buprenorphine is an opioid medication that is used in the treatment of opioid addiction and pain management.[130] Buprenorphine is a potent analgesic that is approximately 40 times more potent than oral morphine on a milligram per milligram basis. It is a derivative of thebaine, which is an extract of opium and is sought by opioid abusers.[131] Historically, buprenorphine has been used as an effective analgesic. More recently, buprenorphine has become a preferred agent for opioid-based addiction treatment programs. Buprenorphine is commercially available as pure buprenorphine (Subutex®) or combined with naloxone (Suboxone®, Zubsolv®).

Combining buprenorphine with naloxone is a strategy to prevent IV abuse of these agents since IV administration of naloxone is likely to produce significant withdrawal symptoms. Buprenorphine is also available in a transdermal patch (Butrans®). Buprenorphine is capable of producing significant euphoria in opioid-naive patients and has the same risks of other opioids in this population. Abuse of this product by addicts *not in recovery* may be seen. Buprenorphine has been reported to be a popular substitute for heroin.[132] Active addicts may use these products to limit the level of physiologic withdrawal until they can get their next high.

> ### Clinical Consideration
> Frequently, dental practitioners are targeted by opioid drug seekers. Dental practitioners are encouraged to be familiar with behaviors, schemes, and scams associated with SUD as well as criminal behaviors (see Chapter 8).

Appendix 2.A lists common opioid controlled substances, brand names, and routes of administration.

Tramadol (Schedule IV)

Tramadol is an opioid and aminergic-acting analgesic. Historically, it has a limited indication in dentistry for the management of acute pain (see Chapter 2). Tramadol has approximately one-eighth the potency of morphine on a milligram per milligram basis. The primary use of tramadol is primarily as an alternative when the use of NSAIDs and codeine–acetaminophen combination analgesics are contraindicated.[133] Tramadol is commonly abused by opioid addicts, health-care professionals, and chronic pain patients. For many individuals, tramadol may be their preferred drug of choice for abuse. Maximum daily dosage should not exceed 400 mg. Doing so is associated with an increased risk of seizures. With the exception of seizures, abuse behaviors and clinical findings are similar to opioids.

> ### Clinical Consideration
> Although buprenorphine is a potent analgesic, it should not be assumed that buprenorphine used in opioid maintenance treatment will provide adequate analgesia in patients with acute dental pain (see Chapter 4).

> ### Clinical Considerations
> Many opioid abusers will settle for being prescribed tramadol when denied their opioid of choice. The abuse of tramadol may minimize the opioid withdrawal to some extent until the "drug of choice" can be obtained.

Stimulants: Methylphenidate and Amphetamine/Dextroamphetamine (Schedule II)

Methylphenidate (Ritalin®) and amphetamine/dextroamphetamine (Adderall®) increase the activity of dopamine and dopamine/norepinephrine respectively, block the reuptake of neurotransmitters into neurons, and stimulate the cerebral cortex and subcortical structures. They have a high potential for abuse. Dental professionals must be aware of certain side effects and possible drug interactions in those individuals using methylphenidate. The most common misuse and abuse of these agents appears to be by high school and college students. Common side effects include xerostomia, increase in heart rate and blood pressure, motor tics, and dyskinesias.[134] As methylphenidate is an amphetamine-like drug, local anesthetics *without* vasoconstrictors are recommended. One of the motor and behavioral symptoms of acute overdose or toxicity is bruxism.[135] Treatment considerations for prescription stimulant abuse are similar to methamphetamine abuse (see Tables 6.1 and 6.2).

Central Nervous System Depressants

Benzodiazepines (Schedule IV)

Benzodiazepines produce effects that are the result of its modulation of GABA, which is the main inhibitory neurotransmitter of the CNS. Many craniofacial and dental signs and symptoms are exhibited in those individuals who are experiencing withdrawal from benzodiazepines. These include aching or painful jaw, complaints about a "band around head," dysphagia, painful scalp, migraines, toothaches, twitching of the head, bruxism, increased or decreased salivary flow, and pain in temple[136,137] (see Box 6.6). Table 6.14 lists considerations for dental patients that may be abusing benzodiazepines.

Box 6.6   Common Signs and Symptoms of Benzodiazepine and Barbiturate Withdrawal

- Aches and pains/flu-like symptoms
- Twitching
- Headaches
- Irritability, anxiousness
- Bruxism
- Jaw pain
- Tremor
- Diaphoresis
- Complaints of a "band around the head"

Clonazepam (Schedule IV)

Clonazepam (Klonopin®) is used to treat anxiety disorders and seizure disorders and to alleviate the pain of muscle spasms. Clonazepam is often frequently abused as a street drug.[138] In order to get a greater high, abusers crush the pills and snort it. This can lead to erosion of the nasal lining and nose structure and the slowing of the heart and respiration rates. Death can occur when combining this medication with other illicit and prescription medications, *especially opioids and alcohol.* Care should be taken when using certain dental anesthetics, opioid pain relievers, and sedatives as they have the potential to have a very dangerous effect on the individual who is taking or abusing clonazepam.[138]

Diazepam (Schedule IV)

Diazepam (Valium®) is a benzodiazepine that is used to treat generalized anxiety, muscle spasms, and alcohol withdrawal symptoms. It acts on the GABA receptors in the limbic system, causing a reduced level of consciousness. Diazepam has been used for decades in

Table 6.14   Dental Considerations for "Active" Abusers of Benzodiazepines and Barbiturates

Signs/symptoms	Routes of administration[a]	Common dental findings	Special dental treatment
• Euphoria • Loss of inhibition • Excessive talking • Poor gait • Slurred speech • Nystagmus • Confusion • Sedation	• Oral • Snorting • IV	• Xerostomia • Bruxism	• Patients may be tolerant to traditional doses of sedatives • Caution is warranted in patients taking opioids

[a]Routes of administration vary significantly and are substance specific.

treating patients with dental phobias. It has a long history of safe and effective use in dentistry. It is considered to be useful for appointments where extensive dental treatment is performed. A reduced dosage should be administered to those patients who are taking other drugs that have the ability to influence the metabolism of diazepam.[139] A reduced dosage is also indicated in the elderly, debilitated, and those taking other CNS depressants. The use of Valium® is contraindicated in those individuals who are pregnant, are under 6 months of age, have narrow-angle glaucoma, and have a hypersensitivity to benzodiazepines.[139, 140]

Alprazolam (Schedule IV)

Alprazolam (Xanax®) is an anxiolytic with a very fast onset of action. Its effects are usually felt within 20 min of ingestion. Alprazolam is commonly used in oral conscious sedation. Symptoms of alprazolam overdose include confusion, shallow breathing, coma, slurred speech, and possible death. It should not be administered to patients who are allergic to any benzodiazepines, have difficulty with breathing, or who are taking CNS depressants. Alcohol must also be avoided in patients who are prescribed alprazolam. Alprazolam use can also cause xerostomia.

Lorazepam (Schedule IV)

Lorazepam (Ativan®) is a benzodiazepine that is used to treat anxiety disorders. Lorazepam has the same potential for abuse as other benzodiazepines. It can cause difficulty in maintaining balance, particularly in the elderly. The usual adult dosage for dental sedation ranges from 0.5 to 4 mg.[141–144]

Barbiturates
Amobarbital (Schedule II)

Amobarbital (Amytal®) is a nonselective CNS depressant that is used as a sedative, for treating insomnia, and as a preanesthetic. It depresses the sensory cortex, thus decreasing motor activity. Amobarbital is only available legally in the USA in injection form. Amobarbital is currently listed among the most commonly abused drugs by the US DEA. Dental practitioners must be aware of its CNS depressant effects.

Phenobarbital (Schedule IV)

Phenobarbital (Luminal®) is a nonselective CNS depressant. It increases synaptic inhibition by acting on GABA GABA-A receptors. Phenobarbital abuse is popular with teens, who refer to these drugs as "feenies" or "phennies" (see Box 6.7). Dental practitioners must be aware of potentially dangerous interactions with alcohol and antihistamines. Prolonged use of barbiturates will likely produce signs and symptoms of withdrawal similar to that seen with alcohol or benzodiazepines (see Box 6.6).

Box 6.7   Signs of Barbiturate Abuse

- Drunken behavior
- Difficulty concentrating
- Clumsiness
- Sleepiness
- Contracted pupils

Butalbital (Schedule IV)

Butalbital is the most commonly prescribed barbiturate and is prescribed predominately in combination analgesic products like Fiorinal® or Fioricet® for headaches. Dental practitioners should be aware of these products, the potential for cross-tolerance to other CNS depressants, and risk of abuse and misuse.

Clinical Consideration

Patients with a history of alcohol abuse or benzodiazepine abuse are at a potential risk for cross-addiction or stimulation of cravings with barbiturates. Use of these agents in this population should be limited.

Antipsychotics

Quetiapine

Quetiapine (Seroquel®) is a drug that is used to treat severe mental disorders like schizophrenia, post-traumatic stress disorder and mania. It is an antipsychotic medication whose exact mechanism of action is unknown but is thought to reduce dopaminergic neurotransmission in the mesolimbic pathway.[145] Common side effects of the use of quetiapine that are of importance to the dental practitioner are dry mouth, sudden drop in blood pressure upon standing, and swelling of the sinuses and pharynx. Misuse of quetiapine has been reported in the prison system, where it is known as "baby heroin" or "quell" (see Box 6.8).

Box 6.8   Effects of Abused Antipsychotics, Muscle Relaxants, and Anticonvulsants

- Euphoria
- Loss of inhibition
- Excessive talking
- Poor gait
- Slurred speech
- Nystagmus
- Confusion

Ziprasidone

Ziprasidone (Geodon®) is used to treat schizophrenia and bipolar disorder. It is thought that ziprasidone's efficacy is based on its dopamine type 2 and serotonin type 2 antagonism. Some side effects of concern to dental practitioners include bradycardia, buccoglossal syndrome, xerostomia, oral leukoplakia, swollen tongue, and gingival pain[146] (see Box 6.8).

Olanzipine

Olanzapine (Zyprexa®) is an antipsychotic whose action is thought to involve antagonism at serotonin receptors. There are some rare cases of olanzapine abuse in the scientific literature.[147] Dental professionals must be aware that xerostomia and tooth discoloration are side effects of olanzapine use (see Box 6.8).

Muscle Relaxants

Carisoprodol (Schedule IV)

Carisoprodol (Soma®) is a CNS depressant that is used to relieve muscular pain on a short-term basis. The abuse of carisoprodol has increased over the past few years. Individuals who abuse carisoprodol seek its sedative and relaxant effects. A major metabolite of carisoprodol is meprobamate, a well-known benzodiazepine. The benzodiazepine metabolite likely produces the desired anxiolytic, euphoric, and sedative effects. The withdrawal syndrome consists of ataxia, insomnia, vomiting, anxiety, tremors, and muscle twitching[148] (see Box 6.8).

Clinical Consideration

Patients with a history of alcohol, benzodiazepine, or barbiturate abuse should not be prescribed this agent. A major metabolite is the benzodiazepine meprobamate. In reality, there are limited evidence-based studies that clinically justify the use of this medication.

Cyclobenzaprine

Cyclobenzaprine (Flexeril®) is a skeletal muscle relaxant that may be helpful in patients with acute pain from muscle spasms. Structurally, cyclobenzaprine is similar to tricyclic antidepressants, causing anticholinergic side effects. Dental findings in these patients may include xerostomia (see Box 6.8).

Anticonvulsants

Gabapentin

Gabapentin (Neurontin®) is a GABA analogue that is used to treat certain types of seizures and neuropathic pain. Neurontin has recently become a drug of abuse. Some users describe the feeling as a marijuana-like high.[149] It is often used as a "cutting agent" in street heroin.[149]

Xerostomia is seen in gabapentin users (see Box 6.8).

Phenytoin

Phenytoin (Dilantin®) is an anticonvulsant used primarily in the management of epileptic seizures and trigeminal neuralgia resulting from multiple sclerosis. Dental practitioners need to be concerned with possible harmful drug interactions with phenytoin. Gingival overgrowth is a condition that has been widely related to the use of phenytoin.[150]

There are cases in the literature describing phenytoin as a recreational drug. It is usually used in combination with other drugs, such as marijuana, alcohol, and cocaine. It is thought that cannabinoids potentiate the high from phenytoin by receptor cross-reactivity[151] (see Box 6.8.)

Clinical Considerations

Abuse of antipsychotics, anticonvulsants, and muscle relaxants is common for many reasons, including:

1. The side effect profile of these three classes is almost identical to the side effect profile of alcohol.
2. These classes of medications are less regulated, so access is very easy.
3. Combining these medications with other substances of abuse may enhance the high or experience or reduce the need for excessive quantities of substances to achieve the desired effect.

Other Agents

Ketamine (Schedule III)

Ketamine is a dissociative anesthetic. It has been misused recently as a "club drug." Ketamine interacts with N-methyl-D-aspartate, opioid, muscarinic, and monoaminergic receptors. Ketamine has been used for years in dentistry,

Table 6.15   Adverse Effects of Anabolic Steroid Abuse

Males	Females	Both
Reduced sperm count	Mood instability	Heart attack/stroke
Infertility	Menstrual problems	Gingival enlargement
Shrunken testicles	Facial/body hair	Liver/kidney tumors
Baldness	Deepened voice	Hypertension
Breast development	Increased sex drive	Increase in tendon injuries
Increased risk of prostate cancer	Hair loss	Fluid retention
Overgrowth of forehead	Swelling of clitoris	High cholesterol
Splayed teeth	Infertility	Acne
	Breast atrophy	
	Depression	

particularly for pediatric sedation. The illicit use of ketamine can result in a dramatic increase in heart rate, which is of concern in the dental setting.

Anabolic Androgenic Steroids (Schedule III)

Anabolic androgenic steroids refer to the synthetic derivatives of the male sex hormone. They act on the anabolic receptors that control the transcription of target genes involved in muscle growth. Commonly abused anabolic androgenic steroids include oxymetholone, oxandrolone, methandrostenolone, stanozolol, nandrolone, decanoate, nandrolone phenpropionate, testosterone cypionate, and boldenone undecylenate. Dental practitioners need to be familiar with the significant levels of gingival enlargement that are associated with anabolic androgenic steroid use[152] (see Table 6.15).

Over-the-Counter Medications

Dextromethorphan

Dextromethorphan is a cough suppressant and expectorant. Individuals who abuse this drug often use it in combination with other drugs, which can produce extremely dangerous synergistic effects. The desired effects of its illicit use are altered time perception, visual hallucinations, and a heightened perceptual awareness. Dextromethorphan products are commonly combined with antihistamines and decongestants that may promote xerostomia. Dextromethorphan abuse results in four plateaus of intoxication, ranging from mild inebriation to a level of intoxication similar to that of ketamine and PCP.[153–155]

Antihistamines

Antihistamines such as diphenhydramine (Benadryl®) or clorpheniramine (Chlor-Trimeton®) are used to combat allergic symptoms or to intentionally induce sleep. Antihistamines abuse is on the rise, as they are easily obtained, are relatively cheap, and may provide synergistic or additive effects to other substances being abused. High doses of antihistamines are often combined with alcohol in order to obtain a potentially sedative effect.[156] These medications usually have high anticholinergic properties that cause significant xerostomia.

Pseudoephedrine

Pseudoephedrine is a common decongestant that is found in both OTC and prescription products and is used to relieve symptoms caused by sinusitis, flu, colds, and allergies. Pseudoephedrine is the desired precursor for methamphetamine production in clandestine methamphetamine labs. Pseudoephedrine products have been regulated[157] in an effort to curb methamphetamine production.[158] Pseudoephedrine is extracted from cold medications by use of various chemicals including solvents, lithium batteries, and coffee filters using "cookbook" protocols easily found on the Internet. Frequently, abusers will ingest commercial pseudoephedrine tablets or liquids in large quantities to achieve the adrenergic or CNS effects associated with these products.

Clinical Consideration

Excessive dosing of pseudoephedrine is common in students and health professionals trying to stay awake or in stimulant addicts unable to get their prescription drugs of choice.

Clinical Consideration

Disposal of Unused Prescription and OTC Medicines: Information for Patients

Leftover or unused medications are a common source of abused drugs. Any unused medications should be destroyed to avoid accidental ingestion or abuse/misuse. Medication take back programs are available in many communities, and patients should be urged to contact their local government health agency or antidrug coalition for more information. Chapter 8 reviews disposal methods to prevent drug diversion.

Summary

The lists of abused illicit drugs, prescription medications, and OTC medications that have the potential for causing harmful situations in the dental setting are ever changing. Dental practitioners must be aware of the many possible drug interactions, oral and dental manifestations, and modifications to dental treatment that result from a patient's abuse of these substances. Knowledge of the dental significance of drug abuse enables dental practitioners to provide safe and effective dental treatment.

References

1. National Institute on Drug Abuse. Prescription drugs: abuse and addiction. Research Report Services. 2011. NIDA, Bethesda, MD. http://www.drugabuse.gov/sites/default/files/rrprescription.pdf. Accessed January 1, 2015.
2. Diagnostic and Statistical Manual of Mental Disorders, 4th ed., text revision, DSM-IV-TR. 2000. American Psychiatric Association.
3. The Diagnostic and Statistical Manual of Mental Disorders, 5th ed., DSM-5. 2013. American Psychiatric Association.
4. National Institute on Drug Abuse. The Neurobiology of Drug Addiction. 6: Definition of tolerance. http://www.drugabuse.gov/publications/teaching-packets/neurobiology-drug-addiction/section-iii-action-heroin-morphine/6-definition-tolerance. Accessed January 1, 2015.
5. Acute Pain Management: Operative or Medical Procedures and Trauma, Clinical Practice Guideline No. 1. AHCPR Publication No. 92-0032; February 1992. Agency for Healthcare Research & Quality, Rockville, MD, pp. 116–17.
6. Phoenix House. Signs and symptoms of substance abuse. http://www.phoenixhouse.org/prevention/signs-and-symptoms-of-substance-abuse/. Accessed January 1, 2015.
7. Treatment4Addiction.com. Stimulant drugs. 2011. www.treatment4addiction.com/drugs/stimulants/. Accessed January 1, 2015.

8. Lineberry TW, Bostwick JM. Methamphetamine abuse: a perfect storm of complications. Mayo Clin Proc 2006;81(1):77–84.

9. National Institute on Drug Abuse. Research Report Series: Methamphetamine Abuse and Addiction. NIH Publication No. 02-4210. 2002. National Institutes of Health, Bethesda, MD.

10. Methamphetamine. 2002. www.hawaii.edu/hivandaids/TeachersGuideonMethamphetamine.pdf. Accessed January 1, 2015.

11. American Dental Association. Oral Health Topics: Meth Mouth. http://www.ada.org/en/member-center/oral-health-topics/meth-mouth. Accessed January 9, 2015.

12. Shaner JW. Caries associated with methamphetamine abuse. J Mich Dent Assoc 2002;84(9):42–7.

13. Duxbury AJ. Ecstasy—dental implications. Br Dent J 1993;175:38.

14. Shetty V, Mooney LJ, Zigler CM, Belin TR, Murphy D, Rawson R. The relationship between methamphetamine use and increased dental disease. JADA 2010;141(3):307–18.

15. Smart RJ, Rosenberg M. Methamphetamine abuse: medical and dental considerations. J Mass Dent Soc 2005;54(2):44–6, 48–9.

16. Padilla R, Ritter AV. Meth mouth: methamphetamine and oral health. J Esthet Restor Dent 2008;20(2):148–9.

17. Saini T, Edwards PC, Kimmes NS, Carroll LR, Shaner JW, Dowd FJ. Etiology of xerostomia and dental caries among methamphetamine abusers. Oral Health Prev Dent 2005;3(3):189–95.

18. Methamphetamine facts. http://casat.unr.edu/docs/fact_sheet_meth_2.pdf. Accessed January 1, 2015.

19. Henry JA. Amphetamines. In: Clinical Toxicology, 1st ed. Ford MD, Delaney KA, Ling LJ, Erickson T, eds. WB Saunders, Philadelphia, pp. 620–7.

20. O'Brien CP. Drug addiction and drug abuse. In: Goodman's & Gilman's The Pharmacological Basis of Therapeutics, 11th ed. Brunton LL, Lazo J, Parker K, eds. McGraw-Hill, New York, pp. 1109–86.

21. University of Utah. Meth in the mouth for oral health care providers. 2007. http://medicine.utah.edu/internalmedicine/infectiousdiseases/uaetc/resources/meth_mouth07.pdf. Accessed January 1, 2015.

22. Maloney W. The significance of illicit drug use to practice. WebmedCentral Dent Drug Abuse 2010;1(7):WMC00455.

23. Hamamoto DT, Rhodus NL. Methamphetamine abuse and dentistry. Oral Dis 2009;15:27–37.

24. Turnispeed SD, Richards JR, Kirk JD, Diercks DB, Amsterdam EA. Frequency of acute coronary syndrome in patients presenting to the emergency department with chest pains after methamphetamine use. J Emerg Med 2003;24:369–73.

25. McGee SM, McGee DN, McGee MB. Spontaneous intracerebral hemorrhage related to methamphetamine abuse: autopsy findings and clinical correlation. Am J Forensic Med Pathol 2004;25:334–7.

26. Little JW, Falace DA, Miller CS, Rhodus NL. Psychiatric disorders. In: Dental Management of the Medically Compromised Patient, 7th ed. 2007. Mosby Elsevier, St Louis, MO, pp. 507–32.

27. Bolla KI, Cade JL. Exogenous acquired metabolic disorders of the nervous system: toxins and illicit drugs. In: Textbook of Clinical Neurology, 3rd ed. Goetz CG, ed. 2007. Saunders Elsevier, Philadelphia, PA, pp. 865–96.

28. Nestler EJ. The neurobiology of cocaine addiction. Sci Pract Perspect 2005;3(1):4–10.

29. Sora I, Hall FS, Andrews AM, Itokawa M, Li X-F, Wei H-B, Wichems C, Lesch KP, Murphy DL, Uhl GR. Molecular mechanisms of cocaine reward: combined dopamine and serotonin transporter knockouts eliminate cocaine place preference. PNAS 2001;98(9):5300–5.

30. Brand HS, Gonggrijp S, Blanksma CJ. Cocaine and oral health. Br Dent J 2008;204:365–9.

31. Villa PD. Midfacial complications of prolonged cocaine snort. J Can Dent Assoc 1999;65:218–23.

32. Blanksma CJ, Brand HS. Cocaine abuse: orofacial manifestations and implications for dental treatment. Int Dent J 2005;55(6):365–9.

33. Parry J, Porter S, Scully C, Flint S, Parry MG. Mucosal lesions due to oral cocaine use. Br Dent J 1996;180:462–4.

34. Brown RS, Johnson CD. Corrosion of gold restorations from inhalation of "crack" cocaine. Gen Dent 1994;42(3)242–6.

35. Johnson CD, Brown RS. How cocaine abuse affects post-extraction bleeding. JADA 1993;124:60–2.

36. Mitchell-Lewis DA, Phelan JA, Kelly RB, Bradley JJ, Lamster IB. Identifying oral lesions associated with crack cocaine use. J Am Dent Assoc 994;125(8):1104–8.

37. Friedlander AH, Gorelick DA. Dental management of the cocaine addict. Oral Surg Oral Med Oral Pathol 1988;65:45–8.

38. Goodger NM, Wang J, Pegrel MA. Palatal and nasal necrosis resulting from cocaine misuse. Br Dent J 2005;198:333–4.

39. Filho PF, Jorge KO, Daiva DC, Ferreira EF, Jorge ML, Zarzar PM. The prevalence of dental trauma and its association with illicit drug use among adolescents. Dent Traumatol 2014;30(2):122–7.

40. TED case studies: qat trade in Africa. http://gurukul.ucc.american.edu/ted/QAT.HTM. Accessed January 1, 2015.

41. Gardiner S. That darned khat: in search of New York's most elusive drug. The Village Voice, November 14, 2006. http://www.villagevoice.com/2006-11-14/news/that-darned-khat/. Accessed January 1, 2015.

42. Yarom N, Epstein J, Levi H, Porat D, Kaufman E, Gorsky M. Oral manifestations of habitual khat chewing: a case–control study. Oral Surg Oral Med Oral Pathol Oral Radiol Endod 2010;109:e60–6. [Erratum: Oral Surg Oral Med Oral Pathol Oral Radiol Endod 2013;115(5):702.]

43. Al-Kholani AI. Influence of khat chewing on periodontal tissues and oral hygiene status among Yemenis. Dent Res J (Isfahan) 2010;7(1):1–6.

44. Prosser JM, Nelson LS. The toxicology of bath salts: a review of synthetic cathinones. J Med Toxicol 2012;8(1):33–42.

45. National Institute on Drug Abuse. DrugFacts: synthetic cathinones ("bath salts"). 2012. http://www.drugabuse.gov/publications/drugfacts/synthetic-cathinones-bath-salts. Accessed January 1, 2015.

46. Rees TD. Oral effects of drug abuse. Crit Rev Oral Biol Med 1992;3(3):163–84.

47. Legal Profession Assistance Conference. A Desk Reference Manual on Drugs and Substances of Abuse for LAP Directors. Chapter 4: Perception Distorting Drugs. http://www.lpac.ca/main/main/Drugmanual_chapter4.aspx. Accessed January 1, 2015.

48. National Highway Traffic Safety Administration. Drugs and Human Performance Fact Sheets. Lysergic acid diethylamide (LSD). 2013. http://www.nhtsa.gov/people/injury/research/job185drugs/lysergic.htm. Accessed January 1, 2015.

49. Cigna. Ecstasy (MDMA). http://www.cigna.com/healthwellness/hw/medical-topics/ecstasy-uq2447. Accessed January 1, 2015.

50. Connor TJ. Methylenedioxymethamphetamine (MDMA, 'ecstasy'): a stressor on the immune system. Immunology 2004;111(4):357–67.

51. Kankaanpaa A, Meririnne E, Lillsunde P, Seppala T. The acute effects of amphetamine derivatives on extracellular serotonin and dopamine levels in rat nucleus accumbens. Pharmacol Biochei Behav 1998;59:1003–9.

52. Koch S, Galloway MP. MDMA induced dopamine release in vivo: role of endogenous serotonin. J Neural Transm 1997;104:135–46.

53. Callaway CW, Wing LL, Geyer MA. Serotonin release contributes to the locomotor stimulant effects of 3,4-methylenedioxymethamphetamine in rats. J Pharmacol Exp Ther 1990;254:456–64.

54. Cole JC, Sumnall HR. The pre-clinical behavioral pharmacology of 3,4-methylenedioxymethamphetamine (MDMA). Neurosci Biobehav Rev 2003;27:199–217.

55. Brand HS, Dun SN, Nievw Amerongen AV. Ecstasy (MDMA) and oral health. Br Dent J 2008;204(2):77–81.

56. Burkhill P, Goodyear A, Hayden P, Walton L. Dental problems. Macalester College. http://www.macalester.edu/academics/psychology/whathap/UBNRP/mdma/dentalproblems.html. Accessed January 1, 2015.

57. Milosevic A, Agrawal N, Redfearn P, Mair L. The occurrence of toothwear in users of ecstasy (3,4-methylenedioxymethamphetamine). Community Dent Oral Epidemiol 1999;27(4):283–7.

58. Green AR, Mechan AO, Elliott JM, O'Shea E, Colado MI. The pharmacology and clinical pharmacology of 3,4-methylenedioxymethamphetamine (MDMA, 'ecstasy'). Pharmacol Rev 2003;55:463–508.

59. Hegadoren KM, Baker GB, Bourin M. 3,4-Methylenedioxy analogues of amphetamine; defining the risks to humans. Neurosci Biobehav Rev 1999;23:539–53.

60. Mechan AO, Esteban B, O'Shea E, Elliott JM, Colado MI, Green AR. The pharmacology of

the acute hyperthermic response that follows administration of 3,4-methylenedioxymetha mphetamine (MDMA, 'ecstasy') to rats. Br J Pharmacol 2002;135:170–80.

61. Nash JF, Jr, Meltzer HY, Gudelsky GA. Elevation of serum prolactin and corticosterone concentrations in the rat after the administration of 3,4-methylenedioxymethamphetamine. J Pharmacol Exp Ther 1988;245:873–9.

62. Liechti ME, Vollenweider FX. Which neuroreceptors mediate the subjective effects of MDMA in humans? A summary of mechanistic studies. Hum Psychopharmacol 2001;16: 589–98.

63. Drug Enforcement Administration. *Salvia divinorum* and salvinorin A. www.deadiversion.usd oj.gov/drug_chem_info/salvia_d.pdf. Accessed October 2013.

64. Wall S. *Salvia divinorum*. 2010. http://www. dentistryiq.com/articles/2010/02/salvia-divin orum.html. Accessed January 1, 2015.

65. Drug Enforcement Administration. Heroin. In: Drugs of Abuse. 2011 Edition: A DEA Resource Guide. http://www.dea.gov/pr/multimedia-library/publications/drug_of_abuse.pdf#page =36. Accessed January 9, 2015.

66. Schlosburg JE, Vendruscolo LF, Bremer PT, Lockner JW, Wade CL, Nunes AAK, Stowe GN, Edwards S, Janda KD, Koob GG. Dynamic vaccine blocks relapse to compulsive intake of heroin. Proc Natl Acad Sci U S A 2013;110(22):9036–41.

67. Hosztafi S. Heroin addiction. Acta Pharm Hung 2011;81(4):173–83 (in Hungarian).

68. Esse K, Fossati-Bellani M, Traylor A, Martin-Schild S. Epidemic of illicit drug use, mechanisms of action/addiction and stroke as a health hazard. Brain Behav 2011;1(1): 44–54.

69. Brand HS, Van Zalingen D, Veerman EC. Heroin and oral health. Ned Tijdschr Tandheelkd 2009;116(9):479–82 (in Dutch).

70. Kinane DF, Johnston FA, Evans CW. Depressed helper-to-suppressor T-cell ratios in early-onset forms of periodontal disease. J Periodont Res 1989;24:161–4.

71. Westerhof WE, Wolters EC, Brookbakker JTW, Boelen RE, Schipper MEI. Pigmented lesions of the tongue in heroin addicts—fixed drug eruption. Br J Dermatol 1983;109(5):605–10.

72. Colon PG, Jr. The effects of heroin addiction on teeth. J Psychedelic Drugs 1974;6(1):57–60.

73. Rosenstein DI. Effects of long-term addiction to heroin on oral tissues. J Public Health Dent 1975;35(2):118–22.

74. Shapiro S, Pollack BR, Gallant D. The oral health of narcotic addicts. J Pub Health Dent 1970;30(4):244–9.

75. Yahya MD, Watson RR. Immunomodulation by morphine and marijuana. Life Sci 1987;41:2503–10.

76. Picozzi A, Dworkin SF, Leeds JG, Nash J. Dental and associated attitudinal aspects of heroin addiction: a pilot study. J Dent Res 1972;51(3):869.

77. National Highway Traffic Safety Administration. Drugs and Human Performance Fact Sheets. Morphine (and heroin). 2013. http://www.nhtsa.dot.gov/people/injury/research/jo b185drugs/morphine.htm. Accessed January 1, 2015.

78. Titsas A, Ferguson MM. Impact of opioid use on dentistry. Aust Dent J 2002;47(2): 94–8.

79. Alliance for Consumer Education. Inhalant abuse. 2012. www.inhalant.org/inhalant-abuse /. Accessed January 1, 2015.

80. National Institute on Drug Abuse. DrugFacts: inhalants. 2012. www.drugabuse.gov/publi cations/drugfacts/inhalants. Accessed January 1, 2015.

81. Williams JF, Storck M, Committee on Substance Abuse, Committee on Native American Child Health. Inhalant abuse. Pediatrics 2007;119(5):1009–17.

82. Balster RL. Neural basis of inhalant abuse. Drug Alcohol Depend 1998;51:207–14.

83. Center for Substance Abuse Research, University of Maryland. Inhalants. 2013. www.cesar. umd.edu/cesar/drugs/inhalants.asp. Accessed January 1, 2015.

84. Lorenc JD. Inhalant abuse in the pediatric population: a persistent challenge. Curr Opin Pediatr 2003;15:204–9.

85. Emmanouil DE, Quock R. Advances in understanding the actions of nitrous oxide. Anesth Prog 2007;54(1):9–18.

86. Narconon International. Effects of sedatives. http://www.narconon.org/drug-abuse/effects -of-sedatives.html. Accessed January 1, 2015.

87. Centers for Disease Control and Prevention. Alcohol-related disease impact (ARDI) software. http://www.cdc.gov/alcohol/ardi.htm. Accessed January 9, 2015.

88. Benson S, Verster J, Alford C, Scholey A. Effects of mixing alcohol with caffeinated beverages on subjective intoxication: a systematic review and meta-analysis. Neurosci Biobehav Rev 2014;47C:16–21.

89. Saitz R, O'Malley S. Pharmacotherapies for alcohol abuse. Med Clin North Am 1997;81(4):881–906.

90. Brown G. The alcohol withdrawal syndrome. Ann Emerg Med 1982;11:276–80.

91. Sanouri I, Dikin M, Soubani A. Critical care aspects of alcohol abuse. South Med J 2005;98(3):372–81.

92. Illinois Department of Health. Facts about date-rape drugs. 2013. www.idph.state.il.us/about/womenshealth/factsheets/date.htm. Accessed January 1, 2015.

93. Maloney WJ. Significance of cannabis use to dental practice. N Y State Dent J 2011;77(3):36–9.

94. Drug Enforcement Administration. Marijuana/cannabis. In: Drugs of Abuse. 2011 Edition: A DEA Resource Guide. http://www.dea.gov/pr/multimedia-library/publications/drug_of_abuse.pdf#page=68. Accessed January 9, 2015.

95. Office of National Drug Control Policy. Street Terms: Drugs and the Drug Trade. http://www.streetlightpublications.net/misc/ondcp.htm. Accessed January 9, 2015.

96. Grotenhermen F. Pharmacokinetics and pharmacodynamics of cannabinoids. Clin Pharmacokinet 2003;42(4):327–60.

97. Lupica CR, Riegel AC, Hoffman AF. Marijuana and cannabinoid regulation of brain reward circuits. Br J Pharmacol 2004;143(2):227–34.

98. Versteeg PA, Slot DE, van der Velden U, van der Weijden GA. Effect of cannabis usage on the oral environment: a review. Int J Dent Hyg 2008;6:315–20.

99. Darling MR. Cannabis abuse and oral health care: review and suggestions for management. SADJ 2003;58:189–90.

100. Darling MR, Arendorf TM. Review of the effects of cannabis smoking on oral health. Int Dent J 1992;42:19–22.

101. Nahas G, Latour C. The human toxicity of marijuana. Med J Aust 1992;6:495–7.

102. Baddour HM, Audemorte TB, Layman FD. The occurrence of diffuse gingival hyperplasia in a patient using marijuana. J Tenn Dent Assoc 1984;64:39–43.

103. Guarisco JL, Cheney ML, LeJeune FE, Jr, Reed HT. Isolated uvulitis secondary to marijuana use. Laryngoscope 1988;98:1309–12.

104. Schwartz R. Uvular edema and erythema. Pediatr Infect Dis 1984;3:187.

105. Almadori G, Paludetti G, Cerullo M, Ottavani F, D'Alatri L. Marijuana smoking as a possible cause of tongue carcinoma in young patients. J Laryngol Otol 1990;104:896–9.

106. Silverstein SJ, Noel D, Heilbron D. Social drug use/abuse and dental disease. J Calif Dent Assoc 1978;6:32–7.

107. Drug Enforcement Agency. Drug schedules. http://www.deadiversion.usdoj.gov/schedules/.

108. Miller N, Greenfield A. Patient characteristics and risk factors for development of dependence on hydrocodone and oxycodone. Am J Ther 2004;11(1):26–32.

109. Chabel C, Erjavek MK, Jacobson L, Mariano A, Chaney E. Prescription opiate abuse in chronic pain patients: clinical criteria, incidence, and predictors. Clin J Pain 1997;13(2):150–5.

110. Singla A, Sloan P. Pharmacokinetic evaluation of hydrocodone/acetaminophen for pain management. J Opioid Manag 2013;9(1):71–80.

111. Barakat NH, Atayee RS, Best BM, Pesce AJ. Relationship between the concentration of hydrocodone and its conversion to hydromorphone in chronic pain patients using urinary excretion data. J Anal Toxicol 2012;36(4):257–64.

112. Samer CF, Daali Y, Wagner M, Hopfgartner G, Eap CB, Rebsamen MC, Rossier MF, Hochstrasser D, Dayer P, Desmeules JA. The effects of CYP2D6 and CYP3A activities on the pharmacokinetics of immediate release oxycodone. Br J Pharmacol 2010;160:907–18.

113. Rodriguez ML. Oxycodone: actions, metabolism, elimination, and detection. Medical Laboratory Observer. 2013. http://www.mlo-online.com/articles/201305/oxycodone-actions-metabolism-elimination-and-detection.php. Accessed January 1, 2015.

114. Meyer M, Maurer H. Absorption, distribution, metabolism and excretion pharmacogenomics of drugs of abuse. Pharmacogenetics 2011;12(2):215–33.

115. Gallego AO, Baron MG, Arranz E. Oxycodone: a pharmacological and clinical review. Clin Transl Oncol 2007;9:298–307.

116. Ramsin B, Trescot A, Datta S, Buenaventura R, Adlaka R, Sehgal N, Glaser SE, Vallejo R. Opioid complications and side effects. Pain Physician 2008;11:S105–20.

117. Kivlehan SM, Collopy KT, Snyder SR. Understanding overdose. EMS World. 2013. http://www.emsworld.com/article/10939148/ems-response-to-opioid-overdose. Accessed January 1, 2015.

118. Perrino PJ, Colucci SV, Apseloff G, Harris SC. Pharmacokinectics, tolerability, and safety of intranasal administration of reformulated OxyContin® tablets compared with original OxyContin® tablets in healthy adults. Clin Drug Investig 2013;33:441–9.

119. Wightman R, Perrone J, Portelli I, Nelson L. Likeability and abuse liability of commonly prescribed opioids. J Med Toxicol 2012;8:335–40.

120. Drug Enforcement Administration. Office of Diversion Control, Drug & Chemical Evaluation Section. Hydromorphone. www.deadiversion.usdoj.gov/drug_chem_info/hydromorphone.pdf. Accessed August 4, 2014.

121. University of Maryland Baltimore Washington Medical Center. Hydromorphone. www.mybwmc.org/library/41/065100. Accessed January 1, 2015.

122. National Institute on Drug Abuse. Fentanyl. www.drugabuse.gov/drugs-abuse/fentanyl. Accessed January 1, 2015.

123. Wyn RL. Actiq®, the sugar-loaded opiate lollipop and the risk for tooth decay. https://www.lexi.com/individuals/dentistry/newsletters.jsp?id=december_10. Accessed January 1, 2015.

124. Gee SS, Cunningham J, Rome J, Reid K. Dental disease and the use of oral transmucosal fentanyl: a case report. American Academy of Pain Medicine, 23rd Annual Meeting, February 7–10, 2007, New Orleans Paper #147. http://aapm.confex.com/aapm/2007am/techprogram/P2037.HTM. Accessed January 1, 2015.

125. Brondani M, Park PE. Methadone and oral health—a brief review. J Dent Hyg 2011;85:92–8.

126. Kreek MJ, Borg L, Ducat E, Ray B. Pharmacotherapy in the treatment of addiction: methadone. J Addict Dis 2010;29(2):200–16.

127. Ciancio S, ed. ADA/PDR Guide to Dental Therapeutics, 4th ed. 2006. ADA/Thompson PDR, Chicago, pp. 31–2.

128. Frei MY, Neilsen S, Dobbin CL. Serious morbidity associated with misuse of over-the-counter codeine–ibuprofen analgesics: a series of 27 cases. Med J Aust 2010;193:294–6.

129. Iedema J. Cautions with codeine. Austr Prescr 2011;34:133–5.

130. The National Alliance of Advocates for Buprenorphine Treatment. What exactly is buprenorphine? www.naabt.org/faq_answers.cfm?ID=2. Accessed January 1, 2015.

131. National Drug Intelligence Center. Intelligence Bulletin: Buprenophine: potential for abuse. 2009. www.justice.gov/archive/ndic/pubs10/10123/index.htm. Accessed January 9, 2015.

132. Drug Enforcement Administration, Office of Diversion Control, Drug & Chemical Evaluation Section. Buprenorphine. www.deadiversion.usdoj.gov/drug_chem_info/buprenorphine.pdf. Accessed July, 2013.

133. Moore PA. Pain management in dental practice: tramadol vs. codeine combinations. J Am Dent Assoc 1999;130(7):1075–9.

134. University of Washington. Oral Health Fact Sheet for Dental Professionals. Children with Attention Deficit Hyperactivity Disorder. ICD9 code 314.01. http://depts.washington.edu/sodent2/wordpress/wp-content/media/sp_need_pdfs/ADHD-Dental.pdf. Accessed January 9, 2015.

135. Morton WA, Stockton GS. Methylphenidate abuse and psychiatric side effects. Prim Care Companion J Clin Psychiatry 2000;2(5):159–64.

136. Benzodiazepines Co-operation Not Confrontation (BCNC). The benzodiazepine withdrawal syndrome. 2012. www.bcnc.org.uk/symptoms.html. Accessed January 1, 2015.

137. Long LP, Johnson B. Addiction: part I. Benzodiazepines—side effects, abuse risk and alternatives. Am Fam Physician 2000;61(7):2121–8.

138. Mayo Clinic. Clonazepam (oral route). 2014. http://www.mayoclinic.org/drugs-supplements/clonazepam-oral-route/precautions/drg-20072102. Accessed January 1, 2015.

139. Goodchild JH, Feck AS, Silverman MD. Anxiolysis in general dental practice. Dent Today 2003;22(3):106–11.

140. Physician's Desk Reference, 56th ed. 2002. Medical Economics Co., Montvalle, NJ, pp. 3047–8.

141. Donaldson M, Gizzarelli G, Chanpong B. Oral sedation: a primer on anxiolysis for the adult patient. Anesth Prog 2007;54(3):118–29.

142. Goodchild JH, Donaldson M. Calculating and justifying total anxiolytic doses of medications for in-office use. Gen Dent 2006;54:54–7.

143. Donaldson M, Goodchild JH. Maximum cumulative doses of sedation medication for in-office oral conscious sedation. Gen Dent 2007;55(2):143–9.

144. O'Boyle CA, Barry H, Fox E, McCreary C, Bewley A. Controlled comparison of a new sublingual lormatazepam formulation and i.v. diazepam in outpatient minor oral surgery. Br J Anaesth 1988;60(4):419–25.

145. Guzman F. Mechanism of action of quetiapine. psychopharmacologyinstitute.com/antipsychotics/quetiapine/mechanism-of-action/. Accessed January 2, 2015.

146. Raghunath A. Gingival pain: an unusual side effect of ziprasidone. BMJ Case Rep 2013; doi: 10.1136/bcr-2012-007577.

147. Kumsarna E. Olanapine abuse. Subst Abus 2013;34(1):73–4.

148. Reeves RR, Burke RS. Carisoprodol abuse potential and withdrawal syndrome. Curr Drug Abuse Rev 2010;3(1):33–8.

149. Smith BH, Higgins C, Baldacchino A, Kidd B, Bannister J. Substance misuse of gabapentin. Br J Gen Pract 2012;62(601):406–7.

150. Corea JD, Queiroz-Junior CM, Costa JE, Teixeira AL, Silva TA. Phenytoin-induced gingival overgrowth: a review of the molecular, immune, and inflammatory features. ISRN Dent 2011;2011:497850.

151. Jessen K. Recreational use of phenytoin, marijuana, and alcohol: a case report. Neurology 2004;62:2330.

152. Ozcelik O, Haytac MC, Seydaoglu G. The effects of anabolic androgenic steroid abuse on gingival tissues. J Periodontol 2006;77(7):1104–9.

153. Center for Substance Abuse Research. Dextromethorphan (DXM). www.cesar.umd.edu/cesar/drugs/dxm.asp. Accessed January 2, 2015.

154. Drug Enforcement Administration, Office of Diversion Control, Drug & Chemical Evaluation Section. Dextromethorphan. http://www.deadiversion.usdoj.gov/drug_chem_info/dextro_m.pdf. Accessed March, 2014.

155. Narconon International. Signs and symptoms of dextromethorphan abuse. http://www.narconon.org/drug-abuse/dextromethorphan-signs-symptoms.html. Accessed January 2, 2015.

156. Over the Counter Drug Addiction. Antihistamine abuse. www.overthecounterdrugaddiction.com/Antihistamine-Abuse.htm. Accessed January 2, 2015.

157. Drug Enforcement Administration, US Department of Justice. Combat Methamphetamine Epidemic Act 2005. www.deadiversion.usdoj.gov/meth/cma2005.htm. Accessed August 4, 2014.

158. Brzecko AW, Leech R, Stark JG. The advent of a new pseudoephedrine product to combat methamphetamine abuse. Am J Drug Alcohol Abuse 2013;39(5):284–90.

Resources and Further Readings

Drug Enforcement Administration. www.DEA.gov. Accessed January 2, 2015.

EROWID. Documenting the Complex Relationship between Humans & Psychoactives. www.erowid.org. Accessed January 2, 2015.

NIDA. Publications. http://www.drugabuse.gov/publications. Accessed January 2, 2015.

RxControl. Awareness and Prevention of Prescription Drug Abuse, Misuse and Diversion. http://rxcontrol.southcollegetn.edu/. Accessed January 2, 2015.

SAMHSA. Publications ordering. http://store.samhsa.gov/. Accessed January 2, 2015.

Streetdrugs. www.streetdrugs.org. Accessed January 2, 2015.

Tobacco Cessation: Behavioral and Pharmacological Considerations

Frank Vitale, MA and Amanda Eades, PharmD

Introduction

Although great strides have been made in reducing the smoking rates in the USA, smoking remains the leading preventable cause of death and disability in the country with over 400,000 deaths and countless illnesses attributed to this behavior each year. Add the next nine highest causes of death together and you get a number that still pales in comparison. Many states have adopted smoke-free workplace laws, taxes have been raised to take the price out of reach of children, advertising has been severely restricted, seven cessation medications have been approved by the US Food and Drug Administration (FDA), and substantial research has been done to determine effective behavioral interventions to help smokers quit permanently. All these efforts have cut the smoking rate by more than half since the early 1960s (Table 7.1). However, the current population of smokers still exerts a profound negative impact on our national health-care costs, and efforts continue to reduce those numbers even further. While the funding for state Quit Lines, local behavioral interventions, and national smoking control policies funding has been withdrawn or significantly reduced, the decline in smoking rates has stagnated, supplemented, unfortunately, by continued numbers of young adults beginning to smoke. While doctors, nurses, pharmacists, and the like have traditionally played a part in helping patients quit, the dental practitioner may play an equally important role. This chapter will provide several practical considerations to aid the dental professional in tobacco cessation counseling and will also discuss the pharmacological treatment options available for tobacco cessation.

Definitions

Cognitive Coping

Cognitive coping is changing how to think before or during a trigger situation so that

The ADA Practical Guide to Substance Use Disorders and Safe Prescribing, First Edition. Edited by Michael O'Neil.
© 2015 American Dental Association. Published 2015 by John Wiley & Sons, Inc.

Table 7.1   Current Cigarette Smoking Among Adults Aged 18 and Over by Sex, Race, and Age: USA, Selected Years 1965–2012

Sex, race, and age	Adults (18 years and over) who were current cigarette smokers (%)										
	1965[a]	1974[a]	1979[a]	1985[a]	1990[a]	2000	2002	2005	2010	2011	2012
All persons	41.9	37.0	33.3	29.9	25.3	23.1	22.3	20.8	19.3	19.0	18.2
Male	51.2	42.8	37.0	32.2	28.0	25.2	24.6	23.4	21.2	21.2	20.6
Female	33.7	32.2	30.1	27.9	22.9	21.1	20.0	18.3	17.5	16.8	15.9
White male	50.4	41.7	36.4	31.3	27.6	25.4	24.9	23.3	21.4	21.4	20.7
Black or African American male	58.8	53.6	43.9	40.2	32.8	25.7	26.6	25.9	23.3	23.2	22.0
White female	33.9	32.0	30.3	27.9	23.5	22.0	21.0	19.1	18.3	17.7	16.9
Black or African American female	31.8	35.6	30.5	30.9	20.8	20.7	18.3	17.1	16.6	15.2	14.2
All males											
18–24	54.1	42.1	35.0	28.0	26.6	28.1	32.1	28.0	22.8	21.3	20.1
25–34	60.7	50.5	43.9	38.2	31.6	28.9	27.2	27.7	26.1	27.5	28.0
35–44	58.2	51.0	41.8	37.6	34.5	30.2	29.7	26.0	22.5	21.2	22.8
45–54	55.9	46.8	42.0	34.9	32.1	28.8	26.9	28.1	25.2	27.0	21.4
55–64	46.6	37.7	36.4	31.9	25.9	22.6	20.7	21.1	20.7	21.4	18.8
≥65	28.5	24.8	20.9	19.6	14.6	10.2	10.1	8.9	9.7	8.9	10.6
All females											
18–24	38.1	24.1	34.7	31.4	25.6	24.5	23.0	21.2	19.1	18.8	16.9
25–34	43.7	38.8	33.7	32.0	28.2	22.3	21.3	21.5	20.6	19.5	19.4
35–44	43.7	39.8	37.0	31.5	24.8	26.2	23.7	21.3	19.0	19.9	16.1
45–54	37.5	36.0	32.6	32.4	28.5	22.2	22.6	20.9	21.3	21.6	21.3
55–64	25.0	30.4	28.6	27.4	20.5	20.9	18.9	16.1	16.5	15.0	16.2
≥65	9.6	12.0	13.2	13.5	11.5	9.3	8.6	8.3	9.3	7.1	7.5

Source: National Center for Health Statistics.[1]
[a]Data prior to 1997 are not strictly comparable with data for later years due to the 1997 questionnaire redesign.

thoughts about cigarettes or other tobacco products do not lead you back to smoking or using; that is, positive visualization, distractions, accepting the thoughts.

Behavioral Coping

Behavioral coping is changing what to *do* before or during typical situations where smoking or tobacco use occurred to prevent being tempted to have a cigarette; that is, rearranging the order of activities, finding alternative behaviors, or avoiding the situations.

Nicotine Replacement Therapy

Nicotine replacement therapy (NRT) provides nicotine in a different form than that of smoking (patches, gum, lozenge, as well as oral and nasal inhaler) to allow smoking cessation slowly and comfortably.

Spit Products

Spit products are any tobacco-based substance that is intentionally chewed, placed buccally, retained orally, or ingested through mucous membranes.

Forms of Tobacco

Historically, many types of tobacco have been available in the USA, but currently the predominant form is machine-made cigarettes. Most are sold in packs of 20 and are manufactured by four major corporations. As of the end of 2103, around 18% of the adult population of the country smoked cigarettes, which is down significantly from nearly half the population in the late 1950s and early 1960s.[2] Flavored cigarettes have been banned in the USA as there is substantial evidence that these products enticed children to begin to smoke. Light and Ultralight designations have also been outlawed as they mislead consumers to think that these types of cigarettes are safer than "regular" ones.[3]

As cigarette consumption has dropped, many other forms of tobacco have taken their place. Chew and snuff, both moist and dry, have been popular in certain sections of the country and with certain populations (rural men, team athletes, farmers) but can now be found in almost all segments of society. Most chew and snuff products consist of the actual tobacco leaf either shredded alone, in pouches, or in plugs, and is meant to be placed between the cheek and gum when used rather than smoked. Many of these products are flavored with sugar and salt as well as various other flavors to make them more palatable. Around 6% of the male population of the USA uses spit products with almost no female use.[4,5] Hookah has become very popular with college students, with many hookah bars located near university campuses. Hookah (shisha, hubble-bubble, or narghile) is flavored tobacco smoked in a water pipe. Young users harbor the misconception that the water somehow makes the smoke safer by "filtering out" all the carcinogens, and so on. But hookah smoke delivers all the same harmful chemicals that cigarette smoking does. In fact, in some cases, the nicotine and carbon monoxide levels are higher than in cigarettes. The water simply reduces irritation and allows the user to inhale more deeply. Cigars remain popular, especially as a symbol of affluence and celebration, but pipe smoking is minimal in the early twenty-first century. Finally, tobacco companies have recently been experimenting with creating new oral tobacco formulations called potentially reduced exposure products or PREPs. These formulations of tobacco are available as small sachets of flavored tobacco, lozenges containing compressed tobacco powder, or dissolvable "pills" of finely grained tobacco with additives. However, it must be noted that *all* forms of tobacco are harmful. All tobacco contains the exact same carcinogens and dangerous chemicals. Likewise, nicotine is present in all tobacco and can engender addiction even with casual use.

> **Clinical Consideration**
>
> Many young adults (e.g., college students) participate in smoking at "hookah" bars under the misperception that smoking hookah pipes is much less dangerous than traditional cigarettes. In fact, in many cases the intake of toxins is actually greater than smoking cigarettes. Asking young adults if they have any experience with hookah may create an excellent educational opportunity.

Oral Effects of Tobacco Use

Smoking has profound oral health effects. About 90% of oral cancer deaths are attributable to smoking.[6] Smokers have increased calculus build up compared to nonsmokers, as well as more loose and shifting teeth. Although the connection is not definite there is increasing evidence that there is a link between increased caries and smoking.[7,8] From the treatment perspective, we know that smokers do not heal as well as nonsmokers following any type of invasive oral procedure. Although data on the oral effects of cigar and pipe use are more limited than for cigarettes, the oral cancer risks are similar. Smoking promotes periodontal disease by depressing polymorphonuclear leukocytes and accelerating the rate of alveolar bone loss, as well as plaque and calculus build-up. It affects treatment of periodontal disease as well by suppressing the immune response, resulting in delay of wound healing.[9] Smoking has other oral effects as well. It contributes to bad breath, discolored teeth, mouth sores, hairy tongue, and an altered sense of taste and smell. Interestingly, second-hand smoke has been shown to have oral effects on children. A study published in JAMA in 2003 showed that second-hand smoke had negative consequences on children's primary teeth: 32% of children who had blood tests verifying consistent exposure to second-hand smoke had caries, as opposed to only 18% of children whose blood work showed a minimal exposure.[10] In addition, smoking promotes a caries-causing bacteria in adults that can be passed to the child via kissing. The use of smokeless tobacco comes with its own set of oral risk factors.[11] Although many of these risks are similar to smoking, especially oral cancers, there is an even greater problem with root caries from smokeless tobacco use due to the extremely high level of sugar found in these products. Some brands are between 30 and 60% sugar by weight. Salt is also used to flavor smokeless tobacco, so there is an increased risk of high blood pressure in users as well.[12] Some 60% of spit users have gingival recession, especially at the site of use, compared with only 14% of nonusers.[13] Smokeless tobacco users have an oral cancer risk between four and six times that of nonusers.[14] In some studies, potential precancerous lesions, or leukoplakia, have been found in over 50% of users, even in adolescents and teens.[15] Furthermore, grit and sand in smokeless tobacco scratches teeth and wears away enamel. Use also impairs the sense of taste, prompting chew users to eat more salty and sugary foods.

> **Clinical Consideration**
>
> Following any dental surgery, dental practitioners and hygienists should stress the importance of smoking cessation during the healing phase of any procedure.

Dental Practitioner Management of Tobacco Use

Dental professionals are in an ideal position to conduct smoking cessation interventions with their patients. In most case, dental practitioners have long-term relationships with patients that have engendered a high degree of trust. In addition, dental practitioners have a practical advantage over many other health-care professionals, since office visits often last for a half hour or more. Finally, dental professionals are the most likely health professionals to see the negative health consequences of spit tobacco products. The Clinical Practice Guideline for Treating Tobacco Use and Dependence clearly shows that even spending 3 min with a patient advising them to quit may have a positive effect on quit rates.[16] Three levels of protocols can be utilized by dental practitioners to help patients quit smoking based on the amount of time available, and these are described in the following subsections.

Brief Intervention: Ask–Advise–Refer

As a basic intervention, dental professionals should ask *every* patient about tobacco use, advise those who use to quit, and then refer interested patients to intensive intervention resources. Simply asking the patient about tobacco use elevates the importance of the issue in the eyes of the patient. Dental practitioners should provide patients with pertinent facts and clear information about how smoking is impacting their dental health. Once patients are advised to quit, refer interested patients to an intensive quitting program where they will receive expert help to create their quit plan. Providing a list of treatment programs with contact information or placing this information in the waiting room may be beneficial. Several helpful programs are listed in Box 7.1. Chapter 8 outlines the Screening, Brief Intervention, and Referral to Treatment (SBIRT) intervention considerations.

Box 7.1   Tobacco Use Quit Program Resources

1 800 QUIT NOW
American Lung Association: www.lung.org
American Heart Association: www.heart.org
www.becomeanex.org
www.quitnet.com

Low Intensity: Motivate–Educate–Refer

Tobacco use is either causing the condition dental practitioners are treating, exacerbating symptoms of that condition, interfering with healing, or producing some combination of these three effects. Better health in general and better dental health in particular can be a profound reason to quit, but it may not necessarily motivate everyone. So it may be helpful to explore other reasons for quitting. As long as the quitter has a strong, legitimate reason, avoid forcing them to find a health motivation. It is important to reinforce whatever motivation is presented. Patients admitting they are not "ready to quit" should be encouraged to notify a health-care professional when they are ready. Most people who fail to quit successfully do so because they do not have a quitting plan. Few patients actually use a cessation medication or frequently do not use them correctly. The Clinical Practice Guidelines clearly shows that

the most efficacious way to quit smoking is to use one of the seven FDA-approved cessation medications along with a program that helps the smoker understand and change the behaviors associated with the habit aspect of smoking.[17]

Clinical Consideration

Once patients are motivated to quit, patients should be educated on two essential aspects of a successful quit: using cessation medication correctly while engaging in a behavior change program.

Moderate Intensity: Create a Plan

Moderate-intensity protocols require more time. If more than 10 min is available to work with a patient then it is beneficial to help create a quitting plan that consists of the following elements:

1. Pick a quit day.
2. Clean house.
3. Understand motivations.
4. Decrease barriers.
5. Learn to cope.
6. Choose a medication.
7. Get support.

It is important to quit on a specific day. The idea of tapering or slowly cutting back generally does not work. Tapering is a good way to get ready to quit but not an especially effective way to quit. There is no prefect day to quit, but doing so during very stressful times may not be appropriate. Suggest to patients to stop smoking when their lives are relatively calm and when they can focus on the quit. Smokers must get rid of *all their cigarettes and smoking-related paraphernalia by their quit day.* There are no exceptions to this advice. If cigarettes are readily available in the first few days of a quit, it is likely that the new nonsmoker will smoke them. Likewise, ashtrays and such simply remind the individual of cigarettes and can trigger strong urges. As long as the quitter has a strong, legitimate, *internal* reason, avoid forcing them to find another motivation. Most smokers will report they smoke to deal with stress or to keep weight down. It is important for these individuals to learn healthy ways to deal with each of these issues, so referral to appropriate resources may be needed. Smokers must be taught to deal with the urges, desires, and triggers to smoke without having to use tobacco. This is known as coping. Coping falls into two categories: changing how to think (cognitive) and changing what to do (behavioral). Changing how to think basically comes down to distracting oneself from thoughts about tobacco. Changing what to do primarily involves rearranging routines that trigger a desire to use tobacco. Many individuals use tobacco absent mindedly throughout the day. A use log can be an effective tool for these individuals to understand their habit. Selecting one of the seven FDA-approved cessation medication choices is recommended at this point. It is advised that patients be referred to an intensive behavior change program to provide ongoing support.

> **Clinical Consideration**
>
> Dental practitioners and dental hygienists have a captured audience for common procedures such as cleanings, whitenings, and so on. This time may allow for moderate-intensity patient education.

Spit Tobacco Interventions

Extensive research has shown that one of the most effect strategies to help spit users stop is to perform an oral cancer screening.[18] Unlike most smoking-related illnesses, conditions caused by spit use are readily visible to the naked eye. Therefore, as part of the screening it is recommend that dental practitioners show the individual any lesions that may be present and discuss the risk of contracting oral cancers. In addition, having pictures of oral cancer lesions can be helpful as a deterrent for those without current visible problems and for younger users who may not know that such problems can develop. This exam, combined with a quitting plan, produces the best long-term quit rates.

Gradual Reduction

Although gradually reducing one's cigarette use (tapering) has not been shown to be especially effective, anecdotally, gradual reduction does seem to help spit users quit. Many brands of spit contain substantially higher amounts of nicotine than cigarettes. Furthermore, the nature of spit use dictates that one leave the spit product in the same place within the buccal mucosa for significant amount of time. As a result, the use of these products tends to deliver high levels of nicotine and abrupt cessation creates rather problematic withdrawal.

> **Clinical Consideration**
>
> None of the seven existing smoking cessation medications has been FDA approved for use with spit cessation, so gradual reduction may be a viable alternative.

When quitting, a chew or snuff user essentially has a choice of three different methods. These methods seem to minimize the withdrawal symptoms by allowing the quitter to slowly lessen the amount of nicotine in the body. In general, this appears to produce more successful quits than stopping abruptly. It is important to emphasize here that it is still recommended that the individual sets a specific day to cease all tobacco use. Without that goal in mind, many individuals will simply settle into a different, less frequent, pattern of use and never actually quit.

- **Brand Switching** This involves going from higher nicotine brands to successively lower level brands until a very low level of nicotine is reached and eventually stopping completely with little withdrawal. If this method is to be used, the individual should determine which brands will be used, how many "steps" it will take to be completely nicotine free, how long it will take on each level, and what the ultimate quit day will be *before* beginning the quit. This method should only be approached as a well thought out plan that has been clearly delineated prior to starting the quit.
- **Nicotine Fading** This involves staying with the same product throughout the quit but slowly reducing the number of chews or dips throughout the day. For this method to be successful, the quitter should also create a specific fading schedule with a planned quit day. Advise the quitter to gradually increase the time between uses until half the usual number of chews or dips is reached. The entire process should be done over a 2 or 3 week period of time. Once the individual reaches half the usage, the product should be discontinued altogether.
- **Blending** This involves taking the user's regular spit product and mixing it with subsequently higher amounts of a herbal, non-tobacco, product such as mint leaves, clover, or licorice. When using the bending method, it is suggested to mix one-third herbal product with two-thirds tobacco. The tobacco product concentration is decreased to a half-and-half blend before moving on to two-thirds herbal–one-third tobacco, with the last step being 100% herbal. This should be done over a 2–3 week period.

For any of these three methods the quitter must be determined not to increase use at any point in the process. Therefore, only recommend one of these methods to those individuals who seem genuinely motivated and well organized. *There is very little formal research to recommend any of these methods. Efficacy has only been shown anecdotally.*

Oral Substitutes

There is abundant evidence to indicate that most spit users miss the oral gratification inherent with chew and snuff when they quit. In some cases, the lack of something in the mouth can lead to relapse. Therefore, it would be prudent to suggest to all quitters to find some type of oral substitute for at least the first few weeks of their quit. Sunflower seeds, hard sugarless candy, a pungent, strong-tasting gum, beef jerky, and mint leaves are some popular suggestions. Some companies are even packaging mint leaves in small teabag-looking pouches and marketing to individuals quitting spit. In any case, caution quitters from substituting some other form of tobacco for the snuff or chew. Eating more should not replace oral gratification.

Social Support/Disapproval

There has been specific clinical research into the vital role of helping smokers quit. Extrapolating that data, we can readily see that social support will also help the spit user quit. Conversely, it is also well known that most spit users have friends who use and who will most likely prove a source of temptation upon cessation. Therefore, quitting with other users increases the chance of success. Interestingly, it appears that disapproval of use by the significant female in a user's life can be a profound motivator to quit. Since most users of spit products are male, the influence of the wife or girlfriend can be quite important.

Medication Management for Smoking Cessation

Current data suggest that a majority of cigarette smokers would like to quit smoking, but have a difficult time breaking the habit on their own. In 2011 it was found that 68.9% of adult smokers wanted to stop smoking and 42.7% had made a quit attempt in the past.[19,20] Unfortunately, only between 4 and 6% of the smoking population is successful at quitting and about one-half of those trying to quit will fail within 1 week.[20] A Cochrane review that examined the effect of combining medication and behavioral support to help treat tobacco dependence found that the chances of a person successfully quitting smoking were increased by 70–100% compared with their chance of success if they just received counseling alone.[21] Consistent with these data, the US Public Health Service recommends pharmacotherapy be discussed with every person making a quit attempt unless the person falls into specific populations for which smoking-cessation agents are contraindicated or have not been adequately studied.[22] Some of these populations include pregnant smokers, light smokers, smokeless tobacco users, and adolescents. Risks and benefits of therapy should be considered before initiating pharmacotherapy in these specific populations.

There are a number of pharmacotherapy options available for treatment of nicotine dependence, and considerations include patient preference, cost of therapy, ease of use, and side-effect profile. FDA-approved first-line smoking-cessation products include NRT, varenicline (Chantix®), and sustained-released (SR) bupropion (Zyban®). Non-FDA-approved second-line therapies for smoking cessation include clonidine and nortriptyline. A Cochrane review that studied the efficacy of these pharmacological interventions found that bupropion therapy and NRT have similar efficacy for treating tobacco dependence, while varenicline is more effective than either of these agents.[23] The review estimates that for every 10 people who quit smoking with placebo, about 18 could be expected to quit with NRT or bupropion and about 28 could be expected to quit with varenicline. Combination NRT was found to have similar efficacy to varenicline therapy. Although there is evidence that clonidine and nortriptyline are effective smoking-cessation options, they are less studied than the first-line agents and generally carry higher risk for adverse effects.

The Role of Nicotine

It is well known that tobacco contained in cigarettes is the main toxin contributing to cancer, lung disease, cardiovascular disease, and various other major health concerns associated with smoking. It is, however, the pharmacologic effects of nicotine that cause a person to become physically dependent on cigarette smoking. Before discussing the pharmacologic treatments of tobacco dependence, it is important to first understand the mechanism behind nicotine addiction and the drug-induced reward system associated with cigarette smoking. Nicotine is a tertiary amine found in tobacco and it is inhaled into the lungs when a person smokes a cigarette. Following inhalation into the lungs, nicotine travels into the systemic circulation and is eventually directed to the brain where it binds to nicotinic cholinergic receptors (nAChRs). The most predominant nAChR subtype in the human brain is the α4β2 receptor subtype, and it is believed to be the main receptor involved in nicotine dependence.[24,25] Stimulation of central nAChRs by nicotine results in the release of a variety of neurotransmitters, including dopamine, norepinephrine, acetylcholine, serotonin, γ-aminobutyric acid, and glutamate.[24]. Dopamine is considered the most important of these neurotransmitters, as it is largely responsible for the reinforcing effects of nicotine, such as stress relief, arousal, increased cognition, and mood control.[24,25] After a person is repeatedly exposed to nicotine, they may experience receptor desensitization and fail to experience the same effects as when initially starting smoking.[24] Additionally, long-term nicotine exposure is believed to cause upregulation of nAChR binding sites in the brain.[24,25] The increase may occur because long exposure of nicotine causes nAChRs to enter states of desensitization much more often, and cell turnover is decreases in the desensitized state.[25] It has been proposed that the nicotinic cholinergic system may enter a state of excess excitability when these nicotine-desensitized nAChRs become unoccupied, eventually leading to the withdrawal effects associated with smoking cessation.[25] Nicotine withdrawal effects include irritability, depressed mood, restlessness, anxiety, difficulty concentrating, increased hunger and eating, insomnia, and craving for tobacco.[24] See Box 7.2.

Box 7.2   Common Nicotine Withdrawal Signs and Symptoms

- Irritability/agitation
- Mild tremor
- Depressed mood
- Inability to focus/concentrate
- Difficulty sleeping
- Increased hunger
- Increased tobacco cravings
- Diaphoresis

Clinical Consideration

Medication-sponsored programs: all seven FDA-approved medications for cessation have free behavioral programs that accompany the medication.

Pharmacotherapy Options

First-Line Agents

Nicotine Replacement Therapy

NRT is designed to reduce motivation to smoke by decreasing physiological and psychomotor withdrawal symptoms often experienced during an attempt to stop smoking.[26] This allows the patient to focus on breaking the psychological dependence to cigarettes while experiencing less nicotine withdrawal effects. As NRT formulations do not deliver nicotine as quickly as a cigarette or cause as large a fluctuation in nicotine blood levels, they carry less abuse potential than nicotine inhaled from a cigarette.[26] There are currently five NRT formulations available in the USA that have been approved by the FDA. These include the nicotine patch, gum, lozenge, nasal spray, and inhaler. The transdermal patch is formulated for absorption through the skin, and all other formulations are absorbed through either the oral or nasal mucosa. Owing to first-passed metabolism, an NRT taken as an oral tablet would have to be dosed too high and would likely cause significant gastrointestinal adverse effects.[26] All NRTs have been proven effective at promoting smoking cessation and carry minimal risk of severe adverse effects; hence, they are considered a first-line treatment of tobacco dependence for those 18 years and older. Although NRT is considered a very safe treatment option, patients should be counseled on signs and symptoms of toxicity. See Box 7.3.

> **Box 7.3 Signs and Symptoms of Nicotine Toxicity[27-31]**
>
> - Pallor
> - Cold sweat
> - Nausea/vomiting
> - Salivation
> - Diarrhea
> - Headache
> - Tremor
> - Confusion

Nicotine Patch

The nicotine patch is the only long-acting NRT designed to release nicotine slowly and passively throughout the day. Patients should be initiated on a dose of either 21 mg or 14 mg daily depending on how many cigarettes they currently smoke per day.[28] Refer to Figure 7.1. The patch may be worn for 16–24 h based on patient preference. Those who get cigarette cravings immediately upon waking should be advised to wear the patch for 24 h, whereas patients who complain of vivid dreams or sleep disturbance while wearing the patch may prefer to remove it prior to bedtime.[26] Recommended treatment duration is 8–10 weeks, and is dependent on patient's starting dose of the nicotine patch. Although patients may desire to use the patch for longer than the recommended 10 weeks, clinical data do not suggest a significant difference in treatment effect between those treated for 8 weeks when compared with those who received extended therapy.[26] These data, however, are derived from indirect comparisons between 8-week trials and extended therapy trials rather than head-to-head comparisons. Therefore, it is advised that the patient speak to their doctor and discuss benefits of continued therapy if they wish to remain on the patch for longer than the recommended treatment period of 10 weeks.

Nicotine Gum

Nicotine gum was the first FDA-approved NRT and has a short and immediate effect compared with that of the nicotine patch.[26] Its short duration of action allows the patient to self-titrate the daily dose based on the frequency and intensity of nicotine cravings.[26] According to a Cochrane review article, most clinical trials testing the efficacy of nicotine gum used a dose of 2 mg; however, trials that compared a dose of 4 mg and 2 mg suggested a significant

	STEP 1 Use one 21 mg patch per day	STEP 2 Use one 14 mg patch per day	STEP 3 Use one 7 mg patch per day
Smoke >10 cigarettes per day	Weeks 1–6	Weeks 7–8	Weeks 9–10
Smoke ≤10 cigarettes per day	SKIP	Week 1–6	Week 7–8

Figure 7.1 Recommended steps for use of nicotine patch.

benefit of the higher dose for those who were highly dependent smokers.[26] In light of these data, the manufacturer recommends a starting dose of 4 mg for those who smoke a cigarette within 30 min of waking up, as this is a sign of severe nicotine dependence.[29] Those who smoke later than 30 min after waking may start at the 2 mg dose.[29] To improve success rate, advise patient to chew at least nine pieces of nicotine gum daily for the first 6 weeks of trying to quit smoking.[29] Patients starting on nicotine gum should be instructed to avoid eating and drinking within 15 min of chewing nicotine gum as acidic foods and beverages can decrease the absorption of nicotine across the buccal mucosa.[29] Patients should be educated to use the "chew and park" method when using nicotine gum. This means the patient should chew the gum until they experience a tingling sensation and then park the gum in the jaw until tingling subsides. The patient should repeat this process until the tingling goes away (usually around 30 min).

> **Clinical Consideration**
>
> Patients should be instructed to read the directions with nicotine gum products carefully. These products are **not** intended be used as typical chewing gum products.

Nicotine Lozenges

Just as the starting dose of nicotine gum is dependent on how long after waking a person smokes their first cigarette, so is the dosing of the lozenge. Initiate the nicotine lozenge at 4 mg if a person smokes within 30 min of waking, and initiate at the 2 mg dose if the first cigarette is later than 30 min after waking.[30] The lozenge should be placed in the mouth and allowed to dissolve; this takes about 20–30 min. Patients should be educated not to chew or swallow the lozenge. Advise patients to use at least nine lozenges per day for the first 6 weeks of therapy to maximize benefits.[30]

> **Clinical Consideration**
>
> Patients should not use more than five lozenges in a 6 h period or more than 20 lozenges in a single day.

Nicotine Inhaler

Unlike the previous NRT formulations discussed, the nicotine inhaler is available by prescription only. It consists of a mouthpiece and plastic cartridge that delivers 4 mg of nicotine to the user, of which about 2 mg is systemically absorbed.[31] The proposed advantage of this formulation is that it provides the hand-to-mouth ritual similar to smoking a cigarette. Ideally, the nicotine inhaler would provide a behavioral coping mechanism while the patient is trying to overcome their nicotine addiction. There is, however, little data to support that this results in improved success in comparison with the other formulations. The initial dosage of the nicotine inhaler is individualized based on patient cravings. It is recommended that a minimum of six cartridges per day be used in those starting the nicotine inhaler, as this is thought to increase chance of success.[31] Patients may then self-titrate to the level of nicotine they require, so long as they do not exceed the maximum dose of 12 cartridges per day. Optimal effects are achieved if the patient continuously puffs on the inhaler for about 20 min. The recommended duration of treatment of the nicotine inhaler is 12 weeks. At this time patients should be weaned off the inhaler by a gradual reduction of the daily dose over 6–12 weeks. It is advised that patients stop smoking upon starting use of the nicotine inhaler. If a patient is unable to stop smoking by the fourth week of therapy, consider discontinuing therapy as it is not likely to be an effective method of smoking cessation.

Nicotine Nasal Spray

Nicotine nasal spray is another prescription-only NRT that is administered as a metered spray to the nasal mucosa. Each actuation delivers 0.5 mg nicotine and one dose is considered two sprays (one in each nostril) for a total dose of 1 mg.[32] Patients should be started on one or two doses per hour, and may increase to a maximum of five doses per hour if necessary. At treatment initiation, patients should be instructed to use at least eight doses per day to help maximize efficacy. In clinical trials, feelings of dependency on the spray were reported by 32% of active spray users.[32] Additionally, 15–20% of patients used the active spray for longer periods than recommended and 5% used the spray at a higher dose than recommended. Some patients also reported cravings for the spray rather than for cigarettes. Properties that cause the nicotine nasal spray to be more addictive than other NRT formulations include its rapid onset of action, greater capacity for self-titration of dose, and its ability to cause rapid fluctuation in plasma nicotine concentrations.

Nasal irritation is the most common side effect of nicotine nasal spray, and was reported by 94% of patients in the first 2 days of treatment.[32] Although the frequency and severity of the irritation declines with prolonged use, it was still experienced by 81% of patients at week 3 of treatment.

Efficacy of Nicotine Replacement Therapy

A Cochrane review article which analyzed 132 trials of NRT concludes there is evidence that all forms of NRT have similar efficacy and increase a person's ability to successfully stop smoking by between 50 and 70%.[26] Findings from this meta-analysis also support the claim that starting NRT for a short period prior to the intended quit date increases the rate of success when compared with starting the NRT on the designated quit date. Another strategy found to increase rate of cessation in clinical trials is using a combination of the nicotine patch and a fast-acting NRT formulation.[26,33] The patch will provide a constant supply of nicotine throughout the day, and the fast-acting NRT formulation will be available to deal with more intense cravings that the patient may experience. See Table 7.2.

Product Selection

Cost of therapy, ease of use, and patient preference should be taken into account when deciding on an appropriate fast-acting formulation. One clinical trial analyzing patient preference between the nicotine gum, inhaler, and nasal spray found that cigarette cravings and withdrawal were reduced with all of these NRT formulations.[34] Nicotine gum, however, ranked above the inhaler and nasal spray on ease of use, safety, and "prefer in public." Study participants also reported more comfort in using the nicotine gum for a period of greater than 3 months versus the nasal spray and inhaler.

Bupropion SR

Bupropion in an atypical antidepressant that was first approved by the FDA for treatment of depression and is now considered a first-line therapy for treating tobacco dependence by the Department of Health and Human Services guidelines.[22] Its mechanism of action for smoking cessation is not completely understood, but it is thought to be related to its inhibition of dopamine and norepinephrine reuptake.[22] It is also known to be a weak antagonist at nicotinic receptors, which may account for some of its effect in smoking cessation.

Bupropion for smoking cessation is formulated as a 150 mg SR tablet. It is recommended to initiate bupropion SR 1 week before the set quit date at a dose of 150 mg daily for 3 days, and then increase to 150 mg twice daily for the duration of therapy.[35] The lower starting dose reduces risk of seizure associated with bupropion. If patients are unable to tolerate a dose of 150 mg twice daily, it is appropriate to treat them at a dose of 150 mg daily. In clinical trials, each of these doses was found to be superior to placebo for treating tobacco dependence, but the higher dose had superior efficacy for causing continuous abstinence throughout the treatment period.[36] Additionally, the 300 mg daily dose resulted in less weight gain in comparison with 150 mg.[36] A dose of 150 mg every other day is suggested for those with hepatic impairment.[35]

> **Clinical Consideration**
>
> It is recommended that treatment with bupropion be continued for at least 7–12 weeks. After this time, health-care providers should reassess the need for continued therapy. If the patient has not quit smoking after 7–12 weeks, *it is unlikely that they will quit during that attempt.*[35]

The most common adverse effects associated with use of bupropion for smoking cessation are insomnia (30–40% of patients) and dry mouth (~10% of patients). Bupropion has also been shown to increase seizure risk and is contraindicated in those considered to have a lower seizure threshold, including patients with bulimia or anorexia nervosa and in those who are undergoing alcohol or sedative withdrawal.[35]

Table 7.2 Comparison of NRT Formulations for Treatment of Nicotine Dependence

Type of NRT	RR[a]	95% CI	No. of studies	No. of participants
Gum	1.49	1.40–1.60	56	10,596/11,985
Patch	1.64	1.52–1.78	43	11,746/7840
Inhaler	1.90	1.36–2.67	4	490/486
Intranasal spray	2.02	1.49–2.73	4	448/439
Tablets/lozenges	1.95	1.61–2.36	7	1808/1597
Choice of product	1.60	1.39–1.84	5	1449/1349
Patch and inhaler	1.07	0.57–1.99	1	136/109
Patch and lozenge	1.83	1.0–3.31	1	267/41

Source: Silagy et al.[26]
RR: relative risk; CI: confidence interval.
[a]Intervention/control.

Efficacy of Bupropion

A Cochrane review of 36 trials investigating bupropion for use in smoking cessation found that bupropion was ~50% more effective than placebo at treating tobacco dependence and resulted in similar quit rates to NRT.[37] Two trials found no difference between bupropion and NRT, whereas one trial comparing cessation rate between bupropion and the nicotine patch modestly favored use of bupropion. There is inconclusive data concerning whether or not therapy with bupropion is effective in patients who have previously failed NRT. One relapse prevention trial randomized smokers who were not able to successfully quit smoking with use of the nicotine patch to bupropion or placebo therapy.[37] The use of bupropion caused one person out of 194 to quit smoking and sustain abstinence at 6 months.[37] There are data to support improved cessation rates with combination therapy of bupropion and NRT. In one clinical trial, patients were randomized to receive either placebo therapy, bupropion SR alone, the nicotine patch alone, or combination therapy with bupropion SR and the nicotine patch.[38] Abstinence rates at 12 months were 15.6% in the placebo group, 16.4% in the nicotine patch group, 30.3% in the bupropion group, and 35.5% in the group given concomitant therapy with the patch and bupropion SR.

Varenicline

Varenicline is a nicotinic receptor partial agonist that is also considered a first-line therapy for treating tobacco dependence.[22] Varenicline has a distinct mechanism of action versus other smoking-cessation agents, and is thought not only to reduce cravings and withdrawal symptoms experienced during a quit attempt, but also to reduce the rewarding effects experienced if a person relapses.[39] It works by acting as an agonist at the $\alpha4\beta2$ nAChR, which is where nicotine binds when it is inhaled into the body from a cigarette.[39]. Activation at the nAChR

causes release of dopamine, ultimately leading to the pleasurable effects of smoking.[39] Similar to bupropion, it is recommended to start varenicline therapy 1 week before the date set by the patient to quit smoking. Starting dose is 0.5 mg once daily for 3 days, titrated to 0.5 mg twice daily for 3 days, and then further titrated to the recommended dose of 1 mg twice daily for at least 12 weeks.[40] An additional 12 weeks of treatment is recommended for successful quitters to increase likelihood of long-term abstinence. For those who are not able to tolerate the maximum dose of varenicline, a dose of 1.0 mg daily or a 0.5 mg twice-daily regimen may be used. A Cochrane meta-analysis found that low-dose varenicline roughly doubled the chances of quitting while reducing side effects.[41] The most common adverse effect of varenicline is nausea, which was experienced by about 30% of patients treated on the recommended dose. Other side effects commonly experienced include insomnia and headache.

Efficacy of Varenicline

One randomized, double-blind trail comparing the efficacy of varenicline versus both placebo and bupropion for smoking cessation found the varenicline treatment group to have higher short-term and long-term cessation rates versus the other treatment groups.[42] At the end of the 12-week treatment period, 43.9% of participants in the varenicline group were abstinent from smoking compared with 17.6% of those in the placebo group and 29.8% in the bupropion SR group. At 1 year, abstinent rates were 23%, 10.3%, and 14.6% respectively. Another study designed to examine the effects on cessation rates of continuing varenicline therapy for 24 weeks rather than 12 weeks found that those who receive an additional 12 weeks of treatment had significantly greater continuous abstinence at both the end of the treatment period and at 52 weeks.[43] Additionally, there were no difference in adverse events between varenicline and placebo.

The effectiveness of varenicline in combination with other tobacco-dependent treatments is not supported by current evidence. A trial designed to study the effectiveness of combination therapy with varenicline and bupropion SR for smoking cessation did not find a significant improvement in cessation rates at 1 year compared with those on monotherapy.[44] In addition, participants receiving combination therapy reported more anxiety and symptoms of depression. One clinical trial observing the effectiveness of combination therapy with varenicline and the nicotine patch found that there was no improvement in abstinence rates with combination therapy versus monotherapy.[45]

Second-Line Agents

Clonidine

Clonidine is an FDA-approved antihypertensive agent that has shown efficacy for treating tobacco dependence. As clonidine is an agonist at the α2 adrenergic receptors, it is known to cause central nervous system effects such as anxiolysis.[46] It is believed that these effects may counterbalance the withdrawal symptoms experienced by persons who are trying to stop smoking.[46] A drawback of clonidine therapy is its adverse effect profile. Its central nervous system activity may result in systemic effects, including hypotension, bradycardia, sedation, dry mouth, and constipation.[46,47]

Nortriptyline

Nortriptyline is a tricyclic antidepressant (TCA) that has shown similar efficacy to bupropion for treatment of tobacco dependence. A Cochrane review that analyzed monotherapy with nortriptyline versus placebo for smoking cessation revealed nortriptyline to be more effective than placebo when the results of six trials were pooled.[37] Data from four trials using nortriptyline as an adjunct to NRT found no benefit with combination therapy.[37] When compared with

bupropion for smoking cessation, there was no significant difference seen between agents, but comparison favored bupropion therapy.[37] Although there is not a specified dose for nortriptyline when used for smoking cessation, the majority of clinical trials used a dose of 75–150 mg daily.[37] TCAs typically carry a worse side effect profile than newer generation antidepressant therapies. Some common adverse effects associated with TCAs are dry mouth, drowsiness, light-headedness, and constipation.[48]

Other Non-FDA-Approved Smoking-Cessation Therapies

Electronic Cigarettes

Electronic cigarettes (e-cigarettes) are battery-operated products that turn nicotine into an aerosol to be inhaled by the user. E-cigarettes have not been fully studied for safety and efficacy by the FDA, so the potential risks of use, as well as the amount of nicotine that is inhaled from their use, remain unknown, as does the efficacy of e-cigarettes as a smoking-cessation agent.[49] One concern with the e-cigarette is that its rapid delivery of nicotine may cause it to have an abuse potential similar to conventional tobacco-containing cigarettes. As e-cigarettes do not have an age requirement, this may act as an avenue for teens and young adults to become addicted to nicotine.[50] At this point in time, there are no quality control processes used to manufacture e-cigarettes.[51] The FDA issued warning letters to five distributors of e-cigarettes for violations of the Federal Food, Drug, and Cosmetic Act (FDCA).[51] These violations included unsubstantiated claims and poor manufacturing practices. Further research is warranted before this product should be recommended to patients as a safe and effective treatment of tobacco dependence.

Table 7.3 lists FDA-approved drug therapy products, doses, adverse reactions, and usage guidelines.

Table 7.3 Pharmacologic Product Guide: FDA-Approved Medications for Smoking Cessation

	Nicotine Replacement Therapy (NRT) Formulations					Bupropion SR	Varenicline
	Gum	Lozenge	Transdermal Patch	Nasal Spray	Oral Inhaler		
Product	**Nicorette[a], Generic** OTC 2 mg, 4 mg original, cinnamon, fruit, mint	**Nicorette Lozenge,[a] Nicorette Mini Lozenge,[a] Generic** OTC 2 mg, 4 mg; cherry, mint	**NicoDerm CQ[a], Generic** OTC (NicoDerm CQ, generic) Rx (generic) 7 mg, 14 mg, 21 mg (24-hour release)	**Nicotrol NS[b]** Rx Metered spray 10 mg/mL aqueous nicotine solution	**Nicotrol Inhaler[b]** Rx 10 mg cartridge delivers 4 mg inhaled nicotine vapor	**Zyban,[a] Generic** Rx 150 mg sustained-release tablet	**Chantix[b]** Rx 0.5 mg, 1 mg tablet
Precautions	• Recent (≤2 weeks) myocardial infarction • Serious underlying arrhythmias • Serious or worsening angina pectoris • Temporomandibular joint disease • Pregnancy[c] and breastfeeding • Adolescents (<18 years)	• Recent (≤2 weeks) myocardial infarction • Serious underlying arrhythmias • Serious or worsening angina pectoris • Pregnancy[c] and breastfeeding • Adolescents (<18 years)	• Recent (≤2 weeks) myocardial infarction • Serious underlying arrhythmias • Serious or worsening angina pectoris • Pregnancy[c] (Rx formulations, category D) and breastfeeding • Adolescents (<18 years)	• Recent (≤2 weeks) myocardial infarction • Serious underlying arrhythmias • Serious or worsening angina pectoris • Underlying chronic nasal disorders (rhinitis, nasal polyps, sinusitis) • Severe reactive airway disease • Pregnancy[c] (category D) and breastfeeding • Adolescents (<18 years)	• Recent (≤2 weeks) myocardial infarction • Serious underlying arrhythmias • Serious or worsening angina pectoris • Bronchospastic disease • Pregnancy[c] (category D) and breastfeeding • Adolescents (<18 years)	• Concomitant therapy with medications/conditions known to lower the seizure threshold • Hepatic impairment • Pregnancy[c] (category C) and breastfeeding • Adolescents (<18 years) **Warning:** • BLACK-BOXED WARNING for neuropsychiatric symptoms[d] **Contraindications:** • Seizure disorder • Concomitant bupropion (e.g., Wellbutrin) therapy • Current or prior diagnosis of bulimia or anorexia nervosa • Simultaneous abrupt discontinuation of alcohol or sedatives/benzodiazepines • MAO inhibitors in preceding 14 days; concurrent use of reversible MAO inhibitors (e.g., linezolid, methylene blue)	• Severe renal impairment (dosage adjustment is necessary) • Pregnancy[c] (category C) and breastfeeding • Adolescents (<18 years) **Warning:** • BLACK-BOXED WARNING for neuropsychiatric symptoms[d]

Nicotine Replacement Therapy (NRT) Formulations

	Gum	Lozenge	Transdermal Patch	Nasal Spray	Oral Inhaler	Bupropion SR	Varenicline
Dosing	*1st cigarette ≤30 minutes after waking: 4 mg* *1st cigarette >30 minutes after waking: 2 mg* Weeks 1–6: 1 piece q 1–2 hours Weeks 7–9: 1 piece q 2–4 hours Weeks 10–12: 1 piece q 4–8 hours • Maximum, 24 pieces/day • Chew each piece slowly • Park between cheek and gum when peppery or tingling sensation appears (~15–30 chews) • Resume chewing when tingle fades • Repeat chew/park steps until most of the nicotine is gone (tingle does not return; generally 30 min) • Park in different areas of mouth • No food or beverages 15 minutes before or during use • Duration: up to 12 weeks	*1st cigarette ≤30 minutes after waking: 4 mg* *1st cigarette >30 minutes after waking: 2 mg* Weeks 1–6: 1 lozenge q 1–2 hours Weeks 7–9: 1 lozenge q 2–4 hours Weeks 10–12: 1 lozenge q 4–8 hours • Maximum, 20 lozenges/day • Allow to dissolve slowly (20–30 minutes for standard; 10 minutes for mini) • Nicotine release may cause a warm, tingling sensation • Do not chew or swallow • Occasionally rotate to different areas of the mouth • No food or beverages 15 minutes before or during use • Duration: up to 12 weeks	*>10 cigarettes/day:* 21 mg/day × 4–6 weeks 14 mg/day × 2 weeks 7 mg/day × 2 weeks *≤10 cigarettes/day:* 14 mg/day × 6 weeks 7 mg/day × 2 weeks • May wear patch for 16 hours if patient experiences sleep disturbances (remove at bedtime) • Duration: 8–10 weeks	1–2 doses/hour (8–40 doses/day) One dose = 2 sprays (one in **each** nostril); each spray delivers 0.5 mg of nicotine to the nasal mucosa • Maximum ~5 doses/hour or ~40 doses/day • For best results, initially use at least 8 doses/day • Do not sniff, swallow, or inhale through the nose as the spray is being administered • Duration: 3–6 months	6–16 cartridges/day Individualize dosing; initially use 1 cartridge q 1–2 hours • Best effects with continuous puffing for 20 minutes • Initially use at least 6 cartridges/day • Nicotine in cartridge is depleted after 20 minutes of active puffing • Inhale into back of throat or puff in short breaths • Do NOT inhale into the lungs (like a cigarette) but "puff" as if lighting a pipe • Open cartridge retains potency for 24 hours • No food or beverages 15 minutes before or during use • Duration: 3–6 months	150 mg po q AM × 3 days, then 150 mg po bid • Do not exceed 300 mg/day • Begin therapy 1–2 weeks **prior** to quit date • Allow at least 8 hours between doses • Avoid bedtime dosing to minimize insomnia • Dose tapering is not necessary • Duration: 7–12 weeks, with maintenance up to 6 months in selected patients	Days 1–3: 0.5 mg po q AM Days 4–7: 0.5 mg po bid Weeks 2–12: 1 mg po bid • Begin therapy 1 week **prior** to quit date • Take dose after eating and with a full glass of water • Dose tapering is not necessary • Dosing adjustment is necessary for patients with severe renal impairment • Duration: 12 weeks; an additional 12-week course may be used in selected patients

(continued)

Table 7.3 (Continued)

	Nicotine Replacement Therapy (NRT) Formulations						
	Gum	Lozenge	Transdermal Patch	Nasal Spray	Oral Inhaler	Bupropion SR	Varenicline
Adverse Effects	• Mouth/jaw soreness • Hiccups • Dyspepsia • Hypersalivation • Effects associated with incorrect chewing technique: – Lightheadedness – Nausea/vomiting – Throat and mouth irritation	• Nausea • Hiccups • Cough • Heartburn • Headache • Flatulence • Insomnia	• Local skin reactions (erythema, pruritus, burning) • Headache • Sleep disturbances (insomnia, abnormal/vivid dreams); associated with nocturnal nicotine absorption	• Nasal and/or throat irritation (hot, peppery, or burning sensation) • Rhinitis • Tearing • Sneezing • Cough • Headache	• Mouth and/or throat irritation • Cough • Headache • Rhinitis • Dyspepsia • Hiccups	• Insomnia • Dry mouth • Nervousness/difficulty concentrating • Nausea • Dizziness • Constipation • Rash • Seizures (risk is 0.1%) • Neuropsychiatric symptoms (rare; see Precautions)	• Nausea • Sleep disturbances (insomnia, abnormal/vivid dreams) • Constipation • Flatulence • Vomiting • Neuropsychiatric symptoms (rare; see Precautions)
Advantages	• Might serve as an oral substitute for tobacco • Might delay weight gain • Can be titrated to manage withdrawal symptoms • Can be used in combination with other agents to manage situational urges	• Might serve as an oral substitute for tobacco • Might delay weight gain • Compared to the gum, nasal spray and inhaler, its use is less obvious to others • Can be titrated to manage withdrawal symptoms • Can be used in combination with other agents to manage situational urges	• Once daily dosing associated with fewer compliance problems • Of all NRT products, its use is least obvious to others • Can be used in combination with other agents; delivers consistent nicotine levels over 24 hours	• Can be titrated to rapidly manage withdrawal symptoms • Can be used in combination with other agents to manage situational urges	• Might serve as an oral substitute for tobacco • Can be titrated to manage withdrawal symptoms • Mimics hand-to-mouth ritual of smoking • Can be used in combination with other agents to manage situational urges	• Once daily oral dosing is simple and associated with fewer compliance problems • Might delay weight gain • Might be beneficial in patients with depression • Can be used in combination with NRT agents	• Once daily oral dosing is simple and associated with fewer compliance problems • Offers a different mechanism of action for patients who have failed other agents

Nicotine Replacement Therapy (NRT) Formulations

	Gum	Lozenge	Transdermal Patch	Nasal Spray	Oral Inhaler	Bupropion SR	Varenicline
Disadvantages	• Need for frequent dosing can compromise compliance • Might be problematic for patients with significant dental work • Proper chewing technique is necessary for effectiveness and to minimize adverse effects • Gum chewing may not be acceptable or desirable for some patients	• Need for frequent dosing can compromise compliance • Gastrointestinal side effects (nausea, hiccups, heartburn) might be bothersome	• When used as monotherapy, cannot be titrated to acutely manage withdrawal symptoms • Not recommended for use by patients with dermatologic conditions (e.g., psoriasis, eczema, atopic dermatitis)	• Need for frequent dosing can compromise compliance • Nasal administration might not be acceptable or desirable for some patients; nasal irritation often problematic • Not recommended for use by patients with chronic nasal disorders or severe reactive airway disease	• Need for frequent dosing can compromise compliance • Cartridges might be less effective in cold environments ($\leq 60°F$)	• Seizure risk is increased • Several contraindications and precautions preclude use in some patients (see PRECAUTIONS) • Patients should be monitored for potential neuropsychiatric symptoms[d] (see PRECAUTIONS)	• Should be taken with food or a full glass of water to reduce the incidence of nausea • Patients should be monitored for potential neuropsychiatric symptoms[d] (see PRECAUTIONS)
Cost/day	2 mg or 4 mg: $1.90–$3.70 (9 pieces)	2 mg or 4 mg: $2.66–$4.10 (9 pieces)	$1.52–$3.48 (1 patch)	$5.00 (8 doses)	$8.51 (6 cartridges)	$2.72–$6.22 (2 tablets)	$8.24 (2 tablets)

[a]Marketed by GlaxoSmithKline.

[b]Marketed by Pfizer.

[c]The U.S. Clinical Practice Guideline states that pregnant smokers should be encouraged to quit without medication based on insufficient evidence of effectiveness and theoretical concerns with safety. Pregnant smokers should be offered behavioral counseling interventions that exceed minimal advice to quit.

[d]In July 2009, the FDA mandated that the prescribing information for all bupropion- and varenicline-containing products include a black-boxed warning highlighting the risk of serious neuropsychiatric symptoms, including changes in behavior, hostility, agitation, depressed mood, suicidal thoughts and behavior, and attempted suicide. Clinicians should advise patients to stop taking varenicline or bupropion SR and contact a healthcare provider immediately if they experience agitation, depressed mood, and any changes in behavior that are not typical of nicotine withdrawal, or if they experience suicidal thoughts or behavior. If treatment is stopped due to neuropsychiatric symptoms, patients should be monitored until the symptoms resolve.

[e]Wholesale acquisition cost from Red Book Online. Thomson Reuters, October 2014.

Abbreviations: MAO, monoamine oxidase; NRT, nicotine replacement therapy; OTC, over-the-counter (non-prescription product); Rx, prescription product.

For complete prescribing information and a comprehensive listing of warnings and precautions, please refer to the manufacturers' package inserts.

Summary

Cigarette smoking remains the single most preventable cause of death in the USA. In the years 2005–2009, cigarette smoking and second-hand smoke were responsible for 87% of deaths from lung cancer, 61% of deaths related to pulmonary disease, and 32% of deaths from coronary heart disease.[20] In hopes of decreasing morbidity and mortality associated with cigarette smoking, the US Public Health Service recommends that all clinicians discuss smoking cessation with every tobacco user seen in a health-care setting.[22] Although it has been proven that the combination of behavioral and pharmacotherapy is the most effective method to help patients stop smoking, simply questioning the patient on their tobacco status and encouraging the patient to consider quitting can cause the patient to question their decision to smoke. It is important to support the recommendation with facts about how the patient's tobacco habit is affecting their dental and overall health. If a patient does express interest in quitting, depending on time and comfort level, dental practitioners may choose to utilize the methods discussed herein to help the patient develop a quit plan. Additionally, all patients should be provided with contact information for more intensive treatment programs which can provide closer follow-up with the patient while they attempt to conquer their addiction.

References

1. Health, United States, 2013: With Special Feature on Prescription Drugs. 2014. National Center for Health Statistics, Hyattsville, MD.

2. Agaku IT, King BA, Dube SR. Current cigarette smoking among adults—United States, 2005–2012. Morb Mortal Wkly Rep 2014;63(2):29–34.

3. Family Smoking Prevention and Tobacco Control Act, Public Law 111-31–June 22, 2009. http://www.gpo.gov/fdsys/pkg/PLAW-111publ31/pdf/PLAW-111publ31.pdf. Accessed January 6, 2015.

4. Substance Abuse and Mental Health Services Administration. Results from the 2012 National Survey on Drug Use and Health: Summary of National Findings. NSDUH Series H-46, HHS Publication No. (SMA) 13-4795. 2013. Substance Abuse and Mental Health Services Administration, Rockville, MD. http://media.samhsa.gov/data/NSDUH/2012SummNatFindDetTables/NationalFindings/NSDUHresults2012.pdf. Accessed January 5, 2015.

5. US Department of Health and Human Services. The Health Consequences of Smoking—50 Years of Progress: A Report of the Surgeon General, 2014. US Department of Health and Human Services, Centers for Disease Control and Prevention, National Center for Chronic Disease Prevention and Health Promotion, Office on Smoking and Health, Atlanta, GA. http://www.surgeongeneral.gov/library/reports/50-years-of-progress/full-report.pdf. Accessed January 11, 2015.

6. US Department of Health and Human Services. 2004 Surgeon General's Report—The Health Consequences of Smoking. US Department of Health and Human Services, Centers for Disease Control and Prevention, National Center for Chronic Disease Prevention and Health Promotion, Office on Smoking and Health, Atlanta, GA. http://www.cdc.gov/tobacco/data_statistics/sgr/2004/index.htm. Accessed January 11, 2015.

7. US Department of Health and Human Services. Oral Health in America: A Report of the Surgeon General. 2000. US Department of Health and Human Services, National Institute of Dental and Craniofacial Research, National Institutes of Health, Rockville, MD.

8. Winn DM. Tobacco use and oral disease. J Dent Edu 2001;65(4):306–12.

9. Mandel I. Smoke signals: an alert for oral disease. JADA 1994;125(7): 872–8.

10. Aligne CA, Moss ME, Auinger P, Weitzman M. Association of pediatric dental caries with passive smoking. JAMA 2003;289:1258–64.

11. The Health Consequences of Using Smokeless Tobacco: A Report of the Advisory Committee to the Surgeon General. 1986. NIH Publication No. 86-2874. US Department of Health and Human Services, Bethesda, MD.

12. Westman EC. Does smokeless tobacco cause hypertension? South Med J 1995;88(7):716–20.

13. Singh P, Rizvi R. Influence of smokeless tobacco on periodontal health status in local population of north India: a cross sectional study. Dent Res J (Isfahan). 2011;8(4):211–20.

14. Boffetta P, Hecht S, Gray N, Gupta P, Straif K. Smokeless tobacco and cancer. Lancet Oncol 2008;9(7):667–75.

15. Taybos G. Oral changes associated with tobacco use. Am J Med Sci 2003;326(4):179–82.

16. Clinical Practice Guideline. Treating Tobacco Use and Dependence: 2008 Update. 2008. US Department of Health and Human Services, Bethesda, MD, p. 12.

17. Clinical Practice Guideline. Treating Tobacco Use and Dependence: 2008 Update. 2008. US Department of Health and Human Services, Bethesda, MD, p. 101.

18. Ebbert J, Montori VM, Vickers-Douglas KS, Erwin PC, Dale LC, Stead LF. Interventions for smokeless tobacco use cessation. Cochrane Database Syst Rev 2007;(4):CD004306. doi: 10.1002/1465 1858.CD004306.pub3.

19. US Department of Health and Human Services. How Tobacco Smoke Causes Disease: What It Means to You. 2010. US Department of Health and Human Services, Centers for Disease Control and Prevention, National Center for Chronic Disease Prevention and Health Promotion, Office on Smoking and Health, Atlanta, GA.

20. US Department of Health and Human Services. The Health Consequences of Smoking—50 Years of Progress: A Report of the Surgeon General. 2014. US Department of Health and Human Services, Centers for Disease Control and Prevention, National Center for Chronic Disease Prevention and Health Promotion, Office on Smoking and Health, Atlanta, GA.

21. Stead LF, Lancaster T. Combined pharmacotherapy and behavioural interventions for smoking cessation. Cochrane Database Syst Rev 2012;(10):CD008286.

22. Fiore MC, Bailey WC, Cohen SJ, et al. Treating tobacco use and dependence: clinical practice guideline. US Department of Health and Human Services, Public Health Service, in press.

23. Cahill K, Stevens S, Perera R, Lancaster T. Pharmacological interventions for smoking cessation: an overview and network meta-analysis. Cochrane Database Syst Rev 2013;(5):CD009329.

24. Benowitz NL. Pharmacology of nicotine: addiction, smoking-induced disease, and therapeutics. Annu Rev Pharmacol Toxicol 2009;49:57–71.

25. Dani J, De Biasi M. Cellular mechanisms of nicotine addiction. Pharmacol Biochem Behav 2001; 70(4):439–46.

26. Silagy C, Lancaster T, Stead L, Mant D, Fowler G. Nicotine replacement therapy for smoking cessation. Cochrane Database Syst Rev 2004; (3):CD0000146.

27. Food and Drug Administration. Nicotine replacement therapy labels may change. 2013. http:// www.fda.gov/forconsumers/consumerupdates/ ucm345087.htm#. Accessed January 6, 2015.

28. Nicoderm CQ (nicotine patch), extended release [package insert]. 2011. GlaxoSmithKline, Research Triangle Park, NC.

29. Nicorette (nicotine polacrilex) [package insert]. 2011. GlaxoSmithKline, Research Triangle Park, NC.

30. Nicorette (nicotine lozenge) [package insert]. 2011. GlaxoSmithKline, Research Triangle Park, NC.

31. Nicotrol (nicotine inhaler) [package insert]. 2007. Pfizer Inc, New York.

32. Nicotrol NS (nicotine nasal spray) [package insert]. 2010. Pfizer Inc, New York.

33. Kornitzer M, Boutsen, M, Dramaix M, Thijs J, Gustavsson G. Combined use of nicotine patch and gum in smoking cessation: a placebo-controlled clinical trial. Prev Med 1995;24(1): 41–7.

34. Schneider NG, Olmstead RE, Nides M, Mody FV, Otte-Colquette P, Doan K, Patel S. Comparative testing of 5 nicotine replacement systems: initial use and preferences. Am J Health Behav 2004;28:72–86.

35. Zyban (bupropion hydrochloride) sustained-release tablets [prescriber information]. 2005. GlaxoSmithKline, Research Triangle Park, NC.

36. Hurt RD, Sachs DP, Glover ED, Offord KP, Johnston JA, Dale LC, Khayrallah MA, Schroeder DR, Glover PN, Sullivan CR, Croghan IT, Sullivan PM. A comparison of sustained-release bupropion and placebo for smoking cessation. N Engl J Med 1997;337:1195–202.

37. Hughes JR, Stead LF, Hartmann-Boyce J, Cahill K, Lancaster T. Antidepressants for smoking cessation. Cochrane Database Syst Rev 2014;(1):CD000031.

38. Jorenby DE, Leischow SJ, Nides MA, Rennard SI, Johnston JA, Hughes AR, Smith SS, Muramoto ML, Daughton DM, Doan K, Fiore MC, Baker TB. A controlled trial of sustained-release bupropion, a nicotine patch, or both for smoking cessation. N Engl J Med 1999;340(9):685–91.

39. Hay JT, Ebbert JO, Sood A. Efficacy and safety of varenicline for smoking cessation. JAMA 2008;121:S32–42.

40. Chantix (varenicline) [prescribing information]. 2006. Pfizer Inc, New York.

41. Cahill K, Stead LF, Lancaster T. Nicotine receptor partial agonists for smoking cessation. Cochrane Database Syst Rev 2012;(4):CD006103.

42. Jorenby DE, Hay JT, Rigotti N, Azoulay S, Watsky EJ, Williams KE, Billing CB, Gong J, Reeves KR. Efficacy of varenicline, an α4β2 nicotinic acetylcholine receptor partial agonist, vs placebo or sustained-release bupropion for smoking cessation: a randomized controlled trial. JAMA 2006;296:56–63.

43. Tonstad S, Tønnesen P, Hajek P, Williams KE, Billing CB, Reeves KR. Effect of maintenance therapy with varenicline on smoking cessation. JAMA 2006;296:64–71.

44. Ebbert JO, Hatsukami DK, Croghan IT, Schroeder DR, Allen SS, Hays JT, Hurt RD. Combination varenicline and bupropion SR for tobacco-dependent treatment in cigarette smokers: a randomized trial. JAMA 2014;311(2):155–63.

45. Hajek P, Myers Smith K, Dhanji A-R, McRobbie H. Is a combination of varenicline and nicotine patch more effective in helping smokers quit than varenicline alone? A randomized controlled trial. BMC Med 2013;11:140.

46. Gourlay SG, Benowitz NL. Is clonidine an effective smoking cessation therapy? Drugs 1995;50:197–207.

47. Catapres (clonidine hydrochloride USP) [prescribing information]. 1998. Boehringer Ingelheim, Ridgefield, CT.

48. Pamelor (nortriptyline HCl) [prescribing information]. 2006. Mallinckrodt Inc, St Louis, MO.

49. US Food and Drug Administration. Electronic cigarettes (e-cigarettes). 2014. http://www.fda.gov/newsevents/publichealthfocus/ucm172906.htm. Accessed January 6, 2015.

50. US Food and Drug Administration. FDA warns of health risks posed by e-cigarettes. 2014. http://www.fda.gov/ForConsumers/ConsumerUpdates/ucm173401.htm. Accessed January 6, 2015.

51. US Food and Drug Administration. E-cigarettes: questions and answers. 2014. http://www.fda.gov/forconsumers/consumerupdates/ucm225210.htm. Accessed January 6, 2015.

Resources and Further Readings

ADA. Smoking and tobacco. 2014. www.mouthhealthy.org/en/az-topics/s/smoking-and-tobacco. Accessed January 6, 2015.

ADA. Smoking and tobacco cessation. http://www.ada.org/en/member-center/oral-health-topics/smoking-and-tobacco-cessation. Accessed January 6, 2015.

CDC. Smoking & tobacco use. 2014. www.cdc.gov/tobacco/. Accessed January 6, 2015.

KillTheCan! http://www.killthecan.org/. Accessed January 6, 2015.

QuitSmokeless. http://www.quitsmokeless.org/. Accessed January 6, 2015.

Detection and Deterrence of Substance Use Disorders and Drug Diversion in Dental Practice

Sarah T. Melton, PharmD, BCPP, BCACP, CGP, FASCP and Ralph A. Orr

Introduction

In order to manage pain for invasive dental procedures or pain from invasive dental pathology, dental practitioners must prescribe medications on a regular basis. Opioid analgesics are associated with physical dependence and risk of addiction. Therefore, it is critical that dental practitioners be able to screen patients for risk factors of substance abuse before prescribing a controlled substance. The dental team must be adept at identifying patients that are drug seeking by evaluating characteristic behaviors and schemes. There are important tools dental practitioners can access to evaluate prescription drug use before prescribing medications. In most states, one of these tools is the prescription drug monitoring program (PDMP). The dental team is primed to serve as educators of patients about the dangers of prescription drug abuse, including tenets of appropriate disposal of prescription medications. When prescribing controlled substances, dental practitioners should use the principles of universal precautions to protect themselves, their practice, and their patients from untoward outcomes from inappropriate prescribing. This chapter will provide education about each of these topics with key questions to ask patients and their other health-care providers before prescribing controlled substances. In addition, special clinical considerations and precautions when managing pain in the dental setting will be discussed.

Definitions

Drug Diversion

Drug diversion may be defined as the intentional transfer of a substance, or possession of a substance, or alteration of legitimate

The ADA Practical Guide to Substance Use Disorders and Safe Prescribing, First Edition. Edited by Michael O'Neil.
© 2015 American Dental Association. Published 2015 by John Wiley & Sons, Inc.

medication orders outside the boundaries designated by the US Food and Drug Administration (FDA), federal Drug Enforcement Administration (DEA), or state regulatory board. Drug diversion may involve prescription or over-the-counter medications or illicit substances. These illegal activities are usually motivated by financial incentives, substance use disorder (SUD) behaviors, or other activities such as sharing medications with the intent to help. Examples include a patient selling or giving their prescription medication to someone else, altering the original information on a prescription without the prescriber's consent, or theft of medications.

Doctor or Dentist Shoppers

Doctor shopping is characterized by the specific intent of a patient to deceive a prescriber to obtain prescription medications. Patients visit multiple treatment providers "shopping" to procure prescription medications illicitly.

Screening Patients for Substance Use Disorder

Dental practitioners are in a unique position to help patients identify unhealthy use of alcohol and drugs and to address these issues before the patient begins engaging in abusive or dependent patterns of use. Dental practitioners are also well positioned to talk with patients about their alcohol or drug use because there is a direct connection between substance use and oral health. Patients with SUD are at increased risk of poor dental health because of limited access to dental care, poor dietary and oral hygiene habits, negative attitudes about oral health and health care, and the direct physical effects of the substance of abuse on oral health.[1] For example, alcohol consumption is a major risk factor for certain head and neck cancers, particularly cancers of the oral cavity, pharynx,

and larynx.[2] Methamphetamine use results in classic problems with oral health that have been termed "meth mouth."

In a recent survey of dentists in West Virginia, 33% of respondents acknowledged they *did not* routinely ask new patients about a current or past history of substance abuse.[3] When health-care professionals do not screen for substance abuse or misuse, key opportunities are missed to intervene and suggest appropriate treatment to patients.

Screening, Brief Intervention, Referral for Treatment

Dental professionals are situated to integrate the Screening, Brief Intervention, and Referral to Treatment (SBIRT) process into daily practice.[4] SBIRT is an evidence-based practice used to identify, reduce, and prevent problematic use, abuse, and dependence on alcohol and illicit drugs.[4] See Box 8.1 for an overview of the SBIRT process. The first component of SBIRT is the screening process, where the dental professional assesses a patient for risky substance use behaviors using standardized screening tools. In the second component, the brief intervention, the dental professional engages a patient showing risky substance use behaviors in a short conversation, providing feedback and advice. The third and final component involves a referral to treatment where the dental professional provides a referral for brief therapy or additional treatment to patients who are in need of additional SUD services.

When the SBIRT process is used in primary care provider offices, it is billable under most insurance plans. In dentistry, however, reimbursement for SBIRT procedure is not universal, resulting in a barrier to integrating the process into the work flow. Dental professionals should check for state grants that provide reimbursement to those who are trained and perform SBIRT in their practice settings. SBIRT screening should be part of every dental practitioner's

> **Box 8.1   Overview of Screening, Brief Intervention, and Referral to Treatment Model[4]**
>
> **Screening** identifies patients who need further assessment or treatment for SUDs. Commonly used screening instruments can be downloaded at http://www.integration.samhsa.gov/clinical-practice/screening-tools#drugs and include:
>
> - Alcohol Use Disorders Identification Test (AUDIT);
> - Alcohol, Smoking, and Substance Involvement Screening Test (ASSIST);
> - Drug Abuse Screening Test (DAST).
>
> **Brief intervention**(s) are session(s) of motivational discussion focused on increasing insight and awareness regarding substance use and motivation toward changing behavior. Intervention can be used as a stand-alone treatment for those at risk, as well as a vehicle for engaging those in need of higher levels of care.
>
> **Brief treatment** is provided to those seeking or already engaged in treatment who acknowledge problems related to substance use. It consists of a limited number of highly focused and structured clinical sessions with the purpose of eliminating hazardous or harmful substance use.
>
> Referral to specialized treatment is provided to those identified as needing more extensive treatment than offered by the screening, brief intervention, and referral to treatment program.

CAGE-AID questionnaire can be used to screen for addiction to alcohol or other substances.[4] The patient should be asked the following four questions in the mnemonic with the answers documented in the dental record.

- **C** Have you felt that you should **CUT** down on your drinking or drug use? *A positive response may indicate the person has lost control of drug use and feels the need to decrease use.*
- **A** Have you ever been **ANNOYED** by others criticizing your alcohol or drug use? *Patients with addiction will often engage in behaviors that cause concern from those that observe them. The addict will often become annoyed when their behaviors are criticized by others.*
- **G** Have you ever felt bad or **GUILTY** about your alcohol or drug use? *Guilt is a common symptom of addiction because of impairment in relationships and social functioning.*
- **E** Have you ever needed an **EYE-OPENER** to steady your nerves or to treat a hangover? *This means that the person needs to use something the next morning to stop withdrawal from occurring or to treat symptoms of overuse of alcohol or other drugs.*

A positive response to any of the four questions is considered a positive screen and the patient should complete more detailed screening, such as the AUDIT or DAST screening tools.[4]

interviewing and counseling regardless of the lack of reimbursement.

CAGE-AID

Quick screening questions can be added into the history a dental assistant or hygienist obtains from the patient. These questions can also be included in new patient paperwork. The screening tools listed in Box 8.1 are more time consuming and should be used when a preliminary screening is positive. For example, the

The National Institute of Drug Abuse Drug Use Screening Tool: NMASSIST

For practices that are interested in screening patients electronically, the National Institute of Drug Abuse (NIDA) developed online resources that allow for quick screening processes.[5] The NIDA Drug Use Screening Tool is an interactive Web-based tool that offers a single question to identify patients with recent substance use.[6] The results can be reviewed with the patient in the examination room. The NIDA-Modified Alcohol, Smoking, and Substance Involvement Screening Test (NMASSIST) is available to fully evaluate drug and alcohol use when the quick screen is positive.[7] The NMASSIST total score is titled the substance involvement (SI) score. The SI is used to rate the patient's level of risk based on a scale of "high," "moderate," and "low" risk.[7] Online resources are available for the dental professional to provide guidance on interventions at each level of risk.[7]

When the dental professional suspects a patient of SUD, they should sensitively express their concerns with the patient and offer referral for treatment. The dental professional can point out the first signs of damage to the teeth that have resulted from drug use. The patient should be shown the damage to the teeth and the professional should explain why they are concerned in a nonjudgmental way.[8]

An example of a brief intervention that encourages a patient to seek help for SUD can be found in the American Dental Association Guide for Talking with Patients About Drug Use:[8]

> "I'm concerned you could be getting in over your head with your drug use. Here's the name of a person at a treatment center. I'd suggest you go talk with them and see if they can help you." It helps if you have a name, and if you know a little about what the patient could expect. For example, "Someone there should be able to see you in the next 24 hours. There's no charge for the first visit. They'll help you find a place you can afford, or that will accept your insurance."

Dental professionals should keep a list of referral resources available at the office. Treatment facilities can be located online at http://findtreatment.samhsa.gov. Local primary-care offices, pharmacies, and emergency rooms typically keep current information on local public and private treatment programs. A list of suggested resources can be found in Box 8.2. For dental professionals interested in working with community members on prescription drug abuse programs, contact your local substance abuse coalitions. These organizations have resources available regarding local treatment for substance abuse.

Box 8.2   Office Ready-Access List for Dental Practitioners

Law Enforcement/Regulatory Agencies
- Local police department
- State drug task force
- DEA
- State Board of Pharmacy
- State dental board

Specialists
- Addiction specialist for methadone or buprenorphine
- Pain specialist
- Community pharmacist
- Substance abuse counselor
- Local addiction treatment centers
- Drug information center/poison center
- Local hospital or emergency department

Schemes and Scams to Obtain Prescription Drugs

Patient Diversion Behaviors in the Office

Dental practitioners have a professional responsibility to prescribe controlled substances appropriately, while guarding against abuse and ensuring that patients have medication available for pain management when indicated. Every dental practice is a potential target for patients wanting to divert controlled substances. Therefore, dental practitioners should be aware of potential situations where drug diversion can occur and develop an action plan to safeguard their practices.

Determining whether a patient is a legitimate patient in need of pain treatment or a potential drug diverter is difficult. New patients may pose challenges, especially if they claim to be on vacation or from "out of town." Other patients may be familiar to the dental team, such as a friend, relative, coworker, or other health-care

---

Box 8.3 Common Characteristics of the Prescription Drug Seeker[9-11]

- Unusual behavior in the waiting room.
- Assertive personality, often demanding immediate attention.
- Unusual appearance—extremes of either slovenliness or being overdressed.
- May show unusual knowledge of controlled substances and/or gives medical history with textbook symptoms OR gives evasive or vague answers to questions regarding medical history.
- Reluctant or unwilling to provide reference information. Usually has no regular doctor and often no health insurance.
- Will often request a specific controlled substance and is reluctant to try a different drug or claims allergies to multiple medications.
- Generally has no interest in diagnosis—fails to keep appointments for further diagnostic tests or refuses to see another practitioner for consultation.
- May exaggerate medical problems and/or simulate symptoms.
- May exhibit mood disturbances, suicidal thoughts, lack of impulse control, or thought disorders.
- Cutaneous signs of drug abuse—skin tracks and related scars on the neck, axilla, forearm, wrist, foot, and ankle. Such marks are usually multiple, hyperpigmented, and linear. New lesions may be inflamed. Shows signs of "pop" scars from subcutaneous injections.

---

professional. Regardless of the category of patient, evaluation of potential "red flags" indicating likelihood of diversion is important. Patients that are dentist or doctor shoppers often have common characteristics. The dental team should work together to design a workflow plan that includes substance abuse screening, including history of addiction and recovery history. During the history-taking process, the team should observe body language and response to questioning. During the physical exam, any evidence of substance abuse effects on the teeth should be documented. In addition, the dental team should take note of other physical signs of substance abuse, which might include pill fragments or dust in the nares or track marks on the antecubital fossa. Common characteristics of prescription drug seekers are listed in Box 8.3.

Prescription drug seekers also tend to have patterns of behavior and operation that should raise awareness of the need to carefully screen the patient for legitimate need of medications. Patterns of behavior that should be of concern in the dental office are included in Box 8.4.

Doctor shopping is a common diversion behavior by patients. Doctor shopping is characterized by the *specific intent* of a patient to deceive a prescriber to obtain prescription medications. Patients visit multiple offices "shopping" for a prescriber to write more prescriptions. The use of PDMP tools (discussed later) has significantly reduced doctor shopping activity. Many states have implemented laws that prosecute individuals for this activity. Patient explanations for doctor shopping relate to clinician-related factors, such as inconvenient office hours or locations, long wait times, interpersonal qualities of the provider, and insufficient time of communication between the patient and provider.[10] Personal factors related to doctor shopping include illness factors (e.g., persistence of symptoms despite treatment, lack of understanding of diagnosis or treatment) and psychological factors (e.g., multiple somatic symptoms, seeking of prescription drugs).[10]

- Must be seen right away.
- Wants an appointment toward end of office hours.
- Calls or comes in after regular hours.
- States they are traveling through town, visiting friends or relatives (not a permanent resident).
- Feigns dental symptoms in an effort to obtain controlled substances.
- Feigns psychological problems, such as extreme anxiety, to obtain sedatives before dental work.
- States that specific noncontrolled analgesics do not work or that they are allergic to them.
- Claims to be a patient of a dental practitioner who is currently unavailable or will not give the name of their primary dentist or primary-care provider.
- States that a prescription has been lost or stolen and needs replacing.
- Uses the "water excuse"—states tablets fell in sink, toilet, or washing machine.
- Attempts to deceive the dental practitioner, such as by requesting refills more often than originally prescribed.
- Tries to pressure the dental practitioner by eliciting sympathy or guilt or by direct threats.

Clinical Consideration

The dental office can be a target for a prescription drug abuser as they may be seeking prescriptions from the prescriber. Paying special attention to medications listed on the medical history may not be sufficient for the patient suspected of abusing prescription drugs as the patient may downplay their use of substances in order to obtain new prescriptions. A key indicator that a patient may be "prescription seeking" is if they ask for drugs by name, dosage, and number of tablets. This should alert the dental team to perform further investigation.

Prevention Practices

In order to not fall victim to a drug diversion, the dental professional should routinely perform a thorough examination appropriate to the presenting condition. The examination results should be documented in the dental record and include answers from the patient on specific inquiries you made of the patient during the history-taking process.

The front-office staff should request picture identification upon initial presentation. A copy of the identification should be placed in the medical record. If possible, a picture of each patient should also be included in the record. At presentation to each appointment, the front-office staff should confirm the patient's current address and telephone number.

The dental provider should contact previous dental practitioners, primary-care provider, hospital, or pharmacist to confirm details in the patient's history. With any suspicious behaviors that raise a red flag, do not take the "patient's word for it." Never prescribe a controlled substance to get the patient to leave the office. Do not prescribe, dispense, or administer any controlled substance outside the scope of dental practice or in the absence of a formal dentist–patient relationship (see Chapter 10).

Finally, if the dental practitioner feels that a patient is inappropriately asking for medications, there are key questions that should be asked and answered by the dental team. These questions can be found in Box 8.5.

Patient Diversion Behaviors Outside the Office

Dental practitioners are likely victims of prescription drug-related crimes occurring outside of the dental office. In a state-wide survey by O'Neil, one-third of dental practitioners suspected they were victims of drug diversion characterized by prescription forgeries, alterations in prescription refills or doses, stolen prescription pads, or reports of stolen

---

Box 8.5 Key Questions to Ask If You Think a Patient May Be Inappropriately Asking You for Medications[12]

- How often does this patient present?
- Has the patient told you that he has moved, but does not want you to talk to his previous dental practitioner or doctor?
- Is the patient paying with cash?
- Does the person have a last known address?
- Have you had trouble contacting the patient between visits?
- Are your prescription pads disappearing?
- Does the patient say that only a particular drug will work, or that no other drug he has tried has worked?
- Does the patient refuse to go to one dental practitioner or primary-care physician?
- Does the patient frequently report losing medications?
- Does the patient demand drugs with high street value?
- Does the patient have prescriptions from multiple doctors or have prescriptions filled at multiple pharmacies?

Clinical Consideration

If the dental practitioner knows or suspects a prescription pad has been stolen from their office, it should be immediately reported to law enforcement and local pharmacies as well as to state pharmacy organizations that can alert pharmacists across the state. Dental practitioners should keep all prescription pads *locked* in safe areas and not left in examination rooms.

---

medications.[3] Common methods of prescription forgery include changing quantities of tablets prescribed, altering refills on prescriptions, or adding an additional medication to a newly written prescription. Many of these illegal activities have become preventable because of the development of tamper-resistant prescription pads. Tamper-resistant or tamper-proof prescription pads incorporate several features that limit the ability to alter or photocopy the prescription. These features usually include a watermark, photocopy paper/ink that "voids" the prescription after photocopying, and written numbers of refills or drug quantities instead of traditional numerical designated quantities of refills. Historically, a prescriber's DEA number was considered confidential information. However, with the development of the Internet, DEA numbers may be easily found and used when forging prescriptions.

More advanced prescription diversion behaviors involve illegitimate phone-in prescriptions. In this scheme, individuals pretending to be dental office staff call in prescription medications using patient aliases or stolen patient information. The perpetrators give a cell phone number as the "office number." When prescribers call later to verify the prescription, the perpetrator is anticipating the call ready to "verify" the prescription. It is not uncommon for these individual to phone in 20–30 false prescriptions per day. Many states have made successful attempts to limit these illegitimate phoned-in prescriptions by requiring pharmacies to verify and document who actually picked up the prescription. The request of photo identification by the pharmacies frequently deters the perpetrators from picking up the prescription. The implementation of electronic transfer of prescription controlled substances will also likely prevent these diversion behaviors.

Dental Practitioner- and Office Personnel-Related Prescription Drug Diversion

Unfortunately, not all prescription drug-related criminal activity in dental offices involves the patient. Dental practitioners and office staff may be implicated in various behaviors or activities that may lead to sanctions by dental boards, fines, and in many cases prosecution and arrests by law enforcement. Common sanctions or reprimands from dental boards usually involve investigations for perceived "excessive prescribing" of controlled substance analgesics to patients, failure to maintain appropriate controlled substance/patient records, or prescribing outside the scope of dental practice. Frequently, the latter two violations may lead to prosecution by federal and state law enforcement agencies. Self-medicating with prescription drugs as a coping mechanism for dealing with the high stress of dental practice can contribute to the development of prescription drug addiction. Chapter 11 discusses SUD and impairment in the dental professional.

Federal regulatory agencies (e.g., DEA) have strict requirements for writing prescriptions, distributing/dispensing, storing, and documenting prescription drug-related activities. Failure to maintain records, such as purchase invoices for controlled substances, DEA 222 transfer forms, and biennial inventories, can lead to sanctions and or fines by federal law enforcement and regulatory boards. Scope of practices violations usually involve prescriptions written by the dental practitioner for treatment that is not part of routine dental care. For example, prescribing anxiolytics or analgesics that are not related to any dental pathology and/or clinical finding or prescribing *chronic medications* (for a duration lasting significantly longer than the acute event) can lead to investigations and possible sanctions. Casual "hallway" prescribing to office personnel without documentation in official patient records or medical records should be avoided.

One common diversion activity that is frequently undetected or overlooked in the office setting is self-prescribing and self-medicating with *sample medication*. The practice of "helping one's self" to products at the employee's work without reimbursement for the products is known as "grazing." These medications commonly include antibiotics, analgesics,

cough and cold products, and muscle relaxants. Because these medications are not controlled substances, record keeping may be lax, so detection of this type of drug diversion is difficult to detect. See Chapter 10 for controlled substance regulations.

Prescription Drug Monitoring Programs

PDMPs have existed in some manner in a few states since 1973. These original programs were generally found in law enforcement agencies and used duplicate or triplicate serialized prescription blanks as the means to track the prescribing and dispensing of controlled substances, generally restricted to Schedule II medications. In the mid-1990s, additional states began programs to address rising abuse of diversion of controlled substances. By 2003, there were approximately 17 states with authority to implement programs with access for health-care providers becoming more prevalent.[13]

In 2014, 49 states and the District of Columbia have authorizing legislation and there are 48 operational programs.[13] Today, most programs allow access for prescribers and dispensers, provide 24/7 access with auto-response software, and collect information for prescriptions in Schedules II–IV (may vary from state to state). Several states are interoperable with other state programs, and there is a great deal of exploration into the integration of PDMP information with health information technology systems.

PDMPs are systems in which selected prescription drug data are collected in a database, centralized by each state, and administered by an authorized state agency to promote the appropriate use of controlled substances for legitimate medical purposes, while deterring the misuse, abuse, and diversion of these substances.[14] Prescribers and/or pharmacists are authorized access to these systems to obtain prescription-related information on patients they are providing or considering initiating treatment for to assist them to make informed prescribing, treatment decisions, or dispensing of controlled substances.

The use of PDMP information is generally voluntary, although there are a number of states that require prescribers to register to use their state PDMP, and in some cases mandate the requesting of PDMP information under certain circumstances. Whether required or not, PDMPs are an excellent risk management tool to use when prescribing controlled substances, and access is available to prescribers and pharmacists at no charge. In addition to applicable state law requirements, prescribers should have a plan and policy concerning the use of the PDMP. A comprehensive policy should address, at a minimum, that a query to the PDMP will be made when considering prescribing an opioid for a new patient, when renewing a prescription, or for an existing patient that has not received an opioid in a set period of time. The policy should reflect any unique requirements of the state's PDMP, such as notification requirements, the placing of PDMP reports, or documenting the review of PDMP information in the patient record and procedures to insure PDMP reports are not further disclosed or accessed unless specifically authorized.

PDMP information can be a very useful addition to the tools a prescriber has to assist in making prescribing decisions.[14] Careful consideration should be given as to the choices available as a result of the review of a PDMP report. These can include, but are not limited to:

- *Prescribe as planned.* The PDMP revealed no issues for concern.
- *Contact pharmacy.* If there is a question about specific information on the report, contact the pharmacy that dispensed the prescription.
- *Contact a previous prescriber.* If there is a question about a previous prescription such as a possible overlap in prescriptions contact a previous prescriber.

- *Discuss concerns.* Have a conversation with the patient to resolve or clarify questions about the report.
- *Change the treatment plan.* The planned prescription is not written and treatment takes a different course.
- *Refer to a specialist.* This could be a pain management specialist or other specialist depending on the issues a patient is experiencing.
- *Refer to substance abuse treatment.* For resources, contact your state or local professional organization.
- *Discharge from practice.* But first, make sure applicable laws are reviewed and regulations (including those concerning patient abandonment) that may apply for discharging patients from a practice.

Dental practitioners should determine whether applicable law requires or permits reporting the information to law enforcement, and whether such disclosure is permitted by applicable privacy laws such as the Health Insurance Portability and Accountability Act (HIPAA). PDMP reports may differ slightly in appearance or arrangement based on the vendor a state has contracted with to provide PDMP services. However, the basic components of the prescription information contained in a report are generally standardized and include patient information, prescriber information, dispenser information, name of drug, strength and form (tablet, capsule), quantity dispensed, days' supply, date filled, and date written. In some states, refill, gender, and method of payment information are also provided. Other specialized information may be provided, such as a morphine equivalent dosing score.

PDMP reports may be short or long depending on the patient and the type of treatment the patient is receiving. Generally, reports will post the most recent prescriptions at the top of the report and then go back in time. Reviewing the fill date, quantity dispensed, and days' supply is a quick way to determine a patient's usage of controlled substances. Additional important factors for consideration include whether the information on the PDMP report matches what the patient discloses, whether the prescribers and pharmacies utilized are in close proximity to where the patient resides, and whether the date written and method of payment information indicates no need for further research. It is important to note that PDMP reports may contain erroneous information, such as the wrong prescriber. If there is conflicting information on a report, it is highly recommended that the prescriber contact the dispensing pharmacy for clarification, as that is where the original prescription information is kept.

The following case details a practical approach to interpreting PDMP reports.

Case Study: Review of a Prescription Drug Monitoring Program Report

A 35-year-old female patient presents at your dental practice complaining of severe tooth pain attributed to an abscessed tooth. This is a new patient to the practice and, therefore, a PDMP report is requested according to practice policy (see Figure 8.1).

A quick review of the PDMP reports reveals that the patient has received 10 prescriptions for controlled substances in the past 30 days; all but two were for opioids. It appears that there *is limited overlap* of prescriptions when comparing quantity dispensed to days' supply for prescriptions reported.

Reviews of prescribers and pharmacies reveal that the patient has been seen and prescribed controlled substances by a family physician, prescribers at three urgent care centers (or emergency departments), and by four dental practitioners. Only the family physician and one of the dental practitioners were reported by the patient on the medical history portion of the intake paperwork. Additionally, the patient used four different pharmacies and three of the 10 prescriptions were paid for with private funds (cash, check, credit card) instead of insurance. All of the prescriptions were new and not refills.

Physical and diagnostic examinations reveal an abscessed tooth. How should the dental practitioner manage this patient?

Possible actions:

1. Prescribe as usual protocol. Patient requires more scrutiny than normal protocols.
2. Contact pharmacy. Probably not required in this case unless some other information comes to light that requires confirmation from a dispenser.
3. Contact the most recent dental practitioner that prescribed an opioid for the patient. The dental practitioner reports that yes they did see the patient and prescribed a short course of pain reliever to last until an appointment to correct the issue can be scheduled. The patient cancelled the follow-up appointment 24 h before treatment was scheduled.
4. Discuss concerns with the patient. Explain dangers of continued behavior and consequences of delaying treatment of abscess.
5. Change the treatment plan. Instead of an opioid, consider prescribing an anti-inflammatory agent or other course of treatment for pain, inflammation and infection until patient comes in for treatment. No opioid prescriptions until after treatment.
6. Refer to a specialist. Does the patient need referral for specialized dental care or other treatment provider?
7. Refer to substance abuse treatment. Have resource contact information on hand.
8. Discharge from practice. Should the dental practitioner discharge the patient from practice?
9. Should the dental practitioner file complaint with law enforcement?

Reporting of Violations or Suspected Criminal Behavior

Laws and regulations regarding the prescriber duty to report a doctor shopper to local law

Sample

Patient RX History Report

Last Name = Patient First Name = Test and Request Period = 6/1/2014 12:00:00 AM to 6/30/2014 12:00:00 AM

Patients that match search criteria

Pt ID	Name	DOB	Address
1660	Patient, Test	06/04/1979	Columbia VA 23114
3799	Patient, Test	06/04/1979	Columbia VA 23114

Prescriptions

Fill Date	Product, Str, Form	Quantity	Days	Pt ID	Prescriber	Written	Rx #	N/R	Pharm	Pay
6/27/2014	OXYCODONE AND ACETAMINOPHEN, 10 MG;650 MG, TABLET	25.00	6	1660	SC79	6/27/2014	1969808	N	B00	04
6/21/2014	OXYCODONE AND ACETAMINOPHEN, 10 MG;650 MG, TABLET	30.00	7	1660	SC79	6/21/2014	1967921	N	B00	04
6/19/2014	OXYCODONE AND ACETAMINOPHEN, 325 MG;7.5 MG, TABLET	8.00	4	1660	JE50	6/19/2014	173328	N	F12	01
6/16/2014	OXYCODONE AND ACETAMINOPHEN, 10 MG;325 MG, TABLET	30.00	8	3799	KI34	6/16/2014	02237262	N	B01	01
6/11/2014	OXYCODONE AND ACETAMINOPHEN, 10 MG;325 MG, TABLET	15.00	3	3799	SC94	6/11/2014	1122608	N	B23	04
6/10/2014	ZOLPIDEM TARTRATE, 10 MG, TABLET, FILM COATED	30.00	30	3799	WI60	6/10/2014	1122282	N	323	04
6/10/2014	ALPRAZOLAM, 1 MG, TABLET	90.00	30	3799	WI60	6/10/2014	1122283	N	B23	04
6/07/2014	OXYCODONE AND ACETAMINOPHEN, 10 MG;325 MG, TABLET	15.00	2	3799	ER41	6/07/2014	172580	N	B23	01
6/05/2014	OXYCODONE AND ACETAMINOPHEN, 10 MG;325 MG, TABLET	15.00	2	3799	JO87	6/05/2014	172365	N	F12	04
6/01/2014	HYDROCODONE BITARTRATE AND ACETAMINOPHEN, 10 MG;660 MG, TABLET	20.00	5	3799	IV23	6/01/2014	1961340	N	B00	04

N/R: N=New R=Refill

Pay:01=Private Pay 02=Medicaid 03=Medicare 04=Commercial Ins. 05=Military Inst. and VA 06=Workers Comp 07=Indian Nations 99=Other   **Total Prescriptions:** 10

Prescribers for prescriptions listed

ER41	DDS 3 VA 23235
IV23	Urgent Care 2 VA 23235
JE50	DDS 2 VA 23225
JO87	DDS 1 VA 23225
KI34	Urgent Care 3 VA 23831
SC94	DDS 4 VA 23236
SC79	Urgent Care1 VA 23235
WI60	Family Physician1 VA 23112

Pharmacies that dispensed prescriptions listed

B01	Chain1 PHARMACY VA 23831
B00	Chain2 VA 23235
B23	Chain3 Pharmacy VA 23113
F12	Chain4 VA 23235

Figure 8.1 Sample PDMP report.

enforcement agency varies from state to state. It is the professional obligation of each dental practitioner to be aware of pertinent laws regarding reporting a patient for doctor shopping in each state where he or she is licensed. Almost all states have a "general" fraud statute that adopts verbatim or with slight alteration the provision in the Uniform Narcotic Drug Act of 1932 or the Uniform Controlled Substances Act of 1970. These statutes prohibit obtaining drugs, including through "doctor shopping," by any or all of the following means: fraud, deceit, misrepresentation, subterfuge, or concealment of material fact.[15]

Patient Privacy

Many prescribers question the release of protected health information to law enforcement when reporting doctor shopping behavior. If doctor shopping is illegal and the doctor shopping occurred at the dental practitioner's office, the dental practitioner should report the patient for doctor shopping in accordance with the laws of the state. If the dental practitioner discerns a doctor shopping pattern through review of a prescription monitoring program for a patient but the doctor shopping actually occurred at another provider's practice, that provider should report the doctor shopping in accordance with applicable law. Although laws regarding disclosure of such information to other providers for mutual patients vary from state to state, if permitted, it is advisable to discuss concerns with other providers so that the patient can receive appropriate intervention.

An example of a state with a specific doctor shopping law is Tennessee. This law states that "any physician, dentist, optometrist, veterinarian, pharmacist, advanced practice nurse with a certificate of fitness, or physician assistant who has actual knowledge that a person has knowingly, willfully and with intent to deceive obtained or attempted to obtain a controlled substance must report that information within

five (5) business days to the local law enforcement agency."[16] An exception to this law is provided for prescribers that are providing treatment to a person with mental illness where they are not required to report the information to law enforcement personnel.[16]

A list of states with general and specific laws regarding doctor shopping can be located online at the Centers for Disease Control and Prevention located at http://www.cdc.gov/homeandrecreationalsafety/Poisoning/laws/dr_shopping.html.

When interviewing a patient who presents for a painful condition that may require prescription for a controlled substance, the dentist may ask the key questions listed in Box 8.6 and document answers in the medical record.[15] After making these inquiries, the dental practitioner should check the state PDMP to verify the answers. Available data indicate the use of prescription monitoring programs decreases the prevalence of doctor shopping.[10,14]

Box 8.6   Key Questions to Ask Patients[15]

- Are you seeing or have you been seen by any other provider for this problem?
- If so, by whom and when?
- What medications are you currently taking for this problem?
- When did you receive the most recent prescription for this?
- Who prescribed it and where was the prescription filled?

Clinical Consideration

PDMP profiles are a tool to deter and possibly detect aberrant controlled-substance-related behavior. Information provided in these databases *is not direct evidence of a crime.* All information should be confirmed with the patient, other prescribers, or pharmacies before definitive action is taken.

Access to Prescription Drug Monitoring Program Database

Access to the PDMP is very restricted regardless of the state. Generally, access is limited to the prescriber and the pharmacist for a specific patient being treated or receiving controlled substances. Law enforcement agencies often in collaboration with drug task forces may have access as part of an active diversion investigation. It is prohibited for any person or agency to query the PDMP database for *anyone that is not an active patient or simply for "curiosity" purposes.*

Prescriber Controlled-Substance Reports

Most PDMP databases are able to be queried for individual prescriber *histories* by the supervising PDMP agency or in many cases the actual prescriber. Frequently, these records are evaluated to determine specific prescribing patterns or trends of prescribing by law enforcement agencies or regulatory boards. Prescribers are encouraged to run reports or request reports every 6 months to a year and review the records with their office manager. This activity may be helpful in detecting fraudulent patients (or prescriptions) that are using prescribers' DEA numbers to obtain controlled substances.

Disposal of Controlled Substances

The American Dental Association and the DEA promote safe disposal of unused, unwanted, and expired medications at participating collection sites throughout the country. Dental professionals should educate patients about appropriate disposal of medications.

The FDA and the White House Office of National Drug Control Policy developed federal guidelines regarding appropriate drug disposal.[17] A summary of these recommendations includes the following:

- Follow any specific disposal instructions on the prescription drug labeling or patient information that accompanies the medicine. Do not flush medicines down the sink or toilet unless this information specifically instructs you to do so.
- Take advantage of community drug take-back programs that allow the public to bring unused drugs to a central location for proper disposal.
- If no disposal instructions are given on the prescription drug labeling and no take-back program is available in your area, throw the drugs in the household trash following these steps.
  - Remove medications from the original container and mix them with an undesirable substance, such as used coffee grounds or kitty litter (this makes the drug less appealing to children and pets, and unrecognizable to people who may intentionally go through the trash seeking drugs). Do not crush tablets or capsules before mixing them in the undesirable substance.
  - Place the mixture in a sealable bag, empty can, or other container to prevent the drug from leaking or breaking out of a garbage bag.

Educate the patient that, before throwing out a prescription vial, it is advisable to make all identifying information on the prescription label unreadable. Taking these precautions will help protect the identity of the patient and the privacy of their personal health information.[17]

Some medications should be disposed of by flushing instead of being placed in the trash. A list of medications that should be flushed can be found online at the FDA website located at http://www.fda.gov/ForConsumers/Consum erUpdates/ucm101653.htm.

Dates of the DEA National Take Back Initiatives can be located online at http://www. deadiversion.usdoj.gov/drug_disposal/takeba ck/.

Universal Precautions in Prescribing Controlled Substances

Many dental practitioners routinely prescribe opioids for patients who have surgical dental procedures. These procedures often include extraction of teeth, root canal, gum surgery, and biopsies. While it is often appropriate for dental practitioners to prescribe opioids after surgical dental procedures, prescribers must use caution each time a prescription is written, keeping in mind the potential for misuse, abuse, and addiction.

In 2002, dental practitioners prescribed about 12% of the opioids in the USA, amounting to about 1 billion doses.[18,19] This placed dental practitioners right behind family medicine physicians, who wrote 15% of the prescriptions.[18,19] The most common opioid medications prescribed were immediate-release formulations of hydrocodone and oxycodone, which are also the most widely abused medications on the street.[18,19] Therefore, dental practitioners who use appropriate prescribing precautions when writing prescriptions for controlled substances will help decrease the amount of opioids and other controlled substances that become drugs of abuse in the community. Chapter 3 discusses acute pain management in dentistry.

Surveys of dental practitioners and maxillofacial surgeons indicate that an average of 20 doses of hydrocodone or oxycodone is prescribed after a dental procedure. Most

dental practitioners surveyed stated they expected patients to have leftover analgesics; indeed, dental practitioners stated that most patients would not require all of the doses dispensed.[19]

It is unclear how often dental practitioners prescribe opioid analgesics for the treatment of moderate to severe chronic orofacial pain. Chronic pain treatment should occur very infrequently, if at all, in dental practice. Little evidence supports use of opioids for the treatment of this type of chronic pain. Therefore, if opioids are used, it should only be after failure of physical therapy, nonsteroidal anti-inflammatory drugs, and adjunctive agents such as anticonvulsants and antidepressant agents. If possible, chronic pain syndromes should be handled by the primary-care physician or pain specialist. If a dental practitioner engages in providing pharmacotherapy for chronic pain orofacial syndromes, they should do so only in collaboration with the other providers caring for the patient.

The principle of universal precautions in prescribing pain medications was developed by Gourlay et al. in 2005.[20] The term "universal precautions" was coined because common groups were identified between those clinicians treating infectious diseases and those who treat chronic pain. In both patient populations, it is nearly impossible to accurately assess risk on the initial visit. Therefore, it necessitates the application of risk management strategies to each and every patient. When opioids are used on a chronic basis, the prescriber must adhere to the 10 principles of universal precautions. By doing so, patient care is improved, stigma is decreased, and overall risk is contained. Adherence to these principals protects patients and the dental practice.

The 10 steps of universal precautions in pain medicine are as follows:[20]

1. **Make a diagnosis with appropriate differential.** The dental practitioner must identify

treatable causes of pain. Any comorbid conditions, including substance SUD and other psychiatric illness, must also be addressed.

2. **Psychological assessment, including risk of addiction.** The dental practitioner must take a complete history of personal and family history of substance abuse. Screening tools integrated into the history-taking process can facilitate this process. If a controlled substance is to be prescribed, discuss use of urine drug screens with the patient as a monitoring tool that is used with every patient to monitor drug therapy. If a patient refuses these assessments, they should be considered unsuitable for pain management using controlled substances.

3. **Informed consent.** Discuss and document the proposed treatment plan with the patient, including benefits and risk of therapy. Specific discussion of issues of addiction, dependence, and tolerance should be provided in language the patient can understand.

4. **Treatment agreement.** If controlled substances are prescribed for chronic pain, a written agreement, combined with the informed consent, should detail expectations and obligations of the patient and the prescriber. This agreement should be signed, dated, and placed in the medical record.

5. **Pre- and post-intervention of pain level and function.** Levels of pain should be documented in the medical record in order to assess success in medication trials. Treatment goals with regard to functioning should also be included in the plan; failure to meet these goals necessitates reevaluation of the treatment plan.

6. **Appropriate trial of opioid with an adjunctive agent.** A trial of an opioid may be appropriate for some patients and the treatment should be individualized based on patient characteristics. In chronic therapy, an adjunctive agent such as an antidepressant or anticonvulsant should be considered.

7. **Reassessment of pain score and level of function.** Patients should be assessed on a regular basis for pain control and functioning. If possible, include family members in the discussion to obtain corroborative support of the patient's report.

8. **Regularly assess the "four As" of pain medicine.** Routine assessment of analgesia, activity, adverse effects, and aberrant behavior will help to direct treatment decisions.

9. **Periodically review pain diagnosis and comorbid conditions, including addictive disorders.** Pain conditions and underlying conditions can change over time. If a patient develops the disease of addiction, referral for treatment is necessary and coordination of care with the addiction provider is needed.

10. **Documentation.** Thorough notes of each visit, along with appropriate risk assessments, should be documented in the medical record. Accurate and complete records should include the following:
    i. medical history and dental examination;
    ii. diagnostic, radiographic, therapeutic, and laboratory results;
    iii. evaluations and consultations;
    iv. treatment objectives;
    v. discussion of risks and benefits;
    vi. treatments;
    vii. medications (date, type, dosage, quantity prescribed);
    viii. informed consent;
    ix. periodic reviews.

Chapters 3, 4, and 6 discuss management of acute dental pain, patients receiving opioid maintenance therapy, patients with SUD, and patients receiving opioids for chronic pain.

Box 8.7 lists a 23-point strategy for preventing drug diversion in dental practice.

Box 8.7   Drug Diversion Prevention Practices

1. Request driver's license or insurance cards of new patients. Insist on a delivery address where the patient actually lives. Patients traveling significant distances should be queried regarding why they chose your office, referral sources, and known patients. Drug seekers frequently travel great distances from within and outside the state.
2. Reinforce "no sharing" of medications with family or friends. Sharing medication is quickly becoming the leading source of prescription drug abuse and misuse.
3. Use a substance abuse/addiction questionnaire (e.g., CAGE, NMASSIST) when considering chronic controlled substance treatment. Document performance of an opioid risk-screening questionnaire at least quarterly.
4. Observe patient records for multiple reports of prescription drug theft or repeated prescription losses.
5. When patients present with family or friends, try to isolate the patient to assess their true needs. Frequently, patients are coerced to request prescriptions by family or friends.
6. Consider tapering medications for patients that have been prescribed controlled substances for greater than 6–8 weeks (e.g., opioids or benzodiazepines). Physiologic withdrawal often leads to further medication abuse, misuse, and prescription requests.
7. Set appropriate goals for pain management. Patients or practitioners with the perception that pain will be completely eliminated with treatment may lead to perceived failure of therapy and prescription misuse.
8. Maintain thorough records of prescribed medications, including drug, date, dose, duration, diagnosis, and refills.
9. Maintain a list of alternative medications for the management of pain, anxiety, and insomnia for patients that are addicts or alcoholics in recovery. Help minimize your patient's risk of relapse.
10. Observe patient records for multiple requests of early refills for controlled substances, muscle relaxants, antipsychotics, gabapentin, and tramadol. Frequently, medications other than controlled substances are abused.
11. Establish a single lock-up site to store tamper-proof prescription pads. Never leave prescription pads in patient rooms.
12. Often, patients that request an increase in dosage early in treatment may not be at therapeutic goal. They may be perceived as drug seekers. This is known as pseudo-addiction and may lead to undertreatment of patients.
13. Always perform thorough background checks on medical and office staff.

Identifying Prescription Drug Seekers

14. You or designated office personnel should perform a prescription monitoring report on new and chronic patients receiving controlled substances. The report alone does NOT prove a crime has been committed and should be used to further questioning or an investigation of prescription drug abuse or diversion.
15. Request reports using your DEA number every 6 months to yearly from PDMPs to identify unknown patients or prescription fraud.
16. Acting immediately on "hearsay" reports from office staff, patients, and patient relatives may jeopardize your practice.
17. If patients report illnesses that are treated with a controlled substance AND a noncontrolled substance such as an antibiotic, follow up with the pharmacy to see if the noncontrolled substance was filled. Frequently, doctor shoppers only fill the controlled substances.

Treatment Considerations and Reporting Strategies

18. Communicate with other practitioners (physicians, dentists, etc.) when mutual patients are doctor shopping.

19. Provide at least a 30-day notice prior to discharging a patient from your practice for contract violations or criminal activities with at least two notifications, one being certified mail. Make certain that any termination is in accordance with all applicable laws, including those related to patient abandonment.

20. Consider referrals to medical or surgical specialists to optimize therapeutic options.

21. Maintain a list of local and regional detox centers, substance abuse treatment facilities, and Alcoholics Anonymous and Narcotics Anonymous meetings. Refer to these organizations when substance abuse or addiction is detected.

22. Report criminal behavior occurring on your premises. Section 164.512(f)(5) of the HIPAA Privacy Rule states, "A covered entity may disclose to a law enforcement official protected health information that the covered entity believes in good faith constitutes evidence of criminal conduct that occurred on the premises of the covered entity."

23. Practitioners lenient toward doctor shoppers will inadvertently attract more doctor shoppers. Respond appropriately to suspected doctor shopping to send the message this behavior is not tolerated in your practice.

Adapted from Ref. 21.

Summary

Dental practitioners play a key role in preventing the diversion, misuse, and abuse of prescription drugs. Dental practitioners should develop office policies and work flow that allow patients to be carefully screened for risk of prescription drug abuse. When SUDs are identified, dental practitioners should be prepared to refer patients to appropriate treatment. It is important for the dental team to recognize red flags in patients that may present seeking controlled-substance prescriptions. Dental practitioners should be registered with the state PDMP and access the program before prescribing any controlled substances for patients. When opioid prescriptions are needed to treat acute or chronic pain following dental procedures, the dental practitioner should use universal precautions in order to protect themselves, their practice, and the patient.

References

1. D'Amore MM, Cheng DM, Kressin NR, Jones J, Samet JH, Winter M, Kim TW, Saitz R. Oral health of substance-dependent individuals: impact of specific substances. J Subst Abuse Treat 2011;41:179–85.

2. Friedlander, AH, Marder SR, Pisegna JR, Yagiela JA. Alcohol abuse and dependence: Psychopathology, medical management and dental implications. JADA 2010;134:731–40.

3. O'Neil M. Dentist's experiences with drug diversion and substance use disorders. Accepted for poster presentation, ADEA Annual Conference, March 2015.

4. SAMSHA-HRSA Center for Integrated Health Solutions. SBIRT: Screening, Brief Intervention, and Referral to Treatment. http://www.integration.samhsa.gov/clinical-practice/SBIRT. Accessed January 2, 2015.

5. National Institute on Drug Abuse. Screening, assessment, and drug testing resources. 2014. http://www.drugabuse.gov/nidamed-medical-health-professionals/tool-resources-your-practice/additional-screening-resources. Accessed January 2, 2015.

6. National Institute on Drug Abuse Drug Screening Tool. Clinician's Screening Tool for Drug Use in General Medical Settings. http://www.drugabuse.gov/nmassist/?q=nida_questionnaire. Accessed January 2, 2015.

7. National Institute on Drug Abuse. Resource Guide: Screening for Drug Use in General Medical Settings. http://www.drugabuse.gov/publications/resource-guide-screening-drug-use-in-general-medical-settings/nida-quick-screen. Accessed January 2, 2015.

8. American Dental Association. Oral Health Topics. Drug Use. Talking With Your Patients. www.

ada.org/2663.aspx#talking". Accessed January 2, 2015.

9. US Department of Justice, Drug Enforcement Agency, Office of Diversion Control. Don't Be Scammed By A Drug Abuser. http://www. deadiversion.usdoj.gov/pubs/brochures/druga buser.htm. Accessed September 1, 2014.

10. Sansone RA, Sansone LA. Doctor shopping: a phenomenon of many themes. Innov Clin Neurosci 2012;9(11–12):42–6.

11. Solaiman T. RM matters: drug seekers. Protect yourself from patients who abuse pain medications. Northwest Dent 2010;89(1):55–6.

12. ACP Internist. 10 questions to identify drug-seeking patients. 2002. http://www.acpinte rnist.org/archives/2002/04/drug_seeking.htm. Accessed January 2, 2015.

13. The National Alliance for Model State Drug Laws (NAMSDL). Prescription Drug Monitoring Programs. http://www.namsdl.org/presc ription-monitoring-programs.cfm. Accessed January 2, 2015.

14. Morgan L, Weaver M, Sayeed Z, Orr R. The use of prescription monitoring programs to reduce opioid diversion and improve patient safety. J Pain Palliat Care Pharmacother 2013;27:4–9.

15. Centers for Disease Control and Prevention. Law: Doctor shopping. http://www.cdc. gov/homeandrecreationalsafety/Poisoning/law s/dr_shopping.html. Accessed January 2, 2015.

16. Tennessee Department of Health. Prescription Safety Act. http://health.state.tn.us/boards/Co ntrolledsubstance/faq.shtml. Accessed January 2, 2015.

17. US Food and Drug Administration. How to Dispose of Unused Medicines. http://www.fda. gov/forconsumers/consumerupdates/ucm1016 53.htm. Accessed January 2, 2015.

18. Denisco RC, Kenna GA, O'Neil MG, Kulich RJ, Moore PA, Kane WT, Mehta NR, Hersh EV, Katz NP. Prevention of prescription opioid abuse: the role of the dentist. JADA 2011;142(7):800–10.

19. Cairns BE, Kolta A, Whitney E, Craig K, Rei N, Lam DK, Lynch M, Sessle B, Lavigne G. The use of opioid analgesics in the management of acute and chronic orofacial pain in Canada: the need for further research. J Can Dent Assoc 2014;80:e49.

20. Gourlay DL, Heit HA, Almahrezi A. Universal precautions in pain medicine: a rational approach to the treatment of chronic pain. Pain Med 2005;6(2):107–12.

21. O'Neil MG. A comprehensive checklist for prevention management of the drug seeking patient. W V Med J 2010;106(4):54–5.

Resources and Further Readings

DEA, Diversion Control. http://www.deadiversion .usdoj.gov/.

Babor TF, McRee BG, Kassebaum PA, Grimaldi PL, Ahmed K, Bray J. Screening, Brief Intervention, and Referral to Treatment (SBIRT): toward a public health approach to the management of substance abuse. Subst Abus 2007;28(3):7–30.

Interviewing and Counseling Patients with Known or Suspected Substance Use Disorders: Dealing with Drug-seeking Patients

George F. Raymond, DDS *and William J. Maloney*, DDS

Introduction

When a patient with a history *or suspected history* of substance abuse presents to the oral health-care provider, a complex and multifaceted relationship often begins. The fact that the patient is dealing or has coped with a substance abuse problem once or many times means there may also be other psychological, social, and medical issues involved. The provider's ethical and moral obligation is to treat the dental needs of the patient, but the provider may at times also offer counseling to assist the patient as well as provide referrals for a variety of services if requested. Patients' previous use of tobacco, alcohol, or other drugs is a predictor for the development of substance use disorder (SUD) across virtually all classes of substances.[1] Educating patients, particularly young adults and adolescents, about the risk of substance abuse can help reduce the rising levels of abuse among the population.

Drug-seeking behavior is a situation any dental provider can encounter. It is important to recognize the difference between a patient legitimately seeking a drug and a drug-seeking patient. This is not an easy task, since it takes a certain degree of objectivity and subjectivity to differentiate between the two types of patients. The provider needs to have good observation skills and should conduct a thorough interview and physical exam and use sound clinical judgment. It may be helpful to utilize various methods, such as screening questionnaires, a visual analog pain scale, and prescription drug monitoring program (PDMP) databases when available to enhance the decision-making process. Chapter 8 reviews screening tools to help identify *at-risk* dental patients.

The ADA Practical Guide to Substance Use Disorders and Safe Prescribing, First Edition. Edited by Michael O'Neil.
© 2015 American Dental Association. Published 2015 by John Wiley & Sons, Inc.

Definitions

Drug-seeking Patient

A drug-seeking patient presents to a health-care provider in person or by phone with the intention of manipulating the provider into prescribing or dispensing a medication that is not needed or one that is in excess quantities.

Motivational Interviewing

Motivational interviewing (MI) is a short-term, direct, patient-centered style of counseling use to help explore and resolve a patient's conflicts involving health decisions.

Patient-centered Approach

The patient-centered approach provides care that is respectful of and responsive to individual patient's preferences, needs, and values and ensures that patient's values guide all clinical decisions.

Active Listening

Active listening is a communication technique that requires the listener to feed back or "mirror" what they hear to the speaker, by way of restating or paraphrasing what they have heard in their own words, to confirm what they have heard and to confirm they understand the speaker.

Prescription Drug Monitoring Programs

Prescription drug monitoring programs (PDMPs) are usually state-hosted Internet databases of prescribed controlled substances that are dispensed from ambulatory practices or community pharmacy practices. These databases provide visual access to dispensing records for various controlled substances (depending on state regulations). Authorized users may use this database to evaluate controlled substance prescribing and dispensing histories. Accessing and utilizing PDMP database information is discussed in detail in Chapter 8.

Preinterview Considerations

Preparing to see "new" patients or patients who visit the practice annually may help identify patient behaviors that can be confirmed through patient interviews and patient screening and ultimately optimize the dental practitioners time. It is recommended that the dental practitioner review the patient's prescription drug monitoring profile if available. *Information in the prescription drug monitoring profile is not evidence of a crime but may direct the line of questioning when interviewing the patient.* Review of past treatment records also should be performed. This brief review should focus on multiple phone-in requests for pain medications, repeat "no-shows" for scheduled procedures after receiving pain medications, and reported aberrant or difficult behaviors by office staff. Caution is recommend in responding to "hearsay" comments by office staff about the patient's social drug or alcohol activities. "Hearsay" comments may inappropriately bias clinical management of patients. Box 9.1

Box 9.1   Common Mistakes Made by Practitioners Prior to Treating Patients

- Making clinical decisions based on staff "hearsay."
- Assuming chronic pain medications will adequately treat acute pain.
- Assuming chronic methadone or buprenorphine-based maintenance programs will adequately treat acute pain.
- Assuming SUD only occurs in low socioeconomic populations.
- Stereotyping patients as drug abusers based on tattoos, piercings, or physical appearances.

lists common mistakes practitioners may make *prior to treating patients*. Dental practitioners may have excellent interview skills but may not acquire accurate information from patients with SUD for various reasons, including fear of receiving inadequate treatment (see Box 9.2).

> **Box 9.2 Why Effective Interviews May Not Happen**
>
> - The patient is fearful of receiving inadequate treatment.
> - The patient is embarrassed to have an SUD diagnosis.
> - The patient is in denial.
> - The patient may be afraid they *might* be reported or arrested.
> - The *true* purpose of the visit is criminal.

Patient Interview Considerations

Asking open-ended questions, questions that cannot be answered with a definitive yes or no, is encouraged, especially at the initiation of the interview. Asking questions to *clarify* answers already given with yes or no responses is acceptable. Use of open-ended questions prevents a patient from effectively shutting down the interview process.

Example:

Closed-ended question: Do you abuse prescription drugs?
Easy patient response: No.

The "no" response quickly shuts the interviewer down. Interviewers who persistently ask questions that that the patient has already answered "no" may appear aggressive or pushy.

Open-ended question: If any, what prescription medications have you ever taken without a prescription?

A patient responding with "I share my back pain medications with my wife when she has kidney stones" or "I occasionally take my pain pill just to relax after a long day" provides important insight into patient misuse or abuse of medications.

A response to this type of question requires a logical thinking path. This type of question also prevents the patient from *easily* making denials about their behavior.

> **Clinical Consideration**
>
> It is critical for dental practitioners to understand that many patients *do not* consider abuse or misuse of prescription substances to be equivalent to abuse of illicit substances like heroin or methamphetamine. Dental practitioners *should not* assume when asking a patient about "substance abuse" issues that the patient knows they also mean prescription medications.

Identifying a substance abuser or a patient displaying drug-seeking behavior is a difficult task. What one provider finds suspicious another may not. Since each patient may use different methods to reach their goal of obtaining a controlled substance or noncontrolled substance (see Chapter 8), it is helpful to identify some behaviors that should raise the provider's level of suspicion (see Box 9.3). Often, the patient will indicate exactly what drug they desire. Statements such as "Only Percocet® works for me" or "Ibuprofen does not work—just give me Vicodin®," are strong indicators of drug-seeking behavior, especially when the patient has no specific contraindications for nonsteroidal anti-inflammatory drugs such as renal insufficiency, gastrointestinal bleeding, or true allergies. This behavior also may be apparent when a patient makes requests by telephone for analgesics or sedatives, requests another prescription because the original was lost or stolen, claims to be allergic to *all* other analgesics, and/or has a history of going from one dental practitioner to another, a behavior known as "doctor shopping."[2] This population of patients has been known to present to the dental office near the end of regular business hours, expressing some sort of dental phobia that prevents receiving treatment that day and just asking for pain medication, or simply waiting to talk to the after-hours or weekend on-call dental practitioner.

Box 9.3   Flag Behaviors Associated with the "Suspicious" Interview

- Friends and family of the *adult* patient are present and are adamant they must be present the whole time.
- Impaired friends or family members accompany the patient.
- The patient refuses to discuss any treatment *except* medications.
- Patients with no allergies to other medications state they are allergic to all narcotics except one.
- The patient exaggerates symptoms.
- The patient changes or adds symptoms during the interview.
- Patients ask for their medication using "street" names or terminology.

Drug-seeking patients often have a pathological dental issue that can or is causing pain. They may defer treatment of that issue until it develops into a problem that the dental practitioner will prescribe the requested medication. Other characteristics of a drug-seeking patient or medication-abusing patient are unusual behavior in the waiting room, unusual appearance, unusual knowledge of controlled substances, reluctance to provide reference or personal information, general disinterest in the diagnosis, exaggerated symptoms, mood disturbances, or cutaneous signs of drug abuse.[3]

Often, the patient's condition will alert the dental practitioner that the patient is a substance or medication abuser. Poor oral hygiene, rampant decay, bruxism, and multiple extraction sites in a young adult can all indicate that the patient is a substance or medication abuser. The patient's primary-care physician should be contacted when a known or suspected substance abuse issue is apparent or confirmed. Primary-care physicians may be able to provide historical information and review the patient's overall health status.[4]

Administering a questionnaire such as the opioid risk tool assessment as part of the patient interview can help the dental practitioner identify a patient who may be less than forthcoming about a substance abuse issue. Questionnaires may be better at obtaining honest answers, as some patients, particularly adolescents, initially may feel embarrassed about discussing an SUD. When patients have or admit to having an SUD, the dental practitioner should ask specific questions targeting the substance or medications abused (see Box 9.4).

Box 9.4   Specific Questions for Known SUD

- What medication or substance was taken?
- When was it last taken?
- How much was taken?
- How was it taken (intravenously, orally, snorted, etc.)?
- Was more than one substance or drug taken (e.g., alcohol plus pain medication)?

Interviewing and Counseling Techniques

There are various methods the provider can use when dealing with a known or suspected substance or medication abuser. MI evolved from the work of clinical psychologist William Miller's work with alcoholics[5,6] and was later elaborated on by Rollnick et al.[7] MI is a patient-centered approach that is used in various health settings.[6] It has gained popularity in the oral health setting. MI seems to have the potential to address the self-care of adolescents and adults and has particular applications to special populations whose oral health status may be related to other health outcomes.[8] Since MI is routinely used for alcohol abusers and other substance abusers, it can be a practical tool for assisting the provider in dealing with a substance-abusing patient. MI is similar to a five-stage model routinely used by psychologists to conduct a well-formed therapy session. These stages include establishing an empathic relationship, story and strengths, goals, restatement, and action.[9]

An assortment of active listening and patient management skills already used by the provider can be helpful when assisting patients with SUDs. Those skills and a variation of MI could be used when managing a substance abuser. If the patient is genuinely interested in assistance, referral to the proper health-care provider is warranted. If the patient is not interested, a nonjudgmental, nonconfrontational approach may establish a rapport that encourages the patient to express their issues with substance abuse. Often, this population will exhibit dental phobias that can also be addressed in a positive communicative atmosphere. See Chapters 2 and 7 for additional information on MI.

The provider should express to the patient that all conversations and responses are confidential. The provider should maintain a nonjudgmental, nonconfrontational tone and allow the patient to talk at will regarding their addiction. The provider should not provoke the patient if open communication regarding substance or medication abuse cannot be accomplished. Offering to listen if the patient wants to discuss their options at future appointments may allow the patient time to gain trust in the provider. *Health-care providers have an ethical obligation to provide assistance or a referral should the opportunity arise.*

What Questions Should Be Asked?

There are several questions that dental practitioners should ask patients with SUDs or suspected SUDs.

1. "Is it OK with you for me to ask you about your medication use, any alcohol use, or other activities?"

   Although this is not an open-ended question, patients who infrequently visit the dental office may not expect to be questioned about drinking or abusing substances. Therefore, it is important to disarm the patient to obtain reliable information, and transparency on the part of the dental practitioner is required. This type of question achieves both goals.

   Patients should be assured that it is OK if they prefer not to discuss these issues.

2. "How many alcoholic drinks, if any, do you have during a week?"

   Determining the quantity of alcohol consumed is an important step. Although many patients tend to underestimate how much they drink, dental practitioners should not "fudge" or change the patient's response.

> ### Clinical Consideration
>
> Generally, patients feel more comfortable discussing alcohol use as opposed to illegal substance use. Asking about alcohol intake before other illicit substances is recommended.

If the patient admits to drinking, an important follow-up question is:

3. "How many drinks might you have at one time, such during as an evening out?"
4. "When was your last drink?"

   When a patient last drank alcohol is a critical question, especially if they require a procedure or medication is necessary.

At this point, administering the CAGE questionnaire (needed to **C**ut down, been **A**nnoyed by criticism, felt **G**uilty, need and **E**ye opener—see Chapter 8) or the Screening, Brief Intervention, and Referral to Treatment (SBIRT) or other screening tools (see the following section) will help determine the line of questioning going forward and inform decision-making about the patient.

The same question can be used when asking about other substances that can be abused. *"When did you last use the medication or substance?"*

5. "What street drugs, if any, have you ever taken; for example, marijuana, bath salts, or methamphetamines?"

Quantities, frequencies, and date of "last use" should always be determined.

After establishing any alcohol and illicit substance use or abuse, the dental practitioner should specifically ask the patient questions about prescription drugs.

Clinical Consideration

Commonly patients do not consider sharing, borrowing, or self-medicating with prescriptions drugs to be illegal, aberrant, or even a dangerous behavior.

Additional questions to ask regarding SUDs can be found in information provided in Resources and Further Readings.

Screening Tools

Screening, Brief Intervention, Referral to Treatment

SBIRT is a tool used to screen and refer at-risk individuals for treatment of SUDs. As defined by the Substance Abuse and Mental Health Services Administration, it is a comprehensive, integrated public health approach to the delivery of early intervention and treatment services for people with SUDs, as well as those who are at risk for developing these disorders. Primary-care centers, office-based practices, and other community settings provide opportunities for health-care practitioners to provide early intervention for at-risk substance users before more serious consequences occur.[10] This theory can also be viewed as an evidence-based approach that was developed to reduce and prevent disease and injury caused by risky health behaviors. SBIRT was initially developed for emergency departments, but it can be used in any health-care setting.[11] It has become an important screening tool and follows other techniques such as the Michigan Alcohol Screening Test, the CAGE questionnaire, and the Drug Abuse Screening Test, all of which are viable approaches to screening substance-abuse patients.[12] The SBIRT screening technique is comprised of three stages:

1. Screening quickly assesses the severity of substance use and identifies the suitable level of treatment.
2. Brief intervention focuses on increasing insight and awareness regarding substance use and motivation toward behavioral change.
3. Referral for treatment provides patients identified as needing more extensive counseling or treatment with access to care.

SBIRT also incorporates MI, and, in the dental setting (and primary-care setting), it is mainly intended to fill the gap between primary prevention efforts and more intensive treatment for persons with serious substance-abuse disorders.[13] This goal can be achieved through interviewing patients or administering questionnaires that can be used at more than one appointment. Some of the patients may not be totally honest at the first meeting, and it would be intuitive to readminister some of the screening tools at future appointments as well. The objective is to establish a relationship that motivates a patient to express their desire to seek further professional help and have the provider recognize this desire and act appropriately. A positive screening should be followed by an intervention that helps prevent the patients from developing disease or by treatment for a diagnosed disease[14] (see Chapter 8).

CRAFFT

CRAFFT is a behavioral health-screening tool that is recommended for use with adolescents (patients under 21 years of age) by the American Academy of Pediatrics' Committee on Substance Abuse (see Table 9.1). It consists of six questions developed to simultaneously screen adolescents for high-risk alcohol and other drug-use disorders. It is a short, effective screening tool used to assess whether a longer conversation about the use, frequency, and other risks and consequences of alcohol and other drug

use is warranted.[15] When screening a young adult or any patient, it is necessary to deal with practical barriers, including limited provider time. Although screening generally can be a quick and easy process, dealing with a positive screening can become time consuming and requires proper office guidelines to address the situation.[14]

Alcohol Use Disorders Identification Test

The alcohol use disorders identification test (AUDIT) questionnaire was developed by the World Health Organization to identify individuals along the full spectrum of alcohol misuse and provide an opportunity for early intervention in nonspecialty settings.[16] This screening is normally used to screen for alcohol abuse, as is the CAGE questionnaire. It may be beneficial to consider administering these screening tools to particular patients, especially as alcohol abuse may lead to abuse of other drugs.

Documentation

Because drug-seeking patients often call after regular office hours or present themselves at the office near the end of normal business hours in hopes that dental practitioners will want to end the meeting quickly and will prescribe the medications they seek, dental practitioners should never prescribe medications to satisfy the needs of a patient who is suspected of drug-seeking behavior or substance abuse regardless of how belligerent they may become. All encounters involving the patient or related to the patient should be thoroughly documented in the dental record in a timely fashion.

The importance of proper chart documentation during every patient encounter cannot be overemphasized. Accurate records are a cornerstone for proper risk management in

Table 9.1   CRAFFT Questionnaire

C   Have you ever ridden in a CAR driven by someone (including yourself) who had been using alcohol or drugs?

R   Do you ever use alcohol or drugs to RELAX, feel better about yourself, or fit in?

A   Do you ever use alcohol/drugs while you are by yourself, ALONE?

F   Do you ever FORGET things you did while using alcohol or drugs?

F   Do your family or FRIENDS ever tell you that you should cut down on your drinking or drug use?

T   Have you gotten into TROUBLE while you were using alcohol or drugs?

the dental practice or clinic. Substance abusers may often miss appointments, and all instances of this should be documented. Any telephone conversations the provider or staff has with a patient should be documented in the chart regardless of how trivial they may seem. A complete record should be kept to document cancellations, missed appointments, prognosis, and treatment plans. Photo identification of the patient should be obtained, copied, and included in the dental record, in addition to a complete health history, dental history, and other pertinent forms normally used.

Summary

Treating a patient who is a substance abuser is a complex undertaking (see Box 9.5). However, it gives dental providers the opportunity to express empathy for the situation and refer the patient to the proper provider if they desire treatment for the addiction. Also, the provider has the chance to be an advocate for the patient in their journey in overcoming the addiction.

Dental practitioners generally are ready to discuss smoking cessation with patients but are reluctant to initiate a conversation about abusing drugs.[2] They need to change that mindset and communicate with patients about their substance abuse. If the patient expresses a desire to stop the addiction or opens a pathway for the provider to guide the patient toward recovery, the provider should act. A multidisciplinary approach is often needed, and a list of local agencies and providers should be available in case a referral needs to be made.

In cases where the patient is not honest about their substance abuse or exhibits drug-seeking behavior, a combination of a thorough patient interview, active listening, and clinical judgment will help providers make efficient clinical decisions concerning the course of treatment for the patient.

> **Box 9.5 American Dental Association Statement on Provision of Dental Treatment for Patients with Substance Use Disorders**[17]
>
> **1.** Dentists are urged to be aware of each patient's substance use history, and to take this into consideration when planning treatment and prescribing medications.
> **2.** Dentists are encouraged to be knowledgeable about substance use disorders—both active and in remission—in order to safely prescribe controlled substances and other medications to patients with these disorders.
> **3.** Dentists should draw upon their professional judgment in advising patients who are heavy drinkers to cut back, or the users of illegal drugs to stop.
> **4.** Dentists may want to be familiar with their community's treatment resources for patients with substance use disorders and be able to make referrals when indicated.
> **5.** Dentists are encouraged to seek consultation with the patient's physician, when the patient has a history of alcoholism or other substance use disorder.
> **6.** Dentists are urged to be current in their knowledge of pharmacology, including: content related to drugs of abuse; recognition of contraindications to the delivery of epinephrine-containing local anesthetics; safe prescribing practices for patients with substance use disorders—both active and in remission—and management of patient emergencies that may result from unforeseen drug interactions.
> **7.** Dentists are obliged to protect patient confidentiality of substances-abuse treatment information, in accordance with applicable state and federal law.
>
> Adopted October 2005.

References

1. Strobbe S. Prevention and Screening, Brief Intervention, and Referral to Treatment for Substance Use in primary care. *Prim Care* 2014;41(2):185–213.

2. Murphy D, Wilmers S. Patients who are substance abusers. *N Y State Dent J* 2002;68(5):24–7.

3. US Department of Justice Drug Enforcement Agency. Don't be scammed by a drug abuser. http://deadiversion.usdoj.gov/. Accessed May 21, 2014.

4. Mohammad A. Substance use disorders. In: The ADA Practical Guide to Patients with Medical Conditions. Patton LL, ed. 2012. Wiley-Blackwell, Ames, IA, p. 335.

5. Miller WR. Motivational interviewing with problem drinkers. *Behav Psychother* 1983;11:142–72.

6. Britt E, Hudson S, Blampied N. Motivational interviewing in health settings: a review. *Patient Educ Couns* 2004;53:147–55.

7. Rollnick S, Heather N, Bell A. Negotiating behavior change in medical settings: the development of brief motivational interviewing. *J Ment Health* 1992;1:25–37.

8. Martins R, McNeil D. Review of motivational interviewing in promoting health behaviors. *Clin Psychol Rev* 2009;29:283–93.

9. Ivey AE, Bradford Ivey M, Zalaquett CP. *Intentional Interviewing and Counseling*, 8th ed. 2014. Brooks/Cole Publishing, Belmont, CA.

10. Substance Abuse and Mental Health Services Administration. Systems-Level Implementation of Screening, Brief Intervention, and Referral to Treatment. 2013. http://www.integration.samhsa.gov/sbirt/tap33.pdf. Accessed January 2, 2015.

11. Bernstein SL, D'Onofrio G. A promising approach for emergency departments to care for patients with substance use and behavioral disorders. Health Aff (Millwood) 2013;32(12):2122–8.

12. Agerwala SM, McCance-Katz EF. Integrating Screening, Brief Intervention, and Referral to Treatment (SBIRT) into clinical practice settings: a brief review. *J Psychoactive Drugs* 2012;44:307–17.

13. Babor TF, McRee BG, Kassebaum PA, Grimaldi PL, Ahmed K, Bray J. Screening, Brief Intervention, and Referral to Treatment (SBIRT): toward a public health approach to the management of substance abuse. *Subst Abus* 2007;28:7–30.

14. Pilowsky DJ, Wu LT. Screening instruments for substance abuse and brief interventions targeting adolescents in primary care: a literature review. *Addict Behav* 2013;38:2146–53.

15. The Center for Adolescent Substance Abuse Research. The CRAFFT screening tool. http://ceasar-boston.org/CRAFFT/index.php. Accessed January 2, 2015.

16. Pradhan B, Chappuis F, Baral D, Karki P, Rijal S, Hadengue A, Gache P. The alcohol use disorders identification test (AUDIT): validation of a Nepali version for the detection of alcohol use disorders and hazardous drinking in medical settings. *Subst Abuse Treat Prev Policy* 2012;7:42.

17. American Dental Association. Statement on Provision of Dental Treatment for Patients with Substance Use Disorders. http://www.ada.org/en/about-the-ada/ada-positions-policies-and-statements/provision-of-dental-treatment-for-patients-with-substance-abuse. Accessed January 2, 2015.

Resources and Further Readings

Babor TF, McRee BG, Kassebaum PA, Grimaldi PL, Ahmed K, Bray J. Screening, Brief Intervention, and Referral to Treatment (SBIRT): toward a public health approach to the management of substance abuse. *Subst Abus* 2007;28(3):7–30.

Martino S, Carroll K, Kostas D, Perkins J, Rounsaville B. Dual diagnosis motivational interviewing: a modification of motivational interviewing for substance-abusing patients with psychotic disorders. *J Subst Abuse Treat* 2002;23(4):297–308. http://www.ncbi.nlm.nih.gov/pmc/articles/PMC3865805/. Accessed January 2, 2015.

National Institute on Drug Abuse. Talking to patients about sensitive topics: communication and screening techniques for increasing the reliability of patient self-report. http://www.drugabuse.gov/nidamed/centers-excellence/resources/talking-to-patients-about-sensitive-topics-communication-screening-techniques-increasing. Accessed January 2, 2015.

Substance Abuse and Mental Health Services Administration (SAMHSA). Enhancing Motivation for Change in Substance Abuse Treatment. Treatment Improvement Protocol (TIP) Series, No. 35. http://www.ncbi.nlm.nih.gov/books/NBK64967/. Accessed January 2, 2015.

The National Alliance of Advocates for Buprenorphine Treatment (NAABT). Substance Use Disorders: A Guide to the Use of Language. 2004. http://www.naabt.org/documents/Languageof addictionmedicine.pdf. Accessed January 2, 2015.

Office Management of Controlled Substances

10

Carlos M. Aquino

Introduction

The use of a controlled substance, whether it is administered, dispensed, or prescribed to a patient by a practitioner, must comply with federal laws and regulations that are enforced by the Drug Enforcement Administration (DEA) through their Office of Diversion Control (Diversion). It is important for both dental practitioners and their office staff to completely understand laws and regulations relating to the dispensing, prescribing, and administering of a controlled substance as part of their professional practice.

Federal Statutes and Regulations

Federal statutes relating to controlled substances are noted in Title 21, United States Code Section 801 et al., also known as the Controlled Substances Act (CSA). Federal regulations are noted under Title 21, Code of Federal Regulations (CFR), sections 1300 to 1316 of which are enforced by DEA personnel.

Statutes and regulations noted in this chapter are found under the "Resources" tab of the DEA Diversion website at www.deadiversion.usdoj.gov and can be printed for use by practitioners.

A more extensive explanation of DEA diversion can also be found in the Practitioner's Manual, which provides a better understanding of federal statutes and regulations. The manual is available at www.deadiversion.usdoj.gov/pubs/manuals/pract/index.html.

Definitions

It is important that dental practitioners understand certain definitions used in federal statutes and regulations.

Prescription

A written direction for the preparation and administration of a medicine. Federal laws and regulations are very clear on defining the purpose of a prescription. Elements include that the prescription must be for legitimate medical purpose and can only be written by a

The ADA Practical Guide to Substance Use Disorders and Safe Prescribing, First Edition. Edited by Michael O'Neil.
© 2015 American Dental Association. Published 2015 by John Wiley & Sons, Inc.

practitioner acting in their usual course of professional practice.

Practitioner

A physician, dentist, veterinarian, or other individual licensed by a state or registered with the DEA to dispense a controlled substance.

Dispense

Delivering a controlled substance *to an ultimate user or the prescribing or administering* of such a controlled substance.

Readily Retrievable

Any purchase of a controlled substance to be administered or dispensed to a patient requires a practitioner to maintain *purchase* and *disposal records*. Such records are required to be maintained for a period of *2 years*. Some states may require such records to be maintained for 5 years.

The term "readily retrievable" means the record is kept or maintained in such a manner that it can be separated out from all other records in a reasonable time or that it is identified by an asterisk, redline, or some other identifiable manner such that it is easily distinguishable from all other records.

Clinical Consideration

Federal law requires the DEA registration-registrant information, authorized power of attorney letters with all DEA Form 222s and the most recent biennial inventory records be kept on site for immediate review. Other records maintained at another location, such as invoices for Schedule III–V purchases, should be retrievable in no less than two business days.

Due Diligence

The practice of performing *reasonable verification* that the information presented is accurate and reliable in order to prevent deceptive or

criminal practices. *Reasonable* implies that the practitioner is doing what any practitioner would and should do in the routine activities of the health-care professional.

Common Violations by Dental Practitioners

Scope of Practice

It is important for a dental practitioner to fully understand the scope of practice of a dental practitioner and their dental staff. Scope of practice is defined the practitioner's state Dental Practice Act and applicable regulations promulgated thereunder. For example, some state regulations may permit the prescribing of a controlled substance or the purchase of controlled substances for dispensing or administering purposes. However, other states may not permit a dental practitioner to dispense the same controlled substance. This is where a dental practitioner may have an administrative or civil action taken against them for *not knowing* the state laws and regulations governing the practice of dentistry. Box 10.1 lists common regulatory violations by dental practitioners associated with controlled substances.

Box 10.1   Common Regulatory Violations by Dental Practitioners

- Prescribing outside the scope of practice.
- Failing to maintain required documents.
- Failing to dispose of controlled substances according to regulations.
- Failing to store controlled substances according to regulation.
- Failing to maintain inventory records according to regulation.
- Prescribing without a *documented* established dental provider–patient relationship.
- Failing to maintain up-to-date registration documentation.
- Health-care or insurance fraud.

Record Keeping

It is important for a dental practitioner to maintain records for the purchase of controlled substances. These records must be maintained, "readily retrievable," and available for inspection by the DEA, state law enforcement, or regulatory entities responsible for these inspections.

Storage of Controlled Substances

It is essential that any controlled substance purchased for office use be stored in a locked, well-constructed metal cabinet or safe, and that access be limited to only a few individuals. The dental practitioner under whose DEA registration number the controlled substances were purchased holds full responsibility for storage. Any diversion of such controlled substances will also be the responsibility of that dental practitioner.

Disposal of Controlled Substances

The DEA has made it clear that any disposal of controlled substances by the dental practitioner should be done by a DEA-registered reverse distributor, who will receive expired, contaminated or defective controlled medications and destroy them. The benefit is that the transfer of

medications to the reverse distributor places the responsibility *on the reverse distributor*.

If a reverse distributor is not used, the DEA requires DEA Form 41 be completed, submitted, and approved BEFORE destruction. Flushing controlled substances or discarding them into the trash are not acceptable disposal techniques.

Documentation

Documentation, or more specifically *lack of documentation*, is one area where the DEA will take administrative or civil action against a dental practitioner. The following are records that need to be maintained in order to comply with federal regulations:

- DEA Form 222 is the form used to purchase or transfer a Schedule II controlled substance to and from a practitioner to their suppliers or reverse distributors. The form is required to have the date of *purchase or transfer* along with the *quantities* that are purchased or transferred by the practitioner (see Figure 10.1).
- Invoices are required for purchases or transfers of Schedule III through Schedule V controlled substances. The same documentation, such as quantity received or shipped and the date received or shipped, is required by those regulations on controlled substances.

DEPICTION of PAGE 1 of DEA FORM-222
U.S. OFFICIAL ORDER FROM-SCHEDULES I & II

See Reverse of PURCHASER'S Copy of Instructions	No order form maybe issued for Schedule I and II substances unless a completed application form has been received (21 CFR 1306.04).	OMB APPROVAL No. 1117-0010

TO: *(Name of Supplier)*   **STREET ADORESS**

CITY and STATE   **DATE**   **TO BE FILLED IN BY SUPPLIER**

SUPPLIERS DEA REGISTRATION No.

LINE No.	No. of Packages	Size of Package	Name of Item	National Drug Code	Packages Shipped	Date Shipped
	TO BE FILLED IN BY PURCHASER					
1						
2						
3						
4						
5						
6						
7						
8						
9						
10						

◀ LAST LINE COMPLETED *(MUST BE 10 OR LESS)*   SIGNATURE OR PURCHASER OR ATTORNEY OR AGENT

Date Issued	DEA Registration No.	Name and Address of Registrant
Schedules		
Registered as a	No. of this Order Form	

DEA Form-222
(Oct 1992)

U.S. OFFICIAL ORDER FORM - SCHEDULES I & II
DRUG ENFORCEMENT ADMINISTRATION
SUPPLIER'S Copy 1

Note: The graphic illustrated above is not intended to be used as an actual order form.

Figure 10.1 DEA Form 222.

- Perpetual inventory is not required by federal laws and regulations, but it may be used to maintain an inventory of controlled substances that are purchased, dispensed, or administered; disposed of as waste; or on-hand. If a dental practitioner purchases controlled substances for office use, the practitioner should maintain such method of inventory. Perpetual implies the "total count" of a controlled substances onsite is known in real time or *near real time*. This is compared with traditional inventories of controlled substances that may be performed and total counts (including discrepancies) that are reconciled only at the time of inventory every 2 years (see Figure 10.2).

- DEA biennial inventory is required every 2 years for all controlled substances on-hand to be dispensed or administered by the practitioner. In some states, the biennial inventory may be required to be done on or about May 1 of all odd years.

> **Clinical Consideration**
>
> It is highly recommended that dental practitioners maintain a perpetual inventory with daily reconciliation of discrepancies. This may help prevent or deter "pilfering" of controlled substances by dental personnel or office staff.

- Prescription records *are documents that should be noted and kept in the patient chart*. When possible, use prescription pads that use a numerical format that would identify a specific patient to a specific number. A carbonless copy or electronic copy should be maintained in the patient chart or electronic records. Any question about a written prescription for a controlled substance can easily be compared with the copy of the original prescription.

It is paramount to maintain complete and accurate records as required by federal laws and regulations. The primary reason for inventory is to determine that no diversion has occurred with the controlled substances used in dentistry.

> **Clinical Consideration**
>
> Should a dental practitioner note a discrepancy in inventory or suspect diversion of controlled substances from their office, this information should be immediately reported to federal and state regulatory agencies. This may protect the dental practitioner, as well as maintain compliance with federal reporting and state requirements.

Surviving a Drug Enforcement Administration Inspection

Every dental practitioner who purchases, administers, or dispenses a controlled substance from their office, to be administered or dispensed to a patient, should be prepared for a state or DEA inspection since controlled substance wholesalers are obligated to report all sales of controlled substances.

The three areas of concern of any inspection by a state regulatory entity and DEA are *required records*, *security* and *storage* of controlled substances, and *due diligence* when administering, dispensing, or prescribing a controlled substance.

The DEA may perform unannounced inspections. All requested information required by federal laws and regulations must be provided in a timely manner. The DEA Diversion personnel will identify themselves and will request the dental practitioner's signature on a Notice of Inspection (DEA Form 81), which permits them to be in the facility. Such inspections occur when a practitioner has purchased controlled substances for office use. Other regulatory agencies, including law enforcement, may request records for inspection based on *suspected* unethical, unprofessional, or possible criminal activities in the course of an investigation of a patient,

SCHEDULE II PERPETUAL INVENTORY

DRUG: _____

DATE	DEA 222 FORM # RX INVOICE #	PURCHASE AMT (+)	PRESCRIPTION TAG WITH RX NUMBER & QUANTITY	BALANCE ON HAND	RPH SIGNATURE

Figure 10.2 Example of a perpetual inventory form.

dental practitioner, or office staff. Disclosures of patient information may be regulated by the Privacy Rule of the Health Insurance Portability and Accountability Act of 1996 (HIPAA), and/or applicable state law. For example, the HIPAA Privacy Rule section 45 CFR 164.512 contains provisions on permissible disclosures:

- that are required by law;
- for judicial and administrative proceedings
- pursuant to process such as court orders and subpoenas; and
- of limited patient information to law enforcement in response to a law enforcement official's request for such information for the purpose of identifying or locating a suspect, fugitive, material witness, or missing person.

The HIPAA "minimum necessary" rule may also apply (see 45 CFR 164.502).

HIPAA does not preempt more stringent state laws, such as laws regulating the confidentiality of dental records. A qualified attorney in the appropriate jurisdiction may be consulted for advice on how to comply with a DEA request for patient information in compliance with applicable federal and state law.

The DEA agent's first action upon arrival to the clinic will be to perform an inventory of all controlled substances on the premise (including expired drugs), followed by a review of dispensing records of those controlled substances. The purpose is to determine that controlled substances have not been diverted by office employees to the illicit market.

During the physical inventory, DEA personnel will evaluate the security of controlled substances. It is essential that a practitioner keep controlled substances in a well-constructed safe or metal cabinet with a key or combination lock to prevent the diversion of those controlled substances. It is highly recommended that an office practice maintain an alarm system that would detect the unauthorized entrance by persons looking for controlled substances or other valuable items. The security of patient charts should

be the second reason for maintaining an alarm system. It is recommended that the practice uses closed-circuit TV cameras to record any unauthorized entrances or an employee theft.

The final purpose for a DEA inspection would be the concern of the DEA to evaluate the practitioner's due diligence policy and their corresponding responsibilities for prescribing a controlled substance as part of a practice. Several steps should be taken to determine that a patient is not a drug seeker or doctor/dentist shopper.

If the practitioner is asked to surrender their DEA registration during a DEA inspection, it is recommended that the practitioner notify legal counsel immediately. Voluntarily surrendering a DEA registration may imply that the practitioner will be acknowledging violation of federal laws and regulations. Such surrender may cause a state dental board to evaluate the practitioner's license to practice dentistry. *It is recommended that a practitioner speak with a lawyer before signing any document used to surrender a DEA registration or license to practice dentistry.*

> **Clinical Consideration**
>
> Dental practitioners performing due diligence with patient records and controlled substance records rarely have to be concerned with federal or state regulatory violations. Many audits or investigations are routine. *Frequently, an individual patient or office staff is the target of these investigations, NOT the dental practitioner.*

Practice Due Diligence Program

There are many different drug-seeking scenarios a prescriber may face. For example, a patient may cut their gums, wait until an infection occurs, and seek an appointment with a dental practitioner, knowing that a controlled substance may be prescribed for pain. The same patient may make multiple visits with as many as 20 dental practitioners to seek an opioid prescription (see Chapter 8). In some cases, a dental practitioner may prescribe a controlled substance for up to 10 days.

These are several recommendations that a dental practitioner can implement to prevent the illicit use of a controlled substance that is dispensed or prescribed to a patient:

- Evaluate first-time patients to determine their past history of dental needs.
- Find out the patient's last dental provider and contact that office for a history chart of services provided.
- If a controlled substance will be dispensed or prescribed to a patient, perform a history check on the state prescription drug monitoring program. Most states will allow a practitioner or pharmacist to review the prescribing history of a patient. In some cases, state regulations will require a practitioner or pharmacist to perform such a search to determine that a patient is not a drug abuser or doctor/dentist shopper.
- Have the patient sign an agreement outlining the practice's requirements when a controlled substance is dispensed or prescribed for pain.
- Use office staff as the first line of defense to determine if patients are seeking controlled substances or truly requesting necessary dental procedures.

Management of Noncontrolled Substances in the Office

Record keeping of all noncontrolled substances prescribed and dispensed from the dental practitioner's office is not required by federal regulations. However, this record keeping should be performed with the same due diligence as controlled substances. Stock medications or sample medications prescribed and dispensed

from the office are frequently diverted, misused, or abused by office staff. *Knowledge about medications does not grant office staff the "privilege" to self-prescribe or self-medicate.*

Summary

The first concern of the DEA, state law enforcement, and other regulatory entities is to prevent the use of controlled substances for illicit purposes. They have placed stringent responsibilities on practitioners, pharmacists, and wholesalers to determine that controlled substances are not being used for purposes other than for legitimate medical reasons. Therefore, any dental practitioners administering, dispensing, or prescribing a controlled substance in an office setting should be familiar with not only federal laws and regulations enforced by the DEA, but with state laws and regulations. Not knowing laws and regulations is not an excuse to avoid civil or administrative action by a federal or state regulatory entity. Noncontrolled substances should also be monitored to prevent office staff misuse and abuse.

Resources and Further Readings

DEA. Diversion Control. www.deadiversion.usdoj .gov.

US Government Publishing Office. Title 45: Public welfare. Part 164—Security and privacy. Subpart E—Privacy of individually identifiable health information. §164.502 Uses and disclosures of protected health information: general rules. http:// www.ecfr.gov/cgi-bin/text-idx?SID=e2c53d18580 1704692edaa0ef1f00ac2&node=se45.1.164_1502&r gn=div8. Accessed January 3, 2015.

US Government Publishing Office. Title 45: Public welfare. Part 164—Security and privacy. Subpart E—Privacy of individually identifiable health information. §164.512 Uses and disclosures for which an authorization or opportunity to agree or object is not required. http://www.ecfr. gov/cgi-bin/text-idx?SID=e2c53d185801704692ed aa0ef1f00ac2&node=se45.1.164_1512&rgn=div8. Accessed January 3, 2015.

11

Addiction and Impairment in the Dental Professional

William T. Kane, DDS, MBA, FAGD, FACD

Introduction

Addiction is a complex disease, chronic in nature, and affects the structure and function of the brain. It also can be *effectively prevented*, treated, and managed by medical and other health professionals. Addiction affects 16% of Americans aged 12 and older—more than one in seven people have an addiction involving nicotine, alcohol, or other drugs. That translates into 40 million people. This is more than the number of Americans with heart conditions (27 million), diabetes (26 million), or cancer (19 million).

Another 31.7% of the population (80.4 million), while not addicted, engage in risky use of addictive substances in ways that threaten health and safety. Addictive diseases remain one of the most serious threats to our nation's public health.[1]

Madden reported the prevalence of substance abuse is so high that every health-care provider in the USA sees patients either at risk themselves or experiencing negative effects of substance use by a friend, family member, or coworker.[2] Practicing

dental professionals should know and recognize both the risk factors and the signs of substance use disorder (SUD) and other impairments in order to adequately treat patients who are either suffering from or in recovery from SUD. Dental patients with addictive diseases are medically compromised, and this may affect the approach and outcome of their dental treatment. Dental practitioners, dental team members, and their families may also have or be at risk for addictions and other impairments. Additionally, dental professionals should begin to take a proactive stance in recognizing, intervening, and referring patients, coworkers, and colleagues for appropriate evaluation and treatment. The information concerning addiction in health-care professionals, and particularly the dental profession, is largely evidence based. However, very few scientific studies exist concerning addiction in dental professionals. The information in this chapter will increase dental practitioners' knowledge of addictive diseases and impairment in dental practitioners and their office personnel. Intervention for these

The ADA Practical Guide to Substance Use Disorders and Safe Prescribing, First Edition. Edited by Michael O'Neil.
© 2015 American Dental Association. Published 2015 by John Wiley & Sons, Inc.

individuals is paramount, since patients are also at immediate risk of potential injury.

Definitions

Addiction

Addiction is a primary chronic disease of brain reward, motivation, memory, judgment, and related circuitry. Dysfunction in these circuits leads to characteristic biological, psychological, social, and spiritual manifestations that frequently result in destructive and life-threatening behaviors. Addiction is influenced by multiple factors, including, but not limited to, genetics, environment, sociology, physiology, and individual behaviors. Addiction is characterized by inability to consistently abstain, impairment in behavioral control, craving, diminished recognition of significant problems in behavior and interpersonal relationships, and a dysfunctional emotional response. Like other chronic diseases, addiction often involves cycles of relapse and remission. Without treatment or engagement in recovery activities, addiction is progressive and can result in disability or premature death.[3]

For the purposes of this book, the term *addiction* may be used to describe alcoholism, drug addiction, chemical dependency, substance use disorders, drug dependence, drug abuse, substance and behavioral addictions. Currently, there are disagreements concerning the use of these terms by scientists, as well as clinicians.[4,5] The term *addiction*, however, is widely accepted by clinicians and treatment professionals.

There are two categories to consider when evaluating addictions: (1) direct or indirect chemical stimulators of the reward pathway (substances such as alcohol, medications, nicotine, or food) and (2) behavioral addictions (such as compulsive gambling, work, sexual activity, problematic Internet use, compulsive exercising, hoarding, or even accumulation of money). For the purposes of this book the term "addiction" will be limited to chemical substance, alcohol, or medication addictions.

Impairment

For the purposes of this book, impairment is defined as the inability to *consistently* think rationally, perform job-related tasks, or communicate *effectively* without reoccurring error while performing job-related activities. *For the purpose of this book, impairment will refer to the disease of addiction.*

Denial

For the purposes of this book, denial is defined as the inability of an individual to rationally recognize *obvious* behaviors or patterns of behaviors that likely are detrimental to personal health, patient care, or dental board licensure. This definition should not be confused with the definition involving lying, which involves *intentional* deception or cover up.

The Complexity of Addiction

Recognition of the disease of addiction is often a difficult and complex process. Common signs and symptoms associated with addiction overlap with those for depression, anxiety disorders, bipolar disorder, sleep disorders, obsessive-compulsive disorders, and schizoaffective disorders. Neurological or endocrine diseases may be seen when comprehensive clinical work-ups or diagnostics are performed. Rarely does an individual with the diagnosis of addiction have *just* the diagnosis of addiction. The side effects or adverse effects of many prescription and over-the-counter (OTC) medications may induce behavioral changes or induce clinical presentations identical to SUD. For many health professionals, self-medicating to treat underlying disorders or to enhance work performance is a frequent pathway to addiction. Social

Table 11.1   Common Signs and Symptoms of Medical Conditions that Overlap with SUD

Depression/anxiety	Neurological or endocrine disorders	Substance or medication addiction	Medication side effects or adverse drug reactions
Labile mood	Labile mood	Labile mood	Labile mood
Cognitive dysfunction/ memory lapses	Cognitive dysfunction/ memory lapses	Cognitive dysfunction/ memory lapses	Cognitive dysfunction/ memory lapses
Unusual diaphoresis, tachycardia, labile blood pressure	Unusual diaphoresis, tachycardia, labile blood pressure	Unusual diaphoresis, tachycardia, labile blood pressure	Unusual diaphoresis, tachycardia, labile blood pressure
Appears oversedated or lethargic	Appears oversedated or lethargic	Appears oversedated or lethargic	Appears oversedated or lethargic
Erratic behavior	Erratic behavior	Erratic behavior	Erratic behavior
Persistent tardiness	Persistent tardiness Slurred speech	Persistent tardiness Slurred speech	Slurred speech

circumstances at home or work further complicate assessments. Table 11.1 compares signs and symptoms of common disorders that may confound the diagnosis of addiction and may lead to inaccurate assessments *or assumptions* about an individual's behavior. Box 11.1 lists common conditions that *may* cause impairment in dental practitioners.

Box 11.1   Potential Causes of Impairment in Dental Professionals

- Psychiatric disorders such as depression, anxiety disorders, or schizoaffective disorders.
- Neurological or endocrine-related disorders such as hormonal imbalances or restless leg syndrome.
- OTC or prescription medication side effects or adverse drug reactions.
- Sleep deprivation.
- SUD.
- Chronic pain syndromes.

The primary or most notable diagnostic feature of addiction is denial. Denial is the addict's unconscious psychological defense system that develops over time through repeated rationalizations. Denial allows addicts to justify their behavior and to avoid painful knowledge of their actions.

Clinical Consideration

The onset of new unusual behaviors, such as slurred speech, sedation, diaphoresis, or mood changes, is a common clinical finding when starting new medications for new diagnosis and should not be automatically *assumed* to be addiction.

The Neurobiology of Addiction

Addiction is a chronic brain disease with underlying neurological pathology.

In the last decade, neuroscientists and clinicians have made significant progress understanding the neurobiology of drug and alcohol addiction. Addiction researchers have collected evidence showing that chronic substance or medication abuse changes the brain in ways that *may* lead to profound behavioral disruptions seen in addicted individuals (see Chapter 2). These disruptions predominately affect areas of the brain responsible for judgment, motivation, and emotion. These changes are long lasting and persist even years after discontinuing the substance or medications abused. New knowledge about drugs' effects on the brain and the role of genetic, developmental, and environmental factors should bring about changes in our approaches to the prevention and treatment of addiction.[6] The neurobiology of addiction is discussed in greater detail in Chapter 2.

The Stigma of Addiction

The American Medical Association (AMA) classified alcoholism and drug addiction as a disease in 1954. Society at large, as well as many medical and dental professionals, may still view it as a moral weakness. The stigma associated with the disease of addiction is so deeply engrained in society that, despite evidence-based studies, patients frequently are denied appropriate, ethical, medical, and dental treatment. At its core, addiction is not a simple social, moral, or criminal problem.[7]

Epidemiology of Addiction in Dentistry

Dental practitioners, like other health-care professionals, are just as susceptible to this disease as others in the general population. Additionally, addiction may affect dental practitioners' family members, members of the dental team, and their families, as well as their patients. The impact of addictive diseases on individual dental practitioners' lives, dental practices, and families' lives is substantial. In no way do statistics capture the human toll of family devastation, broken hearts, broken dreams, and financial ruin.[8]

Kenna and Wood describe the current literature regarding the prevalence of SUD in health care professionals.[9] This information is limited in its scope of generalizability and methodological rigor. The lack of empirical data regarding dental professionals has contributed to the skepticism regarding the actual prevalence of SUD in dental professionals. This statement is best illustrated by contradictory prevalence estimates found in the literature for health professionals.[9] Lifetime rates of SUD among health-care providers are in the range 11–14%. The overall rate of substance abuse among health-care providers is roughly equivalent to that of the general population. However, health-care professionals' patterns of abuse are frequently different than the general population.[10] As an example of this deviation, dental practitioners have historically had easy access to nitrous oxide, which is common in many dental offices and known to be a medication of abuse for dental practitioners. In a study by Clark et al., the data indicated 7.1% of 109 impaired dental practitioners studied were sanctioned for abusing nitrous oxide.[11] The authors concluded that nitrous oxide in particular posed a serious hazard for dental practitioners. Brockman and Able write, "The abuse potential of nitrous oxide coupled with the ease of availability of the drug contributes to its relatively frequent abuse by dentists."[12] According to Kenna and Wood, there is little evidence to suggest that dental practitioners may be at a greater risk of developing alcohol or drug use problems compared with the general population.[9]

Risk Factors for Substance Use Disorder

According to Early, the risk for addiction in physicians is an area rich in speculation and poor in research.[13] This statement could also be made concerning dental practitioners. A substantial number of health-care professionals—including dental practitioners—may report multiple risk factors that may have contributed to their SUD. Box 11.2 lists some of the most common risk factors associated with SUD.

Box 11.2 Common Risk Factors Associated with SUD

- A family history of SUD.
- Significant stress at home, work, or both.
- Emotional problems.
- Using drugs or alcohol at an early age.
- Sensation-seeking behavior.
- Physical or social isolation.
- Ease of substance or medication access.
- Self-prescribing or self-medicating.
- History of childhood trauma.
- History of sexual abuse.

Gender is also considered a risk factor; however, there are often contradictory statements in regard to gender and SUD. Boyd and Knight state that female health-care professionals may have increased risk factors, yet Kenna et al. state male health-care professionals have increased risk factors.[10,13,14] Kenna et al. acknowledge that their results may be the result of the gender imbalance in dentistry since the American Dental Association (ADA) reports that 83% of dental practitioners were male.[10] There are a limited number studies dealing with gender and addiction in the health-care professions.

Family History of Substance Use Disorder

The greatest predictor of substance abuse problems in dental practitioners is the same as that in the general population: a family history of SUD. Several studies have speculated that many dental prac-

titioners perhaps come from dysfunctional families or families with a history of alcohol or drug dependence.[15–18] Sammon et al. reported that 35–39% of students at two dental schools had an alcoholic parent or grandparent.[17] Sandoval et al. reported that 15% of all dental students at the University of Texas had a family history of alcoholism and 17% had a history of illicit drug use.[19] *Current data do not support that dental professionals are at greater risk than other health-care professionals of reporting a family history of alcohol or drug problem.*[20]

Stress

Dentistry is a complex health-care profession. Stressful factors in the workplace may include demanding patients, long work hours, physical and tedious work, financial decisions, personnel issues, and regulatory compliance. Box 11.3 provides a more comprehensive list. For some dental practitioners, these issues may significantly affect their physical health, mental health, or both. Clinical disorders such as burnout, anxiety, and depression may result. These disorders may further influence or complicate dental practitioners' personal relationships, professional relationships, and overarching health and well-being. Stress can indeed have a negative impact on dental professionals' personal and professional lives. One of the possible consequences of chronic occupational stress is professional burnout. Burnout is best described as a gradual erosion of the person.[21] Burnout is defined by three coexisting characteristics. First, the person is exhausted mentally or emotionally. Second, the person develops a negative indifferent or cynical attitude toward patients or coworkers; this is referred to as "depersonalization" or "dehumanization." Third, there is a tendency for individuals to feel dissatisfied with their accomplishments and to evaluate themselves negatively. Some dental practitioners frequently turn to alcohol or medications to self-medicate their burnout.

> **Box 11.3   Common Workplace Stressors in Dentistry**
>
> - Demanding patients.
> - Patients in acute pain.
> - Long work hours.
> - Tedious or meticulous work.
> - Social isolation.
> - Personnel conflicts.
> - Office finance management.
> - Maintaining federal, state, or dental board-related compliance and documentation.
> - Practice management issues (concerns such as staff and overhead).

The stress-related problems associated with dentistry may arise from the work environment and the personality types of the people who choose dentistry as a profession. A study has shown that dentistry tends to attract people with compulsive personalities, who often have unrealistic expectations and unnecessarily high standards of performance, and who additionally require social approval and status. Beginning in dental school, dental practitioners are trained to be both technicians and artists who perform exacting procedures in isolated environments and are determined to achieve the mythical "ideal preparation or restoration."[22] Studies have indicated that both anxiety and depressive disorders are frequently observed in dental practitioners. Depressive disorders often occur with anxiety disorders and substance abuse.[21,22] The relationship between professional stress and suicide, if any, has not been substantiated or quantified.[23] Gropper and Porter, who have treated over 500 addicted dental practitioners, suggest that the relationship between stress in the dental profession and addiction is much more complex.[24] A number of the dental practitioners they have treated have reported elevated levels of fear and dissatisfaction with their career choice.[24] Stress is an elusive concept, and its exact correlation with substance use is unclear. Substance use certainly often occurs in individuals in stressful situations.[13] More commonly today, self-medication with prescription medications may contribute to the disease of addiction.

Other Risk Factors

Additional risk factors include co-occurring or comorbid psychological or psychiatric conditions. Individuals who began using mood-altering drugs at an early age are at greater risk of developing addictive diseases involving substances. Individuals who are thrill seekers are sometimes described as "adrenaline junkies" and are thought to be at a greater risk as well. The isolation of most dental practices combined with the access to drugs and the possibility of self-prescribing create a host of risk factors for dental practitioners. Finally, both men and women who have experienced physical, emotional, or sexual abuse as a child have a significant risk of developing a wider range of psychopathology, particularly eating disorders, alcoholism, and drug addictions.[25]

Substances of Choice

The primary substance of choice for dental practitioners is alcohol. According to Baldwin et al., alcohol abuse is the most common substance abuse issue confronting dentistry, and it can develop during dental school as many students start using alcohol, medications, or substances to cope with stress.[26] In the same study by Baldwin et al., health-care students self-reported that indeed alcohol was by far the most commonly abused substance. An additional study by Kenna and Wood reported that alcohol was the substance abused most frequently by dental practitioners. In their study, dental practitioners reported that alcohol was offered frequently by friends or colleagues in social settings. Other substances of abuse included cigarettes, marijuana, major opioids (such as morphine, fentanyl, meperidine, hydromorphone, and oxycodone), minor opioids (such codeine), and anxiolytics (such alprazolam and diazepam).[9] Nitrous oxide is a medication historically unique to dentistry and anesthesiology. However, commercial availability of nitrous oxide to the general public has increased its abuse (see Chapter 6). Additionally, dental practitioners also report using illegal drugs, such as cocaine and methamphetamine.

Identifying Addiction

Addiction is usually a progressive disease. In dental practitioners, the disease of addiction is frequently in its advanced stages before signs and symptoms become obvious in the office or clinical setting or to patients. Addicted dental professionals often hide their SUD from family, office staff, and patients. As addiction progresses, personal and professional lives deteriorate. A clinical study suggest the order in which addiction-related injury occurs: it starts with family, community, finance, spiritual, emotional health, and physical health and ends with job performance.[27]

Denial and excuses occur not only in the addict but also in their support system. Family members and office staff may protect addicted dental professionals from public embarrassment, regulatory sanctions, or to protect their source of livelihood. The isolation of a solo dental practice further contributes to this process. The disturbances in social and familial functioning can be early predictors of SUD in dental practitioners.[14] Dental professionals with an addiction are commonly in denial of their addiction. *Potential* warning signs of SUDs are listed in Box 11.4. *Additional potential* warning signs for dental practitioners that should be considered in the workplace are listed in Box 11.5.

> ### Box 11.4 Potential Warning Signs of SUD
>
> - Increased difficulty at home, marital conflict, extramarital affairs, problems with children.
> - Repeated appearances of being drunk at social functions.
> - Wide mood swings: anger, depression, nervousness.
> - Frequent unexplained bathroom breaks.
> - Isolation and withdrawal from community and colleagues.
> - Frequently calling in sick or unjustifiable tardiness.
> - Self-medicating.

> ### Box 11.5 Addition Potential Warning Signs in Dental Practitioners
>
> - Self-prescribing.
> - Increased problems with other office staff and patient complaints.
> - Legal and financial problems, lawsuits and debt, arrests for driving under the influence (DUI).
> - Repeatedly and unexplainably leaving the office.
> - Intoxication or the odor of alcohol on the breath at work.
> - Problems with state licensing boards and drug enforcement agencies.
> - Unjustifiable aberrations in office financial records or controlled substance records.

"The Conspiracy of Silence"

Dental practitioners, similar to other professionals and individuals, frequently fail to confront SUD in colleagues even when its presence is undeniable. Colleagues, family, and staff may delay addressing addicted dental professionals in an effort to protect them from adverse consequences, such as shame, social stigmatization, income loss, and licensure actions. Additionally, individuals are often afraid of being wrong or fear potential retaliation from dental professionals or other office staff. "The Conspiracy of Silence" is a common series of behaviors in which family, staff members, and colleagues are wary of bringing addicted dental practitioners' problems to light.[28] Box 11.6 lists common reasons why suspected or known SUDs are not reported.

Box 11.6   Reasons SUDs Are Not Reported

- Inability to recognize aberrant behaviors.
- Lack of *definitive* evidence of SUD.
- Social acceptance of substance or medication misuse or abuse.
- Fear of retaliation from office personnel.
- Fear of losing their job/income.
- Protection of impaired individual from social embarrassment, regulatory sanctions.
- Peer pressure to not report.
- Fear of being the "narc."

Intervention

The ADA's Principles of Ethics and Code of Professional Conduct declares that:[29]

It is unethical for a dentist to practice while abusing controlled substances, alcohol or other chemical agents which impair the ability to practice. All dentists have an ethical obligation to urge chemically impaired colleagues to seek treatment. Dentists with first- hand knowledge that a colleague is practicing dentistry when so impaired have an ethical responsibility to report such evidence to the professional assistance committee of a dental society.

Undoubtedly, one of the most difficult professional decisions a health-care professional can make is to intervene on behalf of a colleague or coworker with an SUD. Despite great difficulties, it is important to recognize that health-care professionals with SUDs, in retrospect, report that an intervention probably saved their lives and protected the public from harm.[9] Often, the initial break in the cycle of denial is the result of some type of intervention. This may come in the form of an investigation from a state dental board, a DUI, an overdose, some type of personal or professional crisis, or even a well-planned professional intervention.

Vernon E. Johnson, considered the father of intervention, stated:[30]

Alcoholism/addiction is a disease, the very nature of which renders the victim incapable of recognizing the severity of the symptoms, the progression of the disease or of accepting any ordinary offers to help. If they are to receive the insight they must have, that insight must come from those around the addicts through conscious, planned and caring acts of intervention.

In years past, it has been assumed that an individual with an addiction had to progress to nearly the end stage of the disease and "hit bottom" before they could be helped. The impact of the disease would have to reach such a significance that the individual would then be willing to ask for help on their own. In the case of the addicted dental professional, many lost their health, families, practices, and licenses to practice; were arrested; left dentistry; or committed suicide. It is now recognized that addicted dental professionals, staff, or family members do not have to "hit bottom" to be directed to help.

Goals of Intervention

The goal of intervention is to direct dental practitioners or individuals to have an evaluation and get treatment, if necessary. An intervention can be described as "the presentation of reality to a dental practitioner or individual with an addictive disease who is unwilling or incapable of accepting 'that reality' on his or her own." An intervention is a process that attempts to disrupt the circle of denial. Formal intervention is a proven, structured process that is the most effective means of helping dental practitioners and others with addictive diseases.[28]

If handled with tact, dental practitioners can generally be "gently coerced" into an evaluation when given the alternatives of possible dental board referral or possible legal actions.[13] Intervention involves direct confrontation with the individual regarding their behaviors and any related concerns. If the intervention is adequately planned and carried out, then, often but not always, the addicted individual begins the process of restoring their personal and professional lives. Persistence of the problem after the intervention should result in it being reported to dental boards.

> ### Clinical Consideration
>
> Dental practitioners who become aware and are certain of a colleague's addictive disease have both a professional and an ethical responsibility to intervene in a constructive manner. Such interventions can involve discussing the issue with the impaired dental practitioner, offering help if possible, and/or involving the state dental association's well-being committee.[28] *Ultimately, an individual who fails to cease practice after an intervention or follow the guidance of a dental peer professional group (when available) must be reported to the state dental board.*

Evaluation/Assessment

Dental professionals vary in their need for an assessment of their addiction. Some dental practitioners' behavior is quickly identified and they agree to cooperate with their treatment needs or at least with an outpatient assessment, or evaluation. Many are more entrenched in their addiction and may have more complex presentations. Several assessment goals are listed in Box 11.7. Owing to the complexity and comprehensive nature of these evaluations, most are conducted in residential or partial hospitalization settings where they can be observed continuously. These evaluations have come to be called a "ninety-six hour evaluation," a term derived from the time usually required to complete this process.[31,32] Usually, certain criteria must usually be met by dentist well-being programs for competent evaluation to be conducted. This includes that the evaluation be performed by a multidisciplinary team composed of an addiction medicine physician and an addiction psychiatrist and that it includes psychological and neuropsychological testing, family assessment, review of previous medical records, and, frequently, the collection of collateral information from coworkers, friends, and any other important sources of information needed. The team involved in a multidisciplinary evaluation meets repeatedly during the course of the evaluation and once again when all data have been collected. The evaluation team is often best served by including a peer assistance representative or other referral source in the summation session; this action decreases confusion regarding the outcome.[13]

> ### Box 11.7   Goals of Addiction Assessment
>
> - Identify substances of abuse, quantities, routes of administration, and duration of use.
> - Identify risks of physiologic withdrawal.
> - Identify possible support networks.
> - Identify risks of other diseases, such as HIV or hepatitis.
> - Identify, when possible, concurrent untreated psychiatric disorders.
> - Identify optimal treatment resources.
> - Refer to capable facilities when necessary.
> - *Give immediate psychiatric support for potential life-threatening circumstances.*

Treatment

The transition from active addiction into recovery involves appropriate treatment. The recovery of dental practitioners with addiction usually involves a long continuum of care. Erickson states that people do not get better without change.[4] Addiction is the only potentially fatal disease wherein the affected person can determine their own outcome once they have been exposed to treatment.[32] Multiple treatment options and combinations of treatment are available to individuals with an SUD. Box 11.8 lists several treatment options available. There are many treatment methods that have been employed with varying degrees of success. It is unlikely that any single treatment method, orientation, or duration can work for every addict or alcoholic. There are approximately a dozen programs in the USA that have experience and special expertise in the treatment of addicted physicians and other health-care professionals; some programs have more than 30 years of experience and have treated thousands of addicted physicians and dental practitioners.[13]

Box 11.8   Common Treatment Modalities Available

- Inpatient treatment.
- Outpatient treatment.
- Residential treatment.
- Faith-based treatment.
- Medication-assisted treatment—pharmacotherapy.
- Support groups such as Alcoholics Anonymous or Narcotics Anonymous.
- Individual and group psychotherapy, cognitive behavioral therapy.

Treatment must be determined based on several factors, including, but not limited to, concurrent psychiatric and medical conditions, financial considerations, family support networks, available treatment options, and previous individual treatments when known. Talbott and Wilson contend that group therapy and treatment with peers are decisive in breaking through denial and dealing with the individual's emerging new identity.[33] Available evidence suggests that physician and dental practitioner treatment programs with the best outcomes employ abstinence-based 12-step principles. These support groups may provide education about addiction, spiritual reconnection, and a psychotherapeutic approach that addresses issues within the individual, the family, and work. Additionally, participation of the family in the therapeutic process is very helpful.[13,34] Also, dental practitioners learn how to better identify stress in the workplace that often comes from sources of stress not recognized in the past. Along with identification and recognition, it is crucial for dental practitioners to develop healthier coping skills to reduce stress in the workplace and all areas of their lives.[32,34]

There is an increasing body of evidence about the safe and effective use of pharmacologic adjuncts in the treatment of alcoholism and opioid dependence. Most physician and dental practitioner treatment programs use one or more medications, including disulfiram, naltrexone, acamprosate, and/or topiramate as adjuncts for alcohol treatment and the opioid blocker naltrexone for opioid-addicted dental practitioners. Chapter 2 discusses this treatment in greater detail.

Family and Staff

When a dental practitioner enters treatment, their family should be involved with both treatment and counseling, as everyone in the family is affected in one way or another. Family and dental staff need to identify, confront, and change the environment that allowed the dental practitioner to maintain their addiction. A great deal has been written about codependency and how family members and/or office staff become part of the additive disease process. These individuals may require education and help in healing and learning how to care for themselves while the addict is learning as part of their own recovery process.[32,34]

Relapse

It is essential that addicts, as well other health professionals, understand that recovery is more than just abstinence. A common myth exists about relapse: *relapse just suddenly occurs without warning*. The reality is that many warning signs precede a relapse.[22,24] The incidence of relapse is inversely related to the duration of recovery, but return to use or abuse (relapse) has been observed in patients with decades of recovery.[34] Slips or very short-term relapses are not uncommon (*particularly in early treatment*). Singular slips are not definitive indicators of complete treatment failure. However, dental practitioners who have difficulty maintaining sobriety and abstinence should be removed from the work force until treatment professionals experienced in recovery feel that they are safe to return to work.[13]

Monitoring

Treatment monitoring is usually associated with dental well-being programs or dental board consent orders. These orders commonly involve weekly group therapy sessions, peer support groups, aftercare groups, individual and family therapy, self-help (12-step) group attendance, random drug testing, and work-site monitoring for 5 years or more. These extensive monitoring efforts allow state dental boards to have the confidence that dental practitioners with an addictive disease are safe to return to

practice.[13] These practice boundaries also act as a deterrent for relapse. See Box 11.9.

> ### Box 11.9 Common Requirements of Peer Assistance or Well-being Contracts
>
> - 5–10-year duration of agreements if no violations.
> - Random urine, hair, or saliva drug or alcohol testing.
> - Mandated treatment.
> - Mandated counseling.
> - Mandated support group attendance.
> - Restrictions in place of work.
> - Restriction in hours of work.

Physicians appear to have a much higher recovery rate (approximately 75%) than the general population. A number of studies have sought to define why physician treatment is so successful and to identify which components of the physician treatment process may also be beneficial to the public at large. It is speculated that these high success rates are likely related to the highly structured nature of the treatment and monitoring programs, along with accountability. The rewards of maintaining sobriety are great, and the costs of relapse are quite high. The high rates of success of dental treatment programs most likely are for the same reasons in physician treatments. No data are available for recovery rates for dental practitioners.

Peer Assistance or Dental Well-being Committee Programs

The beginning of the physician health movement and dental well-being committees can be traced back to the founding of International Doctors in Alcoholics Anonymous by Clarence Pearson in 1949. The AMA has sponsored conferences on physician impairment every other year since 1975. The ADA began doing the same in the early 1980s and has held conferences every other year since 1984. Physicians health programs (PHPs) were a result of this early work. PHPs exist in all states and have worked closely with state medical boards to advocate for physicians suffering from addictive diseases and other well-being issues. Since the late 1970s, state medical boards have developed standards dealing with identification, intervention, treatment, return to practice, relapse, education, prevention, and monitoring. The core concept of PHPs has become clear: "to detect problems that lead to impairment and to intervene and encourage physicians to obtain assistance prior to damaging their careers or harming patients."[13]

The dental profession also formed its own version of a PHP known as dental well-being committees or dental peer assistance committees with similar goals and functions. Virtually all states have recognized dental well-being committees, with varying organizational structures and lines of authorities. Many state well-being committees work closely with their respective state board of dentistry. Dental well-being committees in most states will also serve as a resource to assist family members of dental practitioners and dental team members. Frequently, dental well-being committees provide monitoring of treatment, drug screening, and overall documentation of the recovering dental practitioner's well-being.

Peer assistance or dental well-being committee programs vary from state to state and may not be regulated by the state's dental boards. Three types of programs are described here.

Addiction Support Programs and Information

These programs provide information, resources and nonjudgmental support for dental practitioners with addictive diseases or other well-being issues. These programs allow a colleague, employee, family member, or patient to seek help without reporting the dental professional to the attention of the licensing board. The information gathered is strictly confidential.

Self-report Programs

Self-report programs or diversion programs are available in certain states. Board of dentistry regulations allow dental practitioners to avoid sanctions, provided they follow the programs' recommendations of treatment and mandatory monitoring contracts. These programs may have *memorandum of understanding agreements* with the state dental board.

Consent or Mandated Programs

Consent or mandated programs are formal programs in which a state board of dentistry mandates treatment and monitoring of a dental practitioner with an SUD by an approved treatment plan and treatment facility. Failure of the dental professional to comply with the contract frequently results in sanctioning by the dental board.

Contractual Agreements with Peer Assistance or Well-being Committee Contracts

Various state well-being committees require the dental practitioners to sign and adhere to a formal agreement or contract. These agreements define boundaries that dental practitioners must comply with or else face possible sanctions, including revocation of their dental license. Generally, these contracts allow individuals to return to clinical practice after successful treatment and demonstration that the individual has actively engaged in the recovery process. Box 11.9 lists requirements commonly found in these agreements or contracts.

Clinical Considerations

State dental boards should consider additional limitations or restrictions based on the individual's substance or medication abuse history and relapse record. These considerations should be made on a case-by-case basis and should not be automatically applied to every dental practitioner. Considerations may include the following:

- limitations restricting access to nitrous oxide in office setting;
- limiting prescription authority of controlled substances;
- limiting hours allowed per work week;
- denying dispensing of controlled substances in the office setting.

Summary

Dental professionals are neither immune to nor at a higher risk for addictive diseases. However, patterns of use often reflect both the availability and the knowledge of controlled substances. Multiple risk factors have been identified that may place dental practitioners at increased risk for SUDs. Dental professionals and dental office personnel should learn to recognize and intervene with colleagues with suspected or known SUDs. Referral for evaluation and treatment is frequently warranted.

Dental professionals, family members, and patients whose lives have been affected by addictive diseases frequently recover and lead healthy and productive personal and professional lives. The ADA and state dental associations continue to take a proactive role in assisting those suffering from addictions. The end goal is to get them the proper treatment to enter and maintain their recovery and return to practice.

References

1. CASAColumbia. Addiction Medicine: Closing the Gap between Science and Practice. 2012. The National Center on Addiction and Substance Abuse of Columbia University, New York, p. 1.
2. Madden TE. Coming from all directions: protecting girls and women from the impact of substance use. J Calif Dent Assoc 2008;36(2):119–25.
3. American Society of Addiction Medicine. Definition of Addiction. Public Policy Statement: Definition of Addiction. http://www.asam.org/research-treatment/definition-of-addiction. Accessed January 10, 2015.
4. Erickson CK. Terminology and characterization of "addiction". In: The Science of Addiction: From Neurobiology to Treatment. 2007. WW Norton, New York, pp. 3–5.
5. Gilson AM. The concept of addiction in law and regulatory policy related to pain management. Clin J Pain 2010;26(1):70–7.
6. Volkow ND, Warren KR. Drug addiction: the neurobiology of behavior gone awry. In: The ASAM Principles of Addiction Medicine, 5th ed. Ries RK, Fiellin DA, Miller SC, Saitz R, eds. 2014. Wolters Kluwer Health, Philadelphia, PA, pp. 3–5.
7. Sheff D. Clean: Overcoming Addiction and Ending America's Greatest Tragedy. 2013. Houghton Mifflin Harcourt, Boston, MA, pp. 88–102.
8. CDA, CDRAF. Executive summary. In: On the Road to Wellness: Dealing with Addiction Disease in Dentistry. Final Report. 2012. Canadian Dental Association and The Canadian Dental Regulatory Association, Toronto, Canada, pp. 1–68.
9. Kenna GA, Wood MD The prevalence of alcohol, cigarette and illicit drug use and problems among dentists. JADA 2005;136:1023–32.
10. Kenna GA, Baldwin JN, Trincoff AM, Lewis DC. Substance use disorders in health care professionals. In: Addiction Medicine: Science and Practice. Johnson BA, ed. 2011. Springer, Science+Business Media, pp. 1375–98.
11. Clark JH, Chiodo GT, Cowan FF. Chemically dependency among dentists: prevalence and current treatment. Gen Dent 1988;36:227–9.
12. Brockman CS, Abel PW Drugs of abuse. In: Pharmacology and Therapeutics for Dentistry, 6th ed. Yagiela JA, Dowd FJ, Johnson BS, eds. 2011. Mosby Elsevier, St Louis, MO, p. 811.
13. Early PH. Physician health programs and addiction among physicians. In: The ASAM Principles of Addiction Medicine, 5th ed. 2014. Ries

RK, Fiellin DA, Miller SC, Saitz R, eds. Wolters Kluwer Health, Philadelphia, PA, pp. 602–21.

14. Boyd JW, Knight JR. Substance use disorders among health care professionals. In: Lowinson and Ruiz's Substance Abuse: A Comprehensive Textbook, 5th ed. Ruiz P, Strain E, eds. 2011. Wolters Kluwer Health/Lippincott Williams & Wilkins, Philadelphia, PA, p. 892.

15. Coombs RH. Addicted health professionals. J Subst Misuse 1996;1:187–94.

16. Bowermaster DP. Chemical dependency: are dental students at risk? Ohio Dent J 1989;63:26–30.

17. Sammon PJ, Smith TA, Cooper TM, Furnish G. Teaching an alcohol prevention course in the dental school chemical dependency curriculum: a preliminary report. J Dent Educ 1991;55:30–1.

18. Sandoval VA, Dale RA, Huddleston AM. Abstract from the 67th AADS Conference, March 4–7. J Dent Educ 1990;54:36.

19. Sandoval VA, Hendricson WD, Dale RA. A survey of substance abuse education in North American dental schools. J Dent Educ 1988;52:167–9.

20. Kenna GA, Wood MD. Family history of alcohol and drug use in health care professionals. J Subst Use 2005;10:225–38.

21. Rada ER, Johnson-Leong C. Stress, burnout, anxiety and depression among dentists. JADA 2004;135:788–94.

22. Lange BM, Fung EY, Dunning DG. Suicide rate in the dental profession: fact or myth and coping strategies. Dent Hypotheses 2012;3:164–8.

23. Alexander RE. Stress-related suicide by dentists and other health care workers. Fact or folklore? JADA 2001;132:786–94.

24. Gropper JM, Porter TL. Addiction and progressive self-destructive behavior in dentistry. In: Clark's Clinical Dentistry, vol. 5. Hardin JF, ed. 1997. Mosby, St Louis, MO, pp. 1–13.

25. Zweben JE. Special issues in treatment: women. In: The ASAM Principles of Addiction Medicine, 5th ed. Ries RK, Fiellin DA, Miller SC, Saitz R, eds. 2014. Wolters Kluwer Health, Philadelphia, PA, pp. 524–40.

26. Baldwin JN, Scott DM, Agwral S, Bartec JK, Davis-Hall RE, Reardon TP, DeSimone EM II. Assessment of alcohol and other drug use behaviors in health professions students. Subst Abuse 2006;27(3):27–37.

27. Kane WT. The conspiracy of silence in the dental profession. Dentaltown Mag 2012;(March):81–3. http://www.dentaltown.com/dentaltown/article.aspx?i=276&aid=3729. Accessed January 10, 2015.

28. Johnson VE. Intervention: How to Help Someone Who Doesn't Want Help. 1986. Johnson Institute Books, Minneapolis, MN.

29. American Dental Association's Principles of Ethics and Code of Professional Conduct. 2014. http://www.ada.org/en/about-the-ada/principles-of-ethics-code-of-professional-conduct/. Accessed January 3, 2015.

30. Fung EY, Lange BM. Impact of drug abuse/dependence on dentists. Gen Dent 2011;59(5):356–9.

31. Early PH. Physician health programs and addiction among physicians. In: The ASAM Principles of Addiction Medicine, 4th ed. Ries RK, Fiellin DA, Miller SC, Saitz R, eds. 2009. Wolters Kluwer Health/Lippincott Williams and Wilkins, Philadelphia, PA, pp. 531–47.

32. Walters J. Dentistry: risks for addictive disease. J Am Coll Dent 2007;74(4):24–7.

33. Talbott GD, Wilson PO. Physicians and other health professionals. In: Substance Abuse: A Comprehensive Textbook, 4th edn. Lowinson JH, Ruiz P, Millman RB, Langrod JG, eds. 2005. Lippincott Williams & Wilkins, Philadelphia, PA, pp. 1187–1202.

34. May JA, White HC, Leonard-White A, Warltier DC, Pagel PS. The patient recovering from alcohol or drug addiction: special issues for the anesthesiologist. Anesth Analg 2001;92:1601–8.

Resources and Further Readings

Fenster JM. Ether Day: The Strange Tale of America's Greatest Medical Discovery and the Haunted Men Who Made It. 2001. Harper Collins Publishers, New York.

Scheff D. Clean: Overcoming Addiction and Ending America's Greatest Tragedy. 2014. Houghton Mifflin Harcourt, Boston, MA.

Teitelbaum SA. Addiction: A Family Affair. The University of Florida Guide to Understanding, Prevention and Dealing with Addiction. 2011. University of Florida, Gainesville, FL.

Due Diligence and Safe Prescribing

Michael O'Neil, PharmD

Introduction

Patient care in any health-care environment has become complicated by many factors, such as financial management, management of office personnel, acutely ill patients in pain, and demanding patients. Regulatory boards and law enforcement agencies require dental practitioners to practice due diligence in detecting, deterring, and reporting criminal or suspected criminal activity involving their practice or their prescriptions. In the dental profession, most criminal activity involves patient-related fraud, forgery, or deception in attempts to obtain controlled substances, such as analgesics or anxiolytics. Dental practitioners are required to recognize disease states such as drug and alcohol addiction or other substance use disorders (SUDs) that may have a direct impact on what medications should or should not be prescribed or dispensed to the patient. This chapter will present patient management strategies that will help the dental practitioner identify patients

and discuss reasonable considerations to help direct their care.

Definitions

Due Diligence

Due diligence is the practice of performing "reasonable verification" that the information presented is accurate and reliable in order to prevent deceptive or criminal practices. "Reasonable" implies that the practitioner is doing what any practitioner would and should do in the routine activities of the health-care professional.

Relapse

"Relapse" is defined as the recurrence of behavioral or other substantive indicators of active disease after a period of remission in patients with the disease of addiction. Relapse is not an instantaneous event but a sequence of behaviors leading up to and including reusing a substance of abuse.

The ADA Practical Guide to Substance Use Disorders and Safe Prescribing, First Edition. Edited by Michael O'Neil.
© 2015 American Dental Association. Published 2015 by John Wiley & Sons, Inc.

Prescriber–Patient Analgesic Mismatch

Prescriber–patient mismatch is defined as the inconsistency in treatment goals or expectations of treatment between the prescriber and the patient. Examples include analgesia, sedation, and anxiolysis.

Case Scenarios

For all case scenarios involving analgesia, dental practitioners should discuss goals of postprocedural pain management to prevent mismatch of prescriber–patient analgesic expectations. It is also recommended that dental practitioners evaluate a patient's prescription drug monitoring program (PDMP) profile for any new patient or patients not seen in the previous year. Evidence-based studies in dentistry support nonsteroidal anti-inflammatory drugs (NSAIDs) or NSAIDs+acetaminophen in combination as first-line therapy unless there is a definitive contraindication (see Chapter 3).

Recognition of Diversion Behaviors

See Chapters 8 and 9.

JK is a 34-year-old white female that presents to your dental office unannounced 20 min before the office closes with a chief complaint of excruciating tooth pain. She states she needs something for severe pain and most pain medications do not work. She is accompanied by her boyfriend, who is persistent in stating "she has to stay with him ... she needs him." Cursory review of her medical intake form reveals that she denies any significant past medical history or surgical history. She denies alcohol and illicit substances but admits cigarette smoking. She reports she does not take any medications. Social history reveals she is unemployed, divorced but has two children, 8 and 10 years old. Allergies reported by the patient include Naprosyn®, Toradol®, ibuprofen,
and "codones." The only pain meds that works is Opana® (oxymorphone).*

Based on this patient's clinical presentation what are potential flags that warrant further inquiries and what other information could you or your office staff evaluate to guide your interview and potential treatment?

Possible flags in this patient *may* include:

1. An unannounced visit just prior to office closing.
2. Boyfriend or family member *of an adult patient* adamant about staying with the patient.
3. Multiple allergies to all common prescription and over-the-counter analgesics.
4. Patient directing specific prescription pain medication treatment.

Other accessible information by the dental or office staff includes:

1. The patients address from her driver's license or state-issued ID card should be evaluated. Patient's driving extreme distances (e.g., 50 miles or more) that requires passing several dental practices is a possible flag.
2. Depending on the dental practitioner's state regulations, the PDMP database can be quickly accessed to review controlled substance dispensing records for the patient using name and date of birth from her driver's license. Many states allow the designation of individual staff to access the database on behalf of the dental practitioner. Dental practitioners are urged to utilize staff, when state PDMP laws permit, to access and print PDMP reports *for the dental practitioner to review* prior to prescribing controlled substances.

Follow-up information from the office staff indicates the patient lives 75 miles away in a nearby city. There are at least four dental practitioners in her immediate home town.

Name	Add	Zip	Fill Date	Rx #	medication	strength	QTY	Day sup	RPh	DEA	Pharmacy	DEA	Store
JK	319 LOWER	25526	2 days ago	11222	APAP/HYDRO	300MG-10MG	180	30	SMITH JOE	DH0267890	TOM'S PHARM	GF1234567	25526
JK	319 LOWER	25526	20 days ago	19976	APAP/HYDRO	300MG-10MG	180	30	SMITH JOE	DH0267890	TOM'S PHARM	GF1234567	25526
JK	319 LOWER	25526	30 days ago	23466	APAP/HYDRO	300MG-10MG	180	30	SMITH JOE	DH0267890	TOM'S PHARM	GF1234567	25526
JK	319 LOWER	25526	70 days ago	31111	APAP/HYDRO	300MG-10MG	180	30	SMITH JOE	DH0267890	TOM'S PHARM	GF1234567	25526

Figure 12.1   Sample prescription drug monitoring profile.

The state PDMP revealed the following (see Figure 12.1).

JK's PDMP profile revealed multiple recent prescriptions for opioid analgesics. The sum of the last three prescriptions within the last 30 days should have provided the patient with a *90-day supply*. The PDMP profile information should be confirmed with JK, the pharmacies that filled the prescriptions, or the other prescribers before any definitive action is taken.

What specific questions regarding information reported on the PDMP should be asked when interviewing the patient?

1. Have you been prescribed any pain medications for *any reasons* in the past 1–2 months?
2. Have you been seen by any other medical or dental professionals for any reason in the last 1–2 months?

If the patient answers "no" to either or both questions, sharing information from the PDMP with her is suggested.

If the patient is *lying* about her medication history, this *may be* a "crime." Many states have laws against intentional deception of health-care professionals to obtain treatment

or medications. Federally, prescriptions prescribed under false pretenses are not valid prescriptions.

> **Clinical Consideration**
>
> PDMP reports are a tool. *They are not evidence of a crime.* It is possible for patient or doctor information to be miscoded when the information is entered into the patient's pharmacy computer profile (e.g., wrong patient or prescriber selected). *Generation of this report always requires validation of information before critical decisions are made by the prescriber. Validation should include a call to the pharmacy to verify.*

The oral exam of the patient is significant for a history of multiple extractions and the presence of multiple carious lesions. All teeth were tan to gray in coloration and a nondraining molar abscess was observed.

How can JK's pain be reasonably managed?

Primary treatment involves initial drainage of the abscess and antibiotics to remove the source of the pain. Strategies should include initially treating the abscess and having the patient return for possible extraction.

The patient should be questioned about her allergies to NSAIDs. Patients simply stating "they never work for me" or "I don't like taking them" are not reasons to dismiss NSAID therapy. Conservative treatment would include NSAIDs or NSAIDs+acetaminophen around the clock (see Chapter 3). In the event of a *true* NSAID allergy or contraindication to NSAIDs, tramadol with acetaminophen "'around the clock" is an alternative. If the dental practitioner feels opioids are warranted in this patient, quantities limited to the time necessary for antibiotics to be effective (usually 2–4 days after initial drainage) may be prescribed with schedule doses around the clock. It is recommended that no refills be allowed for this prescription. It is very common for patients to not show up for their scheduled extraction date. Dental practitioners are discouraged from prescribing "multiple rounds of controlled substances" when patients are continually "no shows" for extractions.

Clinical Consideration

It is not uncommon for adult patients to present with other family members, boyfriends, or girlfriends to acquire controlled substances. Dental practitioners should have other adult companions removed from the room during the initial interview since many times patients are being "pressured" or influenced by others to get controlled substances.

Reporting to Law Enforcement

Once the information reviewed on the patients PDMP profile has been confirmed through discussions with the patient, pharmacy, or other prescribers, this patient should be reported to local, regional, or state law enforcement agencies that routinely work with prescription drug diversion. Often times these agencies have titles such as "drug task force."

Ethics and Analgesia

CK is a 33-year-old white male that presents to your clinic for reevaluation of six abscesses evaluated and treated with antibiotics by you 10 days ago. The patient initially presented to your clinic requesting treatment for "mouth sores." The patient admitted that he was a heroin addict but has not used in 2 months. The abscesses are markedly improved and the decision is made to progress to perform the extractions. The patient's past medical history is significant for renal insufficiency (serum creatinine per doctor's office confirmation of 2.4 mg/dL (normal 0.6–1.1 mg/dL) secondary to an infection 2 years ago, history of injection-site-related abscesses, hypertension treated with lisinopril 20 mg daily, and a recent history of a stomach ulcer being treated with omeprazole 20 mg daily. The patient denies current use of heroin, methamphetamine, or cocaine (although he admits he had abused methamphetamine and cocaine years ago.) CK does admit to smoking marijuana. The patient also states he will be getting married next month.

What factors should be considered when determining which analgesic should be prescribed to treat the pain associated with the removal of CK's six abscessed teeth? (See Box 12.1.)

CK should also be specifically asked about use/abuse of prescription opioids.

Renal insufficiency and possible gastric ulcer are contraindications to NSAIDs in CK. Conservative treatment could include acetaminophen around the clock or tramadol in combination with acetaminophen prescribed around the clock.

Clinical Consideration

Patients with a known or suspected history of prescription drug abuse should be specifically asked if they have abused tramadol before prescribing. Tramadol is a commonly abused medication. For many individuals tramadol is a preferred substance of abuse and should be avoided.

> **Box 12.1 Checklist for Optimizing Pain Management in Patients Receiving Opioid Maintenance Treatment or Chronic Opioids for Pain Management**
>
> - Reassure the patient the intent to adequately treat pain **not** deny treatment of pain.
> - Establish specific pain management goals/ expectations *before the procedure* (e.g., pain scores 1–3 not "0").
> - Respect a patient's wishes to **not** receive or be prescribed opioid analgesics or "extra doses" if they are adamant.
> - Educate and emphasize optimal nonpharmacological therapy post procedure (ice packs, oral rinses, hygiene, compliance with eating instructions, smoking discontinuation or reduction, etc.).
> - Consider preemptive strike with NSAID 1 h before the procedure and then *scheduled* NSAID pain treatment around the clock and not "as needed."
> - Consider using the long-acting injectable anesthetic bupivacaine prior to discharge from the office.
> - Use of combination analgesics with NSAIDs or acetaminophen may add additional analgesia. *(Caution is recommended since these agents may be contraindicated in patients with a history of renal or hepatic impairment. Doses of acetaminophen should not exceed 3.0 g/day.)*
> - Do not prescribe excessive doses of medications or in quantities expected to be left over.
> - Consider (with the patient's consent) a responsible family member or friend control pain medications.
> - Document all medications administered or prescribed to the patient and report information to the appropriate treatment facilities.

If the dental practitioner decides to prescribe opioids, what "abuse" factors should be considered?

Other than anecdotal reports, information confirming opioid addicts in recovery receiving opioids for acute pain management causes relapse is not available. *Relapse is a process not an instantaneous event.* The stress of inadequate treatment of acute pain may contribute to the patient's relapse. Ethically, treatment of acute pain in patients with SUD should be managed with the same treatment goals as other patients. Doctor–patient contracts are also an option, along with communication between the patient's sponsor and a reliable family member or friend to dispense the drug to the patient. With only a 2-month history of being "heroin free," the dental practitioner should not assume CK is in recovery.

The state PDMP should be evaluated for patient dispensing history of controlled substances. In a patient with opioid addiction, practitioners are concerned with the patient "taking all their medication in a single dose" to get high. An effective strategy to minimize the risk of a potential large overdose of medications or "dumping" large quantities on the street is to write more than one prescription. Each prescription would provide only a 24–48 h supply of medications (~4–12 pills, depending on the dose and interval). The second prescription should be written with the same date as the initial prescription but with specific directions written on the prescription "DO NOT FILL UNTIL 'X' DATE."

CK is the ideal candidate to encourage addiction treatment. His verbalization of being "drug free for 2 months," intent to start a new life in a marriage, and interest in improving his dental health are positive signs. Asking CK about current participation with an addiction treatment center, counseling support group, or Narcotics Anonymous meetings is critical. Many patients are not receiving addiction treatment or therapy due to inaccurately perceived financial costs, availability of services, or simply lack of encouragement from friends, family, or health-care professionals. Providing CK with a list of local treatment centers (http://findtreatment.samhsa.gov) or support groups may improve CK's chances of addiction recovery.

CK should also be referred to a medical practitioner to be evaluated for possible HIV or hepatitis due to his recent history of intravenous (IV) drug abuse with heroin. Suggesting the patient may possibly infect a spouse or partner with HIV or hepatitis is often an effective motivator for evaluation or treatment.

> **Clinical Consideration**
>
> Patients who have stopped using opioids *for several weeks* have likely lost the opioid tolerance in regard to sedative and respiratory depressant effects. *Aggressive* analgesic treatment is not recommended if opioids are required owing to potential risks of oversedation or respiratory depression. Doses should be titrated carefully on a daily basis when possible.

Alcohol and Benzodiazepines

See Chapter 6.

AB is a 19-year-old female known to your clinic with history of generalized anxiety disorder (GAD), depression, and a history of "high dental chair anxiety." AB calls your clinic and states "she has a problem with 'valium drugs' and alcohol" and requests she not be given them. She has a documented history of benzodiazepine and alcohol abuse/addiction, and a long history of dental anxiety. She requests anxiolysis prior to sleep the night before her procedure and before her root canal scheduled at 10:00 a.m. the next day. Her past medical history includes migraines, GAD, and depression. Other medications include venlafaxine (Effexor XR®) 150 mg daily for GAD and depression, valproic acid (Depakote®) 250 mg b.i.d. for migraine prophylaxis, and sumatriptan (Imitrex®) for acute migraine.

How should AB's anxiolysis be managed?

Multiple nonpharmacological strategies are available to assist in management of AB's anxiet, and utilization of these strategies is recommended.[1–4]

Traditional pharmacological anxiolysis has centered on short-acting benzodiazepines, chloral hydrate, and nitrous oxide. However, use of benzodiazepines is not recommended in AB owing to her history of benzodiazepine and alcohol abuse. Anecdotally, patients with a history of alcohol addiction have reported increased cravings after receiving benzodiazepines or nitrous oxide. Hydroxyzine HCl (Atarax®) 50 mg 1 h before bedtime and at least 1 h prior to the office procedure is a practical consideration. For AB, hydroxyzine HCl has limited risk of anticholinergic side effects in single doses as well as no clinically significant drug interactions with her current medications. AB should be instructed not to drive to and from her procedure.

Are there any special analgesic considerations in AB?

Analgesia in AB may be effectively managed with NSAIDs or NSAIDs+acetaminophen. Tramadol should be avoided in AB owing to the possible drug interactions with Effexor XR® and Imitrex® owing to the potential risk of serotonin syndrome with this combination.

Opioid Maintenance Treatment and Acute Analgesia

See Chapter 4.

LM is a 54-year-old male presenting to your clinic for lower jaw pain. Oral exam reveals two molars requiring extraction. LM informs you that he is receiving Suboxone® (buprenorphine 8 mg–naloxone 2 mg) two strips every morning for his opioid addiction. He states "he has been in recovery for 4 months and is concerned about relapse with pain medications." LM works at a local mill as a supervisor. His past medical history is significant for diabetes, gout, hypertension, chronic renal insufficiency, nonspecific back pain, and opioid addiction. Current medications include insulin (Lantus®) 20 units subcutaneous daily, hydrochlorothiazide 25 mg daily, allopurinol 300 mg daily. Glucoses are well controlled. Serum creatinine is 2.0 mg/dL (normal 0.6–1.1 mg/dL).

How should LM's acute pain post procedure be managed?

Box 12.1 lists considerations in optimizing analgesia for LM. LM is not a candidate for treatment with NSAIDs secondary to his renal insufficiency. Since this is not an emergency procedure, the dental practitioner should contact LM's opioid maintenance treatment (OMT) Suboxone® prescriber for their preference of analgesia. The dental practitioner should recognize that the 16 mg daily dose of buprenorphine *will not provide adequate analgesia as a "one-time" daily dose* since this regimen is prescribed to reduce the cravings associated with opioid addiction. The analgesic effect of buprenorphine requires multiple daily doses or continuously increased serum concentrations that are not provided in single daily doses. Reasonable approaches for the OMT provider may be to divide the 16 mg daily dose into 8 mg––4 mg–4 mg at 6–8 h intervals over 24 h or prescribe, *in addition to the 16 mg daily dose*, Suboxone® 2 mg at 6–8 h intervals. The OMT prescriber may initially prescribe *the higher standard starting dose of short-acting* combination products (e.g., oxycodone 7.5 mg or hydrocodone 10 mg) every 4–6 h around the clock and then titrate doses quickly the following day. Codeine products are not recommended in this patient (see Chapter 4). In the event the dental practitioner must proceed urgently/emergently, adjusting the patient's Suboxone® dosage is not recommended. Adjustment of the Suboxone® dosing regimen without the initial Suboxone® prescriber's authorization in the patient may cause the patient to run out of their daily Suboxone® maintenance therapy, requiring an *early refill* that is likely to be problematic at the pharmacy or dispensing clinic. Initially prescribing the higher standard dosage of hydrocodone 10 mg or oxycodone 7.5 mg–acetaminophen products every 4–6 h around the clock is a reasonable starting point. Follow-up with the patient within 24 h by phone is recommended to optimize dose adjustments. *Anecdotally, lower doses of hydrocodone/oxycodone and acetaminophen combinations provide limited analgesic response.*

Ideally, LM's OMT provider would be able to optimize LM's pain management. LM should be instructed to notify the dental practitioner if pain is *persistently* greater than "4–5" (on a 0–10 scale) since analgesia response is difficult to predict in patients receiving Suboxone®. Development of a provider–patient contract should be considered. The patient could be encouraged to allow a reliable individual to "manage his pain medication" if he is uncomfortable having opioids in his possession. LM should be encouraged to use his addiction support groups, counselors, therapists, and so on to help cope with the stressors of oral surgery, pain, and other addiction-related anxieties during this time. LM could also be given two prescriptions with limited quantities to last only 1–2 days each.

Stimulants and Tooth Pain

See Chapters 6 and 9.

WD is a 31-year-old, thin, white female that presents to the emergency room with complaints of severe tooth pain. WD's oral exam is significant for multiple caries, grossly carious teeth, and multiple previous extractions consistent with methamphetamine abuse. She also has a small draining abscess with mildly inflamed gingiva. All of her vitals are normal. WD states "she wants the tooth out now." WD denies any significant past medical history or medications except oral contraceptives but admits she was a "meth and coke head" but has been clean for 6 months because she almost had her kids taken away.

What special treatment considerations should be taken into account for this patient's extraction procedure and pain management?

It is recommended that *active* methamphetamine or cocaine users not be treated with epinephrine-containing products primarily due to the *potential* of cardiac instability (e.g., hypertension, dysrhythmias, ischemia) from combined methamphetamine (or cocaine) and epinephrine in the patients system.[5] Although WD *claims* to be in recovery from her methamphetamine/cocaine addiction, epinephrine is not absolutely required in this patient and should be avoided.

Table 12.1 lists treatment considerations in patients with a substance abuse history.

How should WD's postprocedure analgesia be managed?

WD has no contraindications for NSAIDs or acetaminophen products, so conservative pain management with these agents is recommended. Although there is no known cross-reactivity with methamphetamine/cocaine products and opioids, the quantity of opioids should be limited to cover only the acute event if the dental practitioner finds it necessary to prescribe opioid analgesia to WD.

What other issues should be addressed by the dental practitioner?

WD should be asked about participation in any treatment center or support groups for her addiction and encouraged to do so if she has not. She should also be asked if she used methamphetamine or cocaine intravenously. If she was an IV drug abuser, the dental practitioner should recommend she be evaluated for potential HIV or hepatitis.

Acute "on" Chronic Pain Management

See Chapter 4.

JJ is a 47-year-old male presenting for evaluation of possible multiple extractions due to persistent lower jaw pain and problems with chewing for the past several weeks. After oral exam, it is determined four extractions are warranted. JJ has a past medical history of hypertension, benign prostatic hypertrophy (BPH), degenerative joint disease (DJD), right knee tendon repair 2 years ago, and spinal fusions at T3–T6 secondary to a motor vehicle accident 6 years ago. Current medications include tamsulosin (Flomax®) 0.4 mg daily for BPH, candesartan 16 mg daily for HTN, cyclobenzaprine (Flexeril®) 10 mg t.i.d. for back spasms, naproxen 500 mg bid for osteoarthritis/spinal surgery, oxymorphone (Opana ER®) 40 mg q 12 h for "back pain," and Opana

immediate release® 10 mg q 4–6 h prn breakthrough pain.

How should JJ's postprocedure analgesia be managed?

JJ is already receiving NSAIDs for osteoarthritis and should be encouraged to continue all his current medications as prescribed. Addition of "extra" NSAIDs is not recommended in this patient. Ideally, the pain specialist or primary-care specialist managing JJ's chronic pain should direct his postprocedure pain management. Reasonable recommendations by JJ's primary prescriber may include using JJ's immediate-release Opana® 10 mg every 4–6 h as already prescribed or scheduled around the clock. The dental practitioner could make the same recommendation to the patient. The patient should be instructed not to exceed the *six* maximum allowable doses per day of the immediate-release Opana® 10 mg tablets. Although prescribing other short-acting opioids to this patient is a reasonable pharmacological consideration, addition of *another* short-acting opioid to the patient's Opana® regimen will likely cause concerns to the pharmacy dispensing his prescriptions. Addition of acetaminophen 500 mg every 4–6 h around the clock may also be helpful in this patient and should be considered.

Alcoholism with Liver Disease

See Chapter 6.

OT is a 65-year-old male presenting to your clinic in extreme pain after falling down the stairs and fracturing three teeth requiring extraction. His past medical history is significant for cirrhosis secondary to long-term alcohol abuse. OT admits to drinking 1 pint per day years ago but does not drink at all now, which is verified by his wife. He appears generally well nourished with no obvious signs of malnutrition. His history also includes a bleed from esophageal varices 1 year ago, hypertension, hypokalemia, and hyperlipidemia. Medications include atorvastatin (Lipitor®) 40 mg daily

Table 12.1 Clinical Findings and Treatment Considerations of Commonly Abused Substances

Abused substances	Psychiatric signs and symptoms	Dental findings	Other physical exam findings	Treatment considerations[a]
Methamphetamine, "bath salts," and prescription stimulants	• Euphoria • Hyperactivity • Paranoia • Dissociation • Insomnia	• Xerostomia • Black rotting teeth • Occlusal wear • Mass caries • Bruxism • Nasal septal necrosis • Powder in nares • Clear mucus discharge from nostrils	• Formication/picking • Track marks • Open or scabbed skin lesions • Cachexia • Burnt fingers • Profound weight loss • Tachycardia • Skin abscess	• Avoid injection or use of local epinephrine products • Occlusive guards • Xerostomia treatment products • Topical fluoride treatments • Avoid treatment at least 24 h from last "use" if possible
Cocaine	• Euphoria • Paranoia • Dissociation • Insomnia	• Xerostomia • Occlusal wear • Mass caries • Bruxism	• Open or scabbed skin lesions • Track marks • Nasal septal necrosis • Powder in nares • Profound weight loss • Dilated pupils • Tachycardia • Skin abscess	• Avoid injection or use of local epinephrine products • Occlusive guards • Xerostomia treatment products • Topical fluoride treatments • Avoid treatment at least 12 h from last "use" if possible
Lysergic acid diethylamide, phencyclidine, mescaline	• Euphoria • Hyperactivity • Dissociation • Insomnia • Paranoia • Agitation • Delusions • Hallucinations • Panic reactions	• Xerostomia • Occlusal wear • Mass caries • Bruxism	• Dilated pupils • Slurred speech • Confusion • Tachycardia	• Xerostomia treatment products • Occlusal guards • Topical fluoride treatments • Avoid treatment at least 12 h from last 'use' if possible

(continued)

Table 12.1 (Continued)

Abused substances	Psychiatric signs and symptoms	Dental findings	Other physical exam findings	Treatment considerations[a]
3,4-Methylenedioxymethamphetamine	• Psychotic episodes • Depression, • Impulsive behavior • Panic reactions • Dissociation • Euphoria	• Jaw-clenching • Jaw soreness • Xerostomia • Occlusal wear • Mass caries • Bruxism	• Dehydration • Dilated pupils • Excessive sweating • Tachycardia	• Avoid injection or use of local epinephrine products • Occlusive guards • Xerostomia treatment products • Topical fluoride treatments • Avoid treatment at least 24 h from last "use" if possible
Heroin, opium and prescription opioids	• Euphoria • Sedation • Dissociation • Delusions • Hallucinations • Slurred speech • Track marks	• Xerostomia • Occlusal wear • Mass caries • Bruxism	• Track marks • Skin erosions • "Pick" marks • Staph sores over skin • Dilated/pinpoint pupils • Goose flesh • Piloerection • Yawning	• Xerostomia treatment products • Occlusal guards • Topical fluoride treatments • Avoid treatment at least 12 h from last "use" if possible
Solvents/paints	• Euphoria • Hyperactivity • Dissociation • Insomnia • Paranoia • Tachycardia • Agitation • Delusions • Hallucinations • Panic reactions	• Paint residue around nose, mouth, teeth, tongue • Redness or irritation around nose, mouth, teeth	• Confusion • Lethargy • Memory lapses • Strong odor of solvents or paints • Tachycardia • Slurred speech	• Delay treatments at least 12 h when possible

Abused substances	Psychiatric signs and symptoms	Dental findings	Other physical exam findings	Treatment considerations[a]
Marijuana and δ-9-tetrahydrocannabinol (including synthetics)	• Euphoria • Hyperactivity • Dissociation • Tachycardia • Paranoia • Delusions • Hallucinations	• Xerostomia • Gingivitis • Alveolar bone loss • Gingival leukoplakia • Gingivitis • Increased caries	• Poor coordination • Irritated conjunctiva	• Avoid injection or use of local epinephrine products • Occlusive guards • Xerostomia treatment products • Occlusal guards • Topical fluoride treatments • Avoid treatment at least 12 h from last acute event
Ethanol	• Euphoria • Hyperactivity • Loss of inhibition • Excessive talking • Poor gait • Slurred speech • Overt odor of alcohol • Nystagmus • Confusion • Coagulopathies • Sedation	• Angular cheilitis • Jaundice • Overt smell of alcohol • Bilateral parotid swelling • Red nose • Spider petechiae on nose	• Confusion • Lethargy • Memory lapses • Slurred speech • Poor coordination • Poor balance • Nystagmus	• Caution with local (e.g., lidocaine) or systemic anesthetics in patients with end-stage liver disease • Patients could be receiving naltrexone that can block effects of opioids

[a]In all patients suspected of substance abuse or addiction, counseling or treatment referrals to specialist involved with substance abuse is recommended. Patients with known or suspected IV drug abuse should also be referred to a medical practitioner for HIV and hepatitis testing.

for lipids, hydrochlorothiazide 25 mg daily for hypertension, spironolactone 200 mg daily for mild ascites/hypokalemia, and potassium chloride 20 mEq daily for hypokalemia. His electrolytes and complete blood count are within normal limits. His coagulation labs, bleeding time, and prothrombin time/international normalized ratio are normal from 2 weeks ago at his last primary care visit.

How should OT's acute pain be managed post procedure?

OT's liver function is significantly compromised *but stable*. He does not appear to have an overt coagulopathy, but coagulation laboratory assessment should be completed prior to any major procedure. *All bleeding risk precautions and interventions are required prior to treating OT.*[6] NSAIDs are contraindicated owing to OT's cirrhosis, history of esophageal varices, and potential risk of causing hepatorenal syndrome. Oxycodone is an effective consideration in OT. Oxycodone in combination with acetaminophen is recommended owing to the additive effects of oxycodone and acetaminophen (see Chapter 3). Initiating oxycodone doses at 5 mg every 4–6 h is recommended. Use of acetaminophen in daily doses less than the previously maximum daily recommended dose of 4.0 g (*current recommended maximum daily dose is 3.0 g acetaminophen*) for acute pain has been shown to not compromise liver disease as long as the duration of acetaminophen treatment is limited to the acute event and no other hepatotoxic medication is taken or alcohol is consumed with acetaminophen.[7-9] A follow-up phone call the day following the procedure may help the dental practitioner direct further dose adjustments of oxycodone products. Codeine should not be prescribed since it requires significant hepatic metabolism to be converted to morphine for its analgesic effect.

Patients with alcoholism not in recovery pose a greater clinical challenge. If OT was actively abusing alcohol, cross-tolerance to benzodiazepines should be anticipated by the dental practitioner. A consideration for sedation

is nitrous oxide. Analgesia should be approached cautiously, similar to the alcoholic in recovery. The quantity of analgesics prescribed should be strictly regulated (e.g., writing two prescriptions with quantities limited to 24–48 h).

Clinical consideration

Sedation inpatients with significant liver disease may be safely accomplished with nitrous oxide, short-acting benzodiazepines or short-acting barbiturates. However, anecdotally many patients in recovery from alcohol addiction have reported increased cravings for alcohol after administration of these agents.

Controlled-Substance Prescribing Regulations

See Chapters 8 and 10.

BT is a 47-year-old male general dental practitioner in private practice for 21 years. Upon opening his office at 07:30 a.m., BT and his office staff are met by the regional Drug Enforcement Agency (DEA) agent and a local law enforcement officer presenting an administrative warrant requesting BT to "produce all requested records and documents." The record request is specifically for all controlled-substance purchase invoices, DEA 222 forms, and patient records for "any and all patients prescribed a controlled substance in the last 3 years." Review of the controlled-substance records from the local pharmacy and the PDMP report indicate that BT has been prescribing alprazolam (Xanax®) 0.5 mg t.i.d. for anxiety and hydrocodone 10 mg–acetaminophen 325 mg for neck pain to his daughter for the last 2 years. BT has been prescribing diazepam 10 mg t.i.d. to his wife for back spasms. Fifteen of BT's patients were found to have received at least 15 prescriptions in the last 3 months from various prescribers in the area, including BT. The total quantity of these prescriptions should have provided each patient with more than a 1 year supply of medications. BT is unable to produce the invoices for controlled substances. *There are no patient records for any of his family members or employees he has prescribed controlled substances to in the past 2 years. Patient records are lacking prescribing information, including indication and quantities dispensed to the patient. Inventories for controlled substances are nonexistent. Controlled substances dispensed by the dental practitioner from his office are kept in an unlocked drawer in one of the open dental bays where four patients may be seen at a time. The dental practitioner acquired the controlled substances by writing a prescription for "bulk bottles" of 100 hydrocodone–acetaminophen tablets that were filled by the local pharmacy.*

What *federal* charges from the DEA is BT possibly facing based on the information provided?

Federal investigations are usually initiated in response to reports from various sources, including, but not limited to, arrest from patients suspected of committing illegal activity, complaints from patients or patient family members, reports from pharmacists for questionable *and usually repeated prescribing practices*, review of purchase records for controlled substances, or PDMP data. BT will possibly be charged with the following:

1. Prescribing/practicing outside his scope of practice (chronic benzodiazepines and opioids for nondental-related issues).

   An order purporting to be a prescription issued not in the usual course of professional treatment or in legitimate and authorized research is not a valid prescription within the meaning and intent of the Controlled Substances Act and the person knowingly filling such a purported prescription, as well as the person issuing it, shall be subject to the penalties provided for violations of the provisions of law relating to controlled substances.[13]

   Prescribing outside the dental practitioner's scope of practice is one of the most common violations committed by

dental practitioners. Scope of practice applies regardless of the relationship of the patient to the prescriber.

2. Failure *to maintain required records* for controlled substances 21CFR 1304.04 Maintenance of records and inventories.[11] Maintenance of all invoices, DEA 222 forms, biennial inventories of controlled substances, patient records of controlled substances dispensed is a must. Records must be "readily retrievable," which *generally means* the dental practitioner must produce all records within two business days. If an individual was arrested selling their opioid pain medications he received from BT *and there are no records of any patient exams, procedures, or known pathology, or rationale for prescribing the medication*, BT may be charged with issuing an invalid prescription.

3. Failure to maintain *required storage* of controlled substances. Title 21, CFR Section 1301.71(a), requires that all registrants provide effective controls and procedures to guard against theft and diversion of controlled substances.

4. Writing illegal prescriptions for controlled substances.

   "A prescription may not be issued in order for an individual practitioner to obtain controlled substances for supplying the individual practitioner for the purpose of general dispensing to patients.[12]

Transfer of a controlled substance to anyone other than the patient requires either a DEA 222 form or invoice depending on the schedule of the controlled substance. The pharmacy should have denied the prescription for the 'bulk medications' the dental practitioner requested in order to dispense individual prescriptions to his patient. The pharmacy is also in violation of this regulation.

What state regulatory violations may have been committed by BT?

In regard to controlled substances, most states have laws *that parallel* federal controlled-substance laws. The state potentially could make similar charges as the DEA. In addition, state dental boards may impose sanctions, suspend licenses, or revoke licensure for additional behaviors depending on the individual state's regulations for prescribing to family members or other "ethical" considerations. In the event that an individual in the community specifically incriminated the dental practitioner (e.g., selling controlled substances to an addict) then local or state law enforcement may be involved.

Regardless of where the investigation originated, the multiple levels of investigation by federal agencies, state boards, and local law enforcement is usually a lengthy, stressful, and costly process.

Impaired Professional

See Chapter 11.

AJ is a 33-year-old male practicing general dentistry. TJ is AJ's 61-year-old father, who is also a dentist. AJ and TJ work together and own their dental practice. AJ is aware that his father was pulled over for drunk driving twice in the past 6 months but was not charged since he knew the officers in his hometown. TJ frequently leaves the office throughout the day to do "multiple errands." Over the last 2–3 months, AJ has overheard office personnel being "scolded" by his father in front of patients and other staff. When AJ asked his father why he smelled like scotch at 7:30 in the morning TJ quickly replied "he was using a new mouthwash." TJ is a prominent community figure, active in his church, and historically participated in his son's little league and high school sports. AJ knows his dad has a medical history of hypertension and hyperlipidemia and takes blood pressure/lipid medications. TJ is married and his wife is a successful accountant. AJ knows his grandfather (TJ's dad) was an alcoholic. Today at the clinic, a patient abruptly left after stating "Dr J smells like a liquor store!"

What are potential flags for significant impairment in TJ?

1. Two "stops" by law enforcement for likely driving under the influence (DUI) in the past 6 months.
2. Leaving the office multiple times throughout the day without reason.
3. Unexplained increase in "belligerent or rude" behavior to family members or office staff.
4. Excuses for "smelling like scotch" in the morning.
5. Biologic parent was an alcoholic.
6. A distressed patient recognizing likely alcohol on TJ.

Boxes 12.2 and 12.3 list common signs of impairment.

Box 12.2 Potential Warning Signs of SUD

- Increased difficulty at home, marital conflict, extramarital affairs, problems with children.
- Repeated appearance of being drunk at social functions.
- Wide mood swings: anger, depression, nervousness.
- Frequent unexplained bathroom breaks.
- Isolation and withdrawal from community and colleagues.
- Frequently calling in sick or unjustifiable tardiness.
- Self-medicating.

Box 12.3 Additional Potential Warning Signs in Dental Practitioners

- Self-prescribing.
- Increased problems with other office staff and patient complaints.
- Legal and financial problems, lawsuits and debt, arrests for DUI.
- Repeated unexplained leaving office.
- Intoxication or the odor of alcohol on the breath at work.
- Problems with state licensing boards and drug enforcement agencies.
- Unjustifiable aberrations in office financial records or controlled-substance records.

What are some reasons TJ has not been confronted with the likely alcohol problem?

1. Denial by TJ's family that a problem exists.
2. Denial by staff that a problem exists.
3. Family and staff are able to "justify" why his drinking is not a problem.
4. "Conspiracy of Silence."
5. Public acceptance of "high alcohol use."
6. General fear of public embarrassment.
7. TJ's family and staff do not know how to intervene.
8. Staff may be worried about their own job security if something happens to TJ.

Who should *ideally* intervene in TJ's situation?

Many states have dental well-being or peer assistance committees as part of the state dental association that will provide information support and direction to family and friends of a potentially impaired dental practitioner. AJ, along with TJ's wife, should reach out to this organization for immediate acceptance. Often times, members in peer assistance committees will direct the intervention to facilitate treatment. Another consideration would be for AJ to notify TJ's primary-care provider to help direct TJ to treatment. Contrary to popular belief, every individual with the disease of addiction does not have to hit "rock bottom" before they agree to get help. In the event that an "intervention" proves to be unsuccessful, TJ should be made aware that the dental regulatory board must be notified since dental patients are at risk. For most health-care practitioners the threat of potential "loss of licensure" by dental boards is a strong motivator to comply and get help. In many other cases the individual needing help may be "relieved" since help is forthcoming.

According to the American Dental Association's "principles of ethics code of professional conduct" 2.D.1 Ability to Practice:

A dentist who contracts any disease or becomes impaired in any way that might endanger patients or dental staff shall, with consultation and advice from a qualified physician or other authority, limit the activities of practice to those areas that do not endanger patients or dental staff. A dentist who has been advised to limit the activities of his or her practice should monitor the aforementioned disease or impairment and make additional limitations to the activities of the dentist's practice, as indicated.[13]

Should TJ enter an appropriate treatment program, how likely is TJ to maintain a life of recovery and successful dental practice?

Recovery data reporting long-term recovery rates of dental practitioners are limited. However, TJ has multiple "motivators" that may influence but not guarantee his success (see Box 12.4). State dental boards and peer assistance programs usually require monitoring that may include random drug testing, counseling, successful completion of a treatment program, and support group attendance. With the appropriate treatment, guidance, and support, TJ should be able to return to dental practice and provide safe dental care (see Chapter 11).

Box 12.4 Factors or Motivators that May Influence Success of Recovery in Health-Care Professionals

- Loss of licensure.
- Loss of financial support (financial incentives).
- Public embarrassment.
- Loss of "perceived role in the community."
- Testing or monitoring by professional boards or peer programs.

Summary

The practice of dentistry is has become increasing complicated by federal/state regulations, medical patients with SUDs, ethical dilemmas, and criminal behaviors of patients. Dental practitioners are frequently required to make many difficult "real-time" decisions in regard to prescribing controlled substances. Frequently, information necessary to make "optimal decisions" regarding controlled substances does not exist. Achieving successful outcomes may require notification of law enforcement, dental boards, or professional peer support groups. Involvement of these organizations is necessary to protect patients, dental practitioners and their staff, and the public.

References

1. Armfield JM, Heaton LJ. Management of fear and anxiety in the dental clinic: a review. Aust Dent J 2013;58(4):390–407; quiz 531. doi: 10.1111/adj.12118.

2. American Dental Association. Guidelines for Teaching Pain Control and Sedation to Dentists and Dental Students. 2007. http://www.ada.org/~/media/ADA/Member%20Center/FIles/anxiety_guidelines.ashx. Accessed January 4, 2015.

3. Dym H. Risk management techniques for the general dentist and specialist. Dent Clin North Am 2008;52(3):563–77, ix. doi: 10.1016/j.cden.2008.02.011.

4. Donaldson M, Gizzarelli G, Chanpong B. Oral Sedation: a primer on anxiolysis for the adult patient. Anesth Prog 2007;54:118–29.

5. American Dental Association. Oral Health Topics: Meth Mouth. http://www.ada.org/en/member-center/oral-health-topics/meth-mouth. Accessed January 7, 2015.

6. Cruz-Pamplona M, Margaix-Muñoz M, Sarrión-Pére MG. Dental treatment in patients with liver disease. J Clin Exp Dent 2011;3(2):e127–34. doi: 10.4317/jced.3.e127.

7. Menashehoff S, Goldstein LB, Brown S, Stickevers S. Safe usage of analgesics in patients with chronic liver disease: a review of the literature. 2013. http://www.practicalpainmanagement.com/treatments/pharmacological/non-opioids/safe-usage-analgesics-patients-chronic-liver-disease-review?page=0,1. Accessed January 4, 2015.

8. Dart RC, Kuffner EK, Rumack BH. Treatment of pain or fever with paracetamol (acetaminophen) in the alcoholic patient: a systematic review. Am J Ther 2000;7(2):123–34.

9. Chandok N, Watt KDS. Pain management in the cirrhotic patient: the clinical challenge. Mayo Clin Proc 2010;85(5):451–8.

10. DEA. Diversion Control. Practitioner's Manual—Section III. http://www.deadiversion.usdoj.gov/pubs/manuals/pract/section3.htm.

11. DEA. Diversion Control. Title 21 CFR—Part 1304—Section 1304.04 Maintenance of records and inventories. http://www.deadiversion.usdoj.gov/21cfr/cfr/1304/1304_04.htm.

12. DEA. Diversion Control. Practitioner's Manual—Section V. http://www.deadiversion.usdoj.gov/pubs/manuals/pract/section5.htm.

13. American Dental Association. Nonmaleficence. 2014. http://www.ada.org/en/about-the-ada/principles-of-ethics-code-of-professional-conduct/nonmaleficence. Accessed January 4, 2015.

The ADA Practical Guide to Substance Use Disorders and Safe Prescribing

Continuing Education Examination

Name: _____

Address: _____

City: _____ State: _____ Zip: _____

Phone (include area code): _____

E-mail: _____

To receive 5 hours of continuing education credit, mail completed test to:

American Dental Association
Lockbox 28094
Network Place
Chicago, IL 60673-1280

A $20 grading fee applies for each test mailed. Please indicate your payment method below:

☐ Check (payable to American Dental Association)

☐ Visa   ☐ MasterCard   ☐ American Express

Credit card number _____ Exp. date (mm/yy) _____

Cardholder signature _____

Tests are graded and responses mailed within a few days of receipt. To check on the status of a test or for other test-related questions, call 800-947-4746.

This test is intended for use by allied dental personnel as well as dentists. Making copies of the blank test for use within a practice is acceptable.

The American Dental Association is an ADA CERP Recognized Provider. Continuing education credits issued for participation in the CE activity may not apply toward license renewal in all licensing jurisdictions. It is the responsibility of each participant to verify the CE requirements of his/her licensing or regulatory agency.

The ADA Practical Guide to Substance Use Disorders and Safe Prescribing, First Edition. Edited by Michael O'Neil.
© 2015 American Dental Association. Published 2015 by John Wiley & Sons, Inc.

Continuing Education Examination

Please circle True or False for each question.

Chapter 1

1.	The four common cultures of prescription drug diversion and substance use disorder based on the "intent" of the individual are: sharing culture, income-driven culture, substance abuse culture, and addiction culture.	TRUE	FALSE

2.	Prescriber–patient mismatch is defined as the inconsistency in treatment goals or expectations of treatment between the prescriber and the patient. Examples include analgesia, sedation, or anxiolysis.	TRUE	FALSE

3.	Medication misuse may be defined as taking a prescribed or over-the counter (OTC) medication for nonprescribed purposes, in excessive doses, shorter intervals than prescribed or recommended, or for reasons other than the original intent of the prescription. Examples include doubling the dosage, shortening dosing intervals, or treating disorders for which the medication was not prescribed.	TRUE	FALSE

Chapter 2

4.	In a patient suspected of having developed tolerance to a substance of abuse, less medication is *usually* required to achieve adequate sedation, analgesia, or anxiolysis, depending on the substance abused.	TRUE	FALSE

5.	Dental practitioners should be cautious when administering benzodiazepines or barbiturates to patients with a history of alcoholism that are in recovery due to the potential to stimulate cravings.	TRUE	FALSE

6.	Common signs and symptoms from withdrawal of stimulants such as methamphetamine and cocaine are seizures, hypertension, and slurred speech.	TRUE	FALSE

Chapter 3

7. Unless contraindicated due to renal disease, allergies, coagulopathies, major drug interactions, and so on, nonsteroidal anti-inflammatory drugs (NSAIDs) are *second-line* agents used in the treatment of acute dental pain.　　**TRUE**　　**FALSE**

8. In patients with liver disease that has been stable for several years, acetaminophen should always be avoided even with total daily doses less than 3 g to treat acute dental pain.　　**TRUE**　　**FALSE**

9. In patients with no contraindications, a "preemptive strike" with NSAIDs 1–2 h before a major dental procedure should be considered for minimizing postprocedure pain and inflammation.　　**TRUE**　　**FALSE**

Chapter 4

10. Patients receiving single daily doses of methadone or buprenorphine for opioid maintenance treatment should not be given additional opioid treatment of any kind since the single daily doses of methadone or buprenorphine provide adequate analgesia for most of the day.　　**TRUE**　　**FALSE**

11. Patients receiving naltrexone (Vivitrol®) 50 mg daily for opioid or alcohol addiction should have their naltrexone stopped 72 h before a procedure that will require treatment with opioids during or post procedure.　　**TRUE**　　**FALSE**

12. In patients receiving daily, around-the-clock opioids for chronic nonmalignant pain, a patient's same daily dosages of opioids will likely treat the acute pain from the dental procedure.　　**TRUE**　　**FALSE**

Chapter 5

| 13. | When performing surgical procedures on a patient with a known or suspected history of recent methamphetamine or cocaine abuse, epinephrine-containing products should be avoided due to the potential for life-threatening cardiovascular events such as dysrhythmias, hypertension, or ischemia. | TRUE | FALSE |

| 14. | Minimal sedation (historically known as anxiolysis) is defined as a drug-induced state during which patients respond normally to verbal commands. Although cognitive function and coordination may be impaired, ventilatory and cardiovascular functions are unaffected. | TRUE | FALSE |

| 15. | Ideally, when selecting anesthesia agents for a patient with a history of substance use disorder those agents should have limited potential to stimulate or provoke cravings. | TRUE | FALSE |

Chapter 6

| 16. | Patients reporting to a dental practitioner that they have recently used "bath salts" should anticipate similar adverse effects seen with stimulants or cannabis substances. | TRUE | FALSE |

| 17. | Prescription medications that are commonly abused include antipsychotics, muscle relaxants, and anticonvulsants owing to their side effect profile being similar to alcohol. | TRUE | FALSE |

| 18. | OTC products like pseudoephedrine or dextromethorphan are not likely to be abused since current commercial products have minimal concentrations of these substances in each tablet or bottle. | TRUE | FALSE |

Chapter 7

19.	All tobacco education occurring at the dental practitioner's office should be done by the dentist.	**TRUE**	**FALSE**
20.	To optimize the likelihood of tobacco cessation quitting success, nicotine replacement therapy should be done in conjunction with counseling and/or behavior modification.	**TRUE**	**FALSE**
21.	Nicotine gum products are easy to use for tobacco cessation since patients should "chew" these products constantly exactly like chewing gum without "parking" the gum between the cheek and teeth when effects of the gum are detected orally.	**TRUE**	**FALSE**

Chapter 8

22.	SBIRT is an evidence-based practice used to identify, reduce, and prevent problematic use, abuse, and dependence on alcohol and illicit drugs.	**TRUE**	**FALSE**
23.	After printing a prescription drug monitoring program patient profile or report, immediate observations of aberrant patterns of prescription refills for opioids are definitive evidence of a crime.	**TRUE**	**FALSE**
24.	One of the most common illegal activities of dental practitioners is prescribing outside the scope of dental practice.	**TRUE**	**FALSE**

Chapter 9

25.	Motivational interviewing is a short-term, directive, patient-centered style of counseling to help explore and resolve ambivalence.	**TRUE**	**FALSE**
26.	When interviewing patients, open-ended questions should be used to help prevent patients from "shutting down the interviewer" with simple yes or no responses.	**TRUE**	**FALSE**
27.	"Disarming the patient" at the beginning of the dental office interview is a strategic goal to minimize a patient's fears of the possible dental practitioner's responses to the patient's answers.	**TRUE**	**FALSE**

Chapter 10

28. If a dental practitioner wants to dispense individual dosages (e.g. 10–12 dosage units) of hydrocodone products to several patients from the dental office, the dental practitioner can legally obtain a bulk bottle of hydrocodone products with a single prescription and then dispense the products to multiple patients.   TRUE   FALSE

29. Due diligence is the practice of performing reasonable verification that the information presented is accurate and reliable in order to prevent deceptive or criminal practices. Reasonable implies that the practitioner is doing what any practitioner would and *should do* in the routine activities of the health-care professional.   TRUE   FALSE

30. According to federal regulations involving controlled substances, the term "Readily retrievable" means records should be able to be produced on site within two business days.   TRUE   FALSE

Chapter 11

31. Drug or alcohol relapse "IS" an *instantaneous event* of reusing a substance of abuse.   TRUE   FALSE

32. Impairment may be defined as the inability to consistently think rationally, perform job-related tasks, or communicate effectively without reoccurring error while performing job-related activities.   TRUE   FALSE

33. "The Conspiracy of Silence" is a common series of behaviors in which family, staff members, and colleagues are wary of bringing the addicted dental practitioner's problem to light.   TRUE   FALSE

Index

Page numbers in *italics* denote figures, those in **bold** denote tables.

The ADA Practical Guide to Substance Use Disorders and Safe Prescribing, First Edition. Edited by Michael O'Neil.
© 2015 American Dental Association. Published 2015 by John Wiley & Sons, Inc.